Ultrasound - The Next Step in Clinical Evaluation

Edited by Dana Liana Stoian

Published in London, United Kingdom

Ultrasound - The Next Step in Clinical Evaluation
http://dx.doi.org/10.5772/intechopen.1001695
Edited by Dana Liana Stoian

Contributors
Aderonke Adesiyan, Aleksandrina Topalova-Shishmanova, Alexandru Popa, Alina Popescu, Anca I. Ciurea, Andreea Bena, Andreea Bena, Andreea Borlea, Arda Kiani, Atefeh Abedini, Carolina Solomon, Corina Paul, Cristina-Laura Sîrbu, Cristina Mihaela Roi, Cătălin-Daniel Căleanu, Dana Liana Stoian, Dana Liana Stoian, Denisa Pescari, Fatemehsadat Rahimi, Flaviu Bob, Florentin Ananu Vreju, Georgiana Simion, Georgi Pavlov, Ghiţă-Adrian Burdan, Ioan Sporea, Iulia Dana Grosu, Kingsley Ufuoma Tobi, Luciana Moisa-Luca, Luciana Moisa Luca, Mehdi Kazempour Dizaji, Monica Simina Mihuta, Pegah Soltani, Rareş Crăciun, Razvan Adrian Ionescu, Siamak Afaghi, Simina Mihuta, Susana González Suárez, Tudor Mocan, Tudor Moga, Valentin Stoilov, Zeno Spârchez

First published in London, United Kingdom, 2025 by IntechOpen
IntechOpen is the global imprint of INTECHOPEN LIMITED, registered in England and Wales, registration number: 11086078, 167-169 Great Portland Street, London, W1W 5PF, United Kingdom

For EU product safety concerns: IN TECH d.o.o., Prolaz Marije Krucifikse Kozulić 3, 51000 Rijeka, Croatia, info@intechopen.com or visit our website at intechopen.com.

British Library Cataloguing-in-Publication Data
A catalogue record for this book is available from the British Library

Ultrasound - The Next Step in Clinical Evaluation
Edited by Dana Liana Stoian
p. cm.
Print ISBN 978-0-85466-452-8
Online ISBN 978-0-85466-451-1
eBook (PDF) ISBN 978-0-85466-453-5

Meet the editor

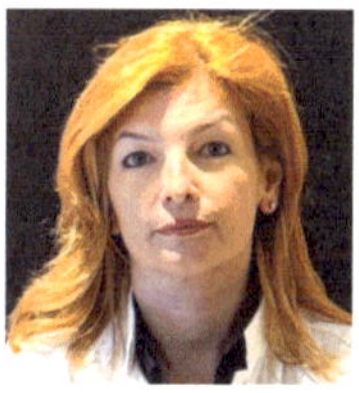

Dana Liana Stoian, MD, Ph.D., is Professor of Endocrinology at the "Victor Babeș" University of Medicine and Pharmacy, Timișoara, Romania, and founder of Dr. D Medical Center. An internationally recognized expert in endocrine and ultrasound diagnostics, she has authored over 150 ISI-indexed papers (H-index 19), more than 10 books, and 14 book chapters published by leading international publishers. Prof. Stoian lectures extensively across Europe on thyroid, adrenal, and breast imaging and plays a key role in postgraduate education, organizing EUROSON Schools and EFSUMB-endorsed ultrasound courses. Her research focuses on integrating imaging into endocrine pathology and advancing the applications of contrast-enhanced ultrasound in clinical practice. She also serves as an Academic Editor and reviewer for leading journals in endocrinology and ultrasound.

Contents

Preface

Ultrasound has evolved far beyond its traditional role as a purely imaging modality. It has become an essential extension of the clinical examination, providing real-time, dynamic insights that bridge the gap between bedside evaluation and complex diagnostic algorithms. *Ultrasound – The Next Step in Clinical Evaluation* aims to reflect this transformation and to inspire clinicians to incorporate ultrasound into their daily practice as an indispensable tool for integrative diagnosis.

This volume gathers contributions from experts across multiple fields, highlighting the versatility and clinical depth of modern ultrasonography. The chapters explore the multiparametric ultrasound assessment of thyroid disease, including both nodular and diffuse forms, as well as the emerging applications of point-of-care ultrasound (POCUS) in breast and lung evaluation. Musculoskeletal ultrasound is presented from both diagnostic and POCUS perspectives, emphasizing its utility in functional and structural assessment.

Further sections address the ultrasound evaluation of hepatic disorders, including fatty liver disease, portal hypertension, and the expanding role of artificial intelligence in multiparametric liver diagnostics. A dedicated section of the book focuses on the vascular consequences of obesity in children and on the practical ultrasonographic approach to arteriovenous anastomoses, highlighting the relevance of vascular ultrasound in understanding systemic disease.

The unifying concept of this book is that ultrasound should not be perceived merely as a descriptive imaging tool, but as a continuation of the clinical examination, an immediate, bedside extension of the physician's senses and reasoning. Through this perspective, the book invites clinicians to incorporate ultrasound into their diagnostic thought process, refine their decision-making, and ultimately enhance patient care.

We hope that this book will ignite curiosity and confidence among beginners, while offering fresh insights to experienced practitioners. As the boundaries between clinical medicine and imaging continue to dissolve, *Ultrasound – The Next Step in Clinical Evaluation* stands as a testament to a new, integrative era of diagnostic medicine.

Dana Liana Stoian
Department of Endocrinology,
County Emergency Hospital "Pius Branzeu",
Timișoara, Romania

"Victor Babes" University of Medicine and Pharmacy,
Timisoara, Romania

Section 1

Neck

Chapter 1

Multiparametric Ultrasound Evaluation of Diffuse Thyroid Disease

Dana Liana Stoian and Andreea Bena

Abstract

This chapter discusses the advanced multiparametric ultrasound (MPUS) evaluation of diffuse thyroid diseases (DTD), including forms with hyperthyroidism, hypothyroidism, and the euthyroid, asymptomatic disease. A complete evaluation, including a combined use of various ultrasound modalities: B-mode, color Doppler, spectral Doppler, elastography, and contrast-enhanced ultrasound, offers improved diagnostic accuracy. This chapter addresses the challenges and innovations in ultrasound technology, providing a step-by-step diagnostic approach that integrates MPUS with other diagnostic tools. This comprehensive overview aims to enhance the accuracy and efficiency of DTD diagnosis, reflecting on the evolving landscape of thyroid disease diagnosis.

Keywords: elastography, thyroid nodules, thyroid cancer, MPUS, thyroid CEUS

1. Introduction

Diffuse thyroid diseases represent a complex spectrum of disorders affecting the thyroid gland including autoimmune conditions like Graves' disease (GD), Hashimoto's thyroiditis (HT), and other types of thyroiditis, each presenting typical challenges in diagnosis and further therapeutic management. The estimated prevalence of autoimmune thyroid disease with clinical thyroid dysfunction (AITD) is 5%, with an even greater number of individuals with positive antithyroid antibodies presenting without clinical disease [1, 2]. All these conditions alter the thyroid's structure and function in multiple ways, leading to typical clinical manifestations. The term thyroiditis refers to a broad range of conditions that result in inflammation of the thyroid gland and diffuse thyroid disease [3].

Biochemical diagnosis plays a crucial role in differentiating between Graves' disease, Hashimoto's thyroiditis, and other forms of thyroiditis, each characterized by distinct hormonal and antibody profiles. Graves' disease is characterized by high thyroid-stimulating immunoglobulins (TSI) and in most cases accompanied by hyperthyroidism [4]. However, Hashimoto's thyroiditis is characterized by high thyroid peroxidase (TPO) and antithyroglobulin antibodies and normal, raised, or reduced thyroid hormone levels depending on the disease stage. Due to their different inflammatory and autoimmune mechanisms, subacute or silent thyroiditis generally has a brief hyperthyroid phase, but no autoantibodies like in Graves' or Hashimoto's. Thus, appropriate diagnosis and treatment of these different thyroid disorders require a complete biochemical study, but sometimes the chemical picture may also overlap [5].

Thyroid scintigraphy remains the reference method for differentiating between destruction and hyperproduction conditions in cases with hyperthyroidism including cases with thyrotoxicosis which may arise due to the release of deposited, pre-synthesized thyroid hormones versus overactive thyroid tissue due to Graves' disease and more rarely, other types of thyroiditis. Precise diagnosis of GD from thyroiditis is essential to prevent the prescription of antithyroid drugs to patients with thyroiditis, as this could result in hypothyroidism or other adverse effects, while a patient with hyperproduction would not benefit from anti-inflammatory medication, with possible progression of the disease [6, 7].

Central to the evaluation of these diffuse thyroid disorders is the use of ultrasound (US) imaging. Ultrasound is a fundamental tool in the field of thyroid diagnosis due to its non-invasive nature, accessibility, and its exceptional ability to provide detailed images of the thyroid's structure and vascularity. In diffuse thyroid disease, ultrasound imaging is particularly valuable, as it can detect subtle changes in the gland's size, echotexture, and blood flow patterns, which are often key indicators of underlying pathology. The introduction of advanced ultrasound techniques has further enhanced our ability to assess these diseases. Doppler ultrasound allows for the evaluation of blood flow within the thyroid gland, aiding in the differentiation between various types of diffuse thyroid diseases based on their vascular patterns. Similarly, elastography provides insights into the stiffness of thyroid tissues, a feature that can vary significantly among different thyroid pathologies [5, 8, 9].

However, while conventional techniques such as B-mode and Doppler provide useful structural and vascular information, they often fall short in confidently differentiating between overlapping DTD phenotypes—particularly in early disease stages or atypical presentations. For instance, both Graves' disease and Hashimoto's thyroiditis may present with diffusely hypoechoic parenchyma, making diagnosis uncertain without additional data.

Multiparametric ultrasound (MPUS), by combining B-mode, Doppler, elastography, contrast-enhanced ultrasound (CEUS), and the emerging modality of viscosity estimation, offers a more comprehensive tissue characterization. This integrated approach allows not only for improved diagnostic accuracy but also for better phenotyping and staging of DTDs, especially when biochemical or nuclear imaging is inconclusive or unavailable.

As such, MPUS holds increasing promise in the non-invasive, real-time differentiation of diffuse thyroid diseases, offering clinicians a powerful adjunct to laboratory and scintigraphic data.

The future of an initial, prompt diagnosis in DTD is likely to meet a shift toward imaging, particularly ultrasound imaging, enhanced by the advantages of multiparametric US-based assessment.

2. Overview of DTDs

2.1 Hashimoto's thyroiditis

Hashimoto's thyroiditis (HT) is the most prevalent form of autoimmune thyroiditis and commonly presents with a hypoechoic, heterogeneous thyroid on ultrasound.

Diagnosing asymptomatic or subclinical thyroiditis does not mean overdiagnosis, but rather an early diagnosis [10]. Screening asymptomatic, euthyroid patients helps in avoiding the complications of untreated thyroid dysfunction. In this condition, the patients show no evident symptoms of thyroid dysfunction at the time of diagnosis, but a significant share will develop hypothyroidism. The markers in its detection are the raised serum concentrations of thyroid antibodies, namely antithyroid peroxidase (TPOAb) and anti-thyroglobulin (TGAb) [4, 5]. These antibodies are also present in other thyroid conditions like Graves' disease, their prevalence increases with age and is more common in women, suggesting a demographic pattern in thyroid autoimmunity [11].

The role of ultrasound imaging emerges as crucial in this scenario, as it can detect changes in thyroid tissue indicative of autoimmunity even before TPOAb positivity, particularly in the 20% of cases where TPOAb may not be detectable despite ultrasound evidence [6, 12]. The ultrasound appearance may vary from slightly hypoechoic (**Figure 1**) to a typical appearance of HT, as well as different pictures of elasticity and vascular patterns [13].

It is believed that a combination of genetic predisposition and environmental influences contributes to the breakdown of immune tolerance, resulting in an autoimmune assault on thyroid tissue and the subsequent development of the disease [14]. The onset of this condition might be linked to the CTL-4 protein or a cytotoxic

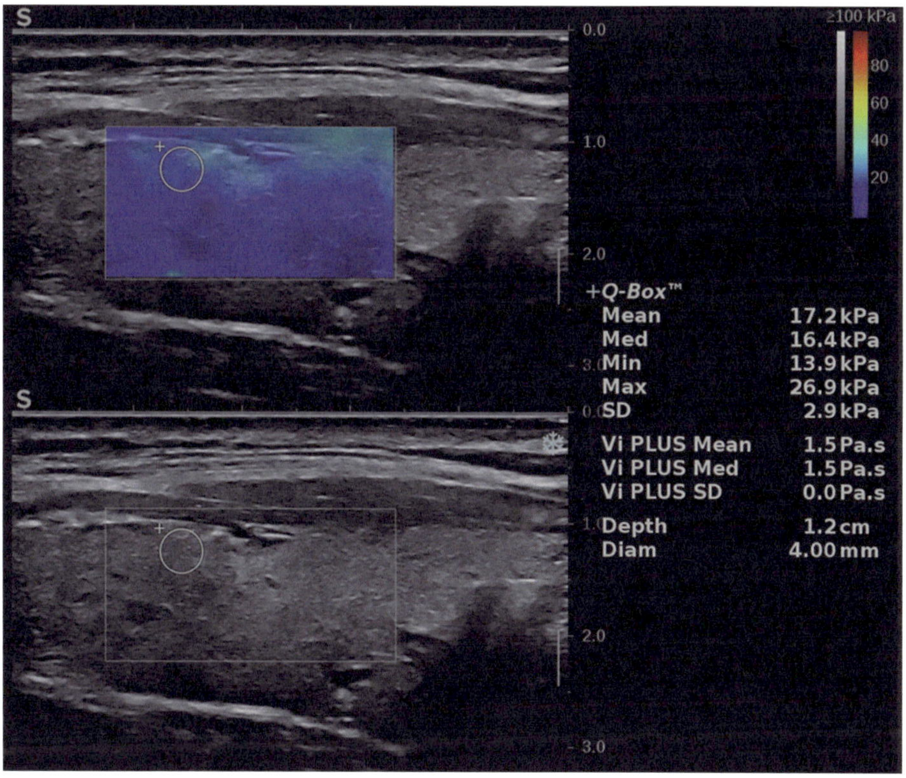

Figure 1.
Longitudinal view of the right thyroid lobe in a patient with asymptomatic autoimmune thyroiditis; moderate diffuse inhomogeneity in B-mode (lower image); mean elasticity index 17.2 kPa, color map – blue and green - showing slightly increased thyroid stiffness in the selected region of interest Q-Box (upper image) – multimodal ultrasound assessment suggests autoimmune diffuse thyroid disease.

T-lymphocyte antigen [15]. Individuals with HT often face challenges like memory lapses and concentration issues, alongside symptoms such as irritability, sleep disturbances, mood fluctuations, and depression. They may associate myopathy, neuropathy, and encephalopathy, though the precise reasons behind these symptoms remain largely unexplained [11, 16].

2.2 Graves' disease

GD is a specific autoimmune disorder targeting the thyroid, primarily caused by circulating autoantibodies that stimulate the thyroid-stimulating-hormone receptor, resulting in hyperthyroidism. This condition arises also from the loss of immune tolerance to thyroid antigens, namely against the TSH receptor (TRAb), with 99% specificity [17]. In cases where classic symptoms like dermopathy or ophthalmopathy and a diffuse goiter are absent, radionuclide scanning becomes essential to confirm a diagnosis of Graves' disease. It also helps differentiate GD from other thyrotoxicosis causes like exogenous thyroid hormone intake or follicular destruction, employing techniques like radioiodine uptake measurement to make this differentiation [4, 17]. GD may be diagnosed in subclinical forms, when thyroid ultrasound appearance may already present the typical features of the disease, before thyroid function alterations or the development of eye disease.

2.3 Destruction thyroiditis

Destructive thyroiditis is a form of thyroid inflammation characterized by the transient release of thyroid hormones due to the destruction of thyroid follicular cells, rather than overproduction. Some destructive conditions such as post-partum thyroiditis or Hashitoxicosis are typically part of a spectrum of autoimmune thyroid disorders and can sometimes be mistaken for Graves' disease due to the initial thyrotoxic phase [18]. However, unlike Graves' disease, destructive thyroiditis usually does not involve an immune response directly stimulating the thyroid to produce excess hormones [19]. Instead, the damage to thyroid cells leads to the leakage of stored thyroid hormones into the bloodstream, causing temporary hyperthyroidism. Other destruction states include iatrogenia, as in the use of amiodarone, immunotherapy, lithium, and radiation therapy [20, 21]. This phase is often followed by a hypothyroid phase as hormone stores are depleted, which can then return to normal thyroid function in many cases. Understanding and identifying destructive thyroiditis is crucial for providing appropriate treatment and avoiding unnecessary interventions like long-term thyroid suppression therapy, which may not be beneficial in this self-limiting condition and may actually harm the patient [18].

3. Role of ultrasound in diffuse thyroid disease diagnosis

3.1 B-mode ultrasound in DTD

Diffuse inhomogeneity and hypoechogenicity can be present in any type of DTD and predict thyroid DTD with great accuracy [3].

In autoimmune thyroiditis, the appearance may vary, and sometimes it shows different pictures from one evaluation to another. Multiple typical features have been described: typically, it presents as a diffusely heterogeneous gland with patchy hypoechoic areas and echogenic bands, creating a micronodular or "giraffe skin" appearance [22, 23]. In the initial phase the thyroid volume is usually increased or normal. As the condition advances with inflammation and fibrosis, the gland develops hyperechoic bands, a more heterogeneous and nodular surface, and may become atrophic (**Figure 2**), occasionally showing "pseudonodules" [24].

The hypoechogenicity seen in Graves' disease is attributed to various histological changes within the thyroid gland, such as lymphocytic infiltration, increased vascularity, and changes in the thyroid's stromal and parenchymal composition, changes which alter the way the thyroid tissue interacts with ultrasound waves [4, 25]. The intense hypoechoic pattern seen in Graves' disease (**Figure 3**) can be a useful diagnostic feature, although the appearance overlaps in many cases with the appearance of HT. The thyroid volume is usually above the upper limit, and less commonly can also be normal [26].

In subacute thyroiditis, the characteristic ultrasound presentation often shows patchy, undefined hypoechoic areas (**Figure 4**), in either one or both lobes, accompanied by notably reduced vascularity in the thyroid tissue. This can sometimes resemble a "lava flow" pattern of diffuse and merging hypoechoic regions. The resolution of these imaging features can take several weeks to months [27].

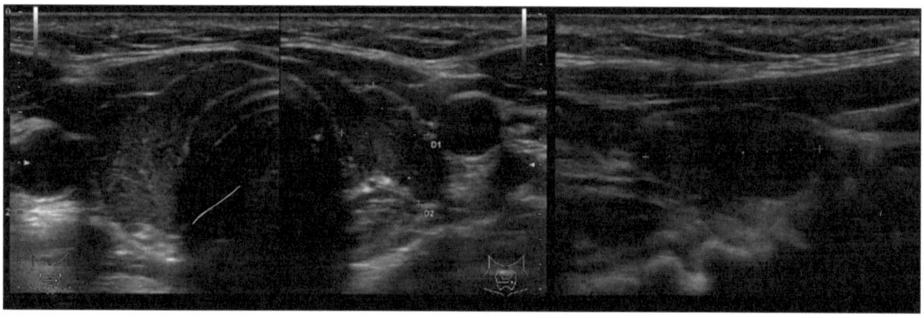

Figure 2.
Atrophic, hypoechoic thyroid gland caused by autoimmune thyroiditis, seen in transverse view (left), and longitudinal view of the right lobe (right).

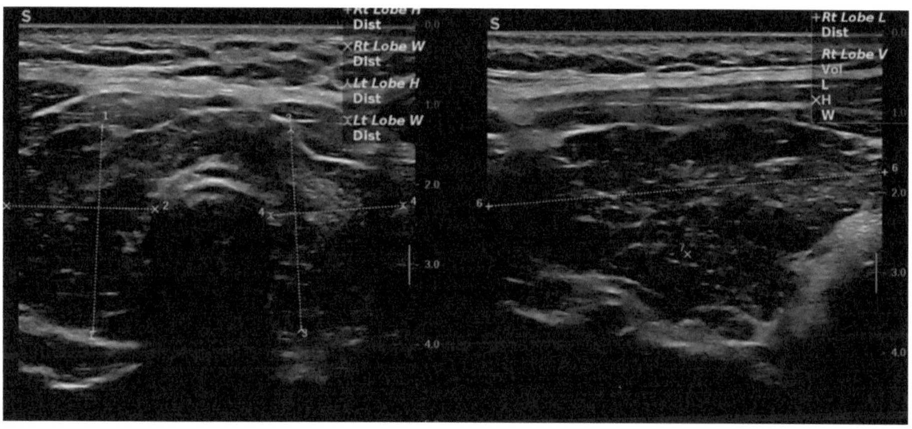

Figure 3.
Diffusely enlarged, intense hypoechoic thyroid parenchyma in a patient with Graves' disease in transverse view (left) and longitudinal view of the right lobe (right).

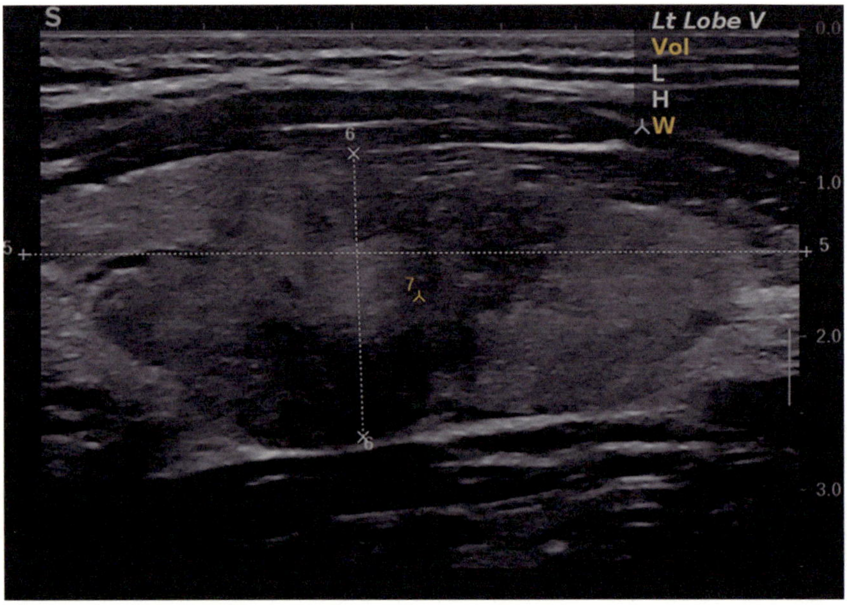

Figure 4.
Longitudinal view, left lobe in a patient with subacute thyroiditis: Hypoechoic areas that alternate with normal appearing thyroid tissue.

4. Color Doppler and spectral Doppler ultrasound

Autoimmune thyroiditis can present with either increased, normal, or decreased vascularity *in Color Doppler*, depending on factors like TSH value or time from onset (**Figure** 5).

Undoubtedly, Graves' disease is marked by abundant intralesional blood flow, as seen in color Doppler ultrasound imaging (**Figure 6**).

In subacute thyroiditis, during the acute phase, increased vascularity might be observed (**Figure** 7), while the subacute phase typically exhibits widespread hypovascularity [3, 18].

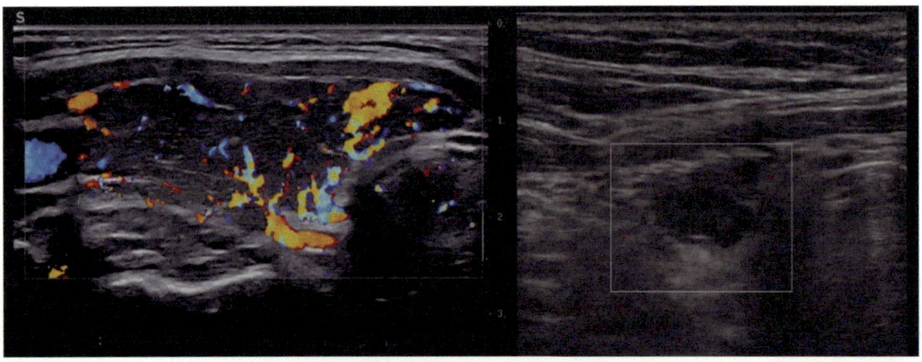

Figure 5.
Color Doppler: Increased vascularity in Hashimoto (left); decreased vascularity in atrophic thyroiditis (right).

DOI: http://dx.doi.org/10.5772/intechopen.1012823

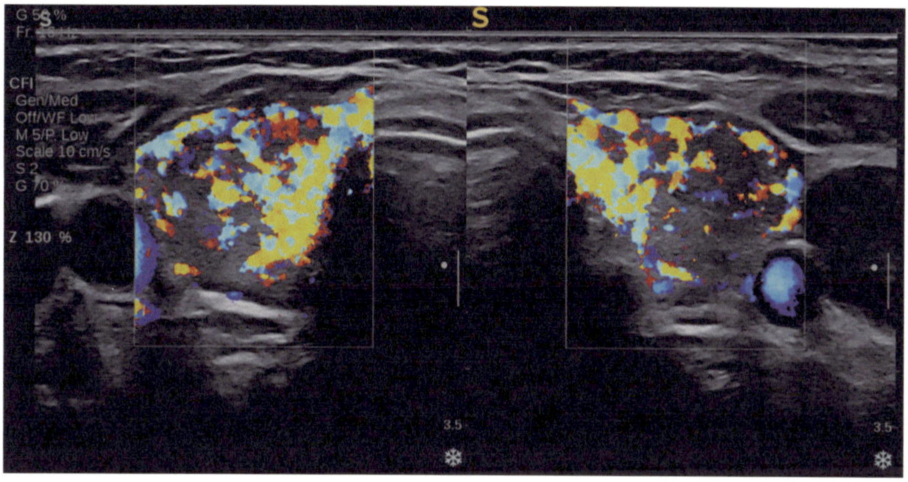

Figure 6.
Color Doppler: Diffusely increased vascular pattern seen in a Graves' disease patient.

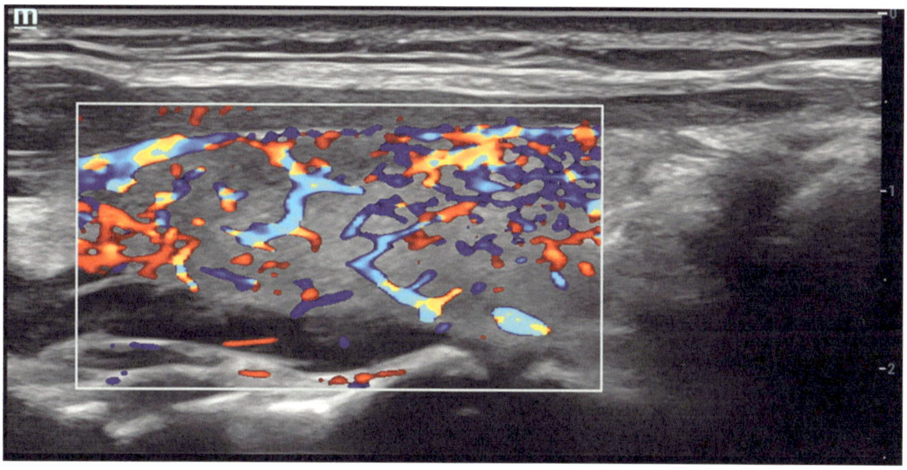

Figure 7.
Power Doppler imaging: Diffuse recovered areas displaying increased vascularity with some decrease in vascular pattern corresponding to the hypoechoic, most affected area in subacute thyroiditis - beginning of resolution phase.

Spectral Doppler (SD) is an advanced technique employed in thyroid artery examinations, particularly useful in distinguishing between GD and other thyroiditis forms. By measuring the peak systolic velocity (PSV) in the superior thyroid arteries on both sides, SD provides a quantitative appraisal of blood flow. The procedure involves maintaining the Doppler angle at or below 60° and adjusting the correction angle parallel to the flow direction. PSV values, measured in centimeters per second, have shown a strong correlation with radioactive iodine uptake recorded both at 3 and 24-hour intervals. This correlation has significantly enhanced the accuracy and reliability of SD in thyroid diagnostics. A PSV cutoff range of 40–50 cm/sec has been proposed to distinguish between GD (**Figure 8**) and other forms of thyroiditis (**Figure 9**) [28, 29].

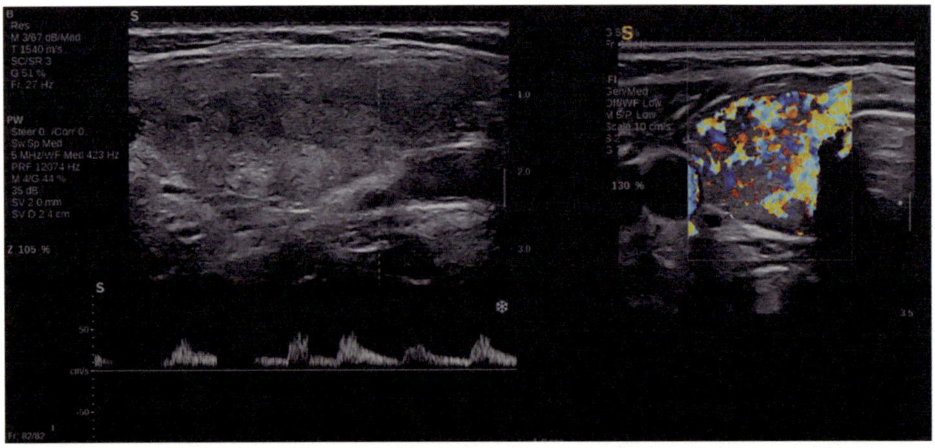

Figure 8.
Spectral and color Doppler assessment in a patient with Graves', with increased vascular pattern Schultz 3 in color Doppler (right) and high peak systolic velocity, suggesting Graves' disease.

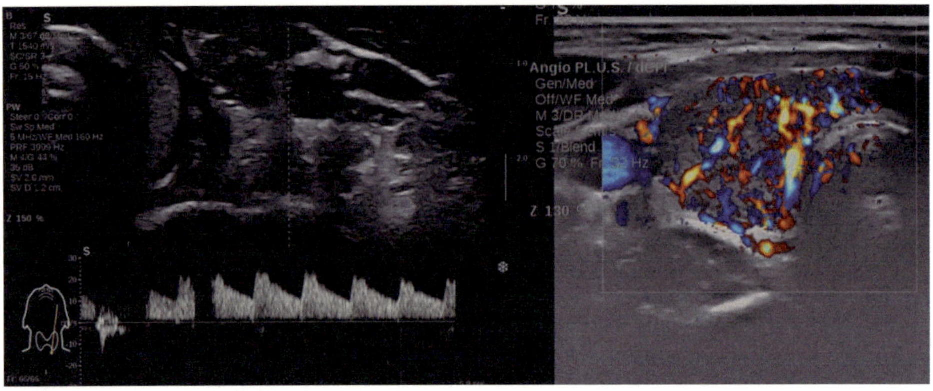

Figure 9.
Spectral and color Doppler assessment in a patient with autoimmune thyroiditis at debut, also with increased vascular pattern Schultz 3 in color Doppler (right), but peak systolic velocity lower than Graves' threshold = 22 cm/sec.

5. Elastography in DTD

Elastography methods, both strain and shear-wave-based, are highly effective for identifying potentially malignant thyroid nodules [30], but they can also detect conditions like autoimmune thyroiditis and Graves' disease, by estimating tissue mechanical properties [31]. Strain elastography measures tissue deformation in response to an applied force, either manual compression or internal movement. It provides qualitative or semi-quantitative information, displaying the relative stiffness of tissues in a color-coded format without offering exact measurements. In contrast, shear wave elastography is a more advanced, quantitative method. It utilizes the generation of shear waves within the tissue by the ultrasound probe; the waves' speed is directly related to tissue stiffness: the faster the waves travel, the stiffer the tissue. Shear wave elastography provides a more objective and reproducible measurement of tissue stiffness, often expressed in kilopascals (kPa) as the elasticity index (EI), enabling more precise and reliable assessments [32]. In DTD, stiffness is an indicator of thyroid fibrosis.

In the literature, normal thyroid elasticity values are approximately 9.0 ± 11.3 kPa; 13.5 ± 3.3 kPa using 2D SWE techniques [33, 34]. It is worth mentioning that all these values are technique- and machine-dependent. There is substantial evidence indicating that in patients with HT, thyroid tissue stiffness is higher compared to normal thyroid tissue, with mean 2D-SWE values ranging between 19.5 ± 6.8 kPa and 36.15 ± 18.7 kPa [27, 33, 35]. Similar findings were also observed in pediatric patients (**Figure 10**) [31].

In Graves' disease (**Figure 11**), the thyroid tissue usually presents a low elastic index, similar to the normal thyroid (mean values ranging between 11.6 and 17.4).

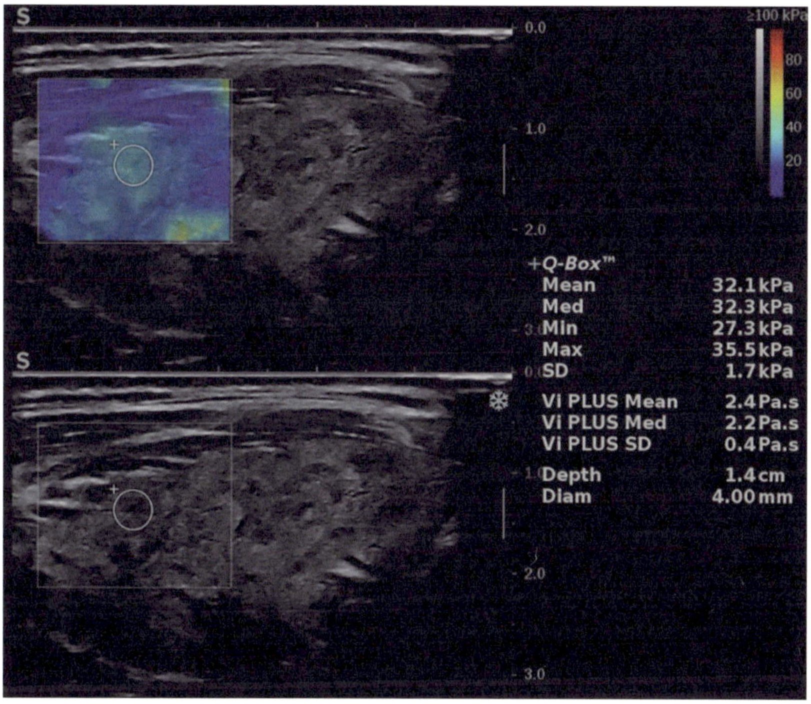

Figure 10.
Increased mean elasticity index (32.1 kPa) in the selected region of interest Q-Box; color map – mostly green - in a patient with Hashimoto's.

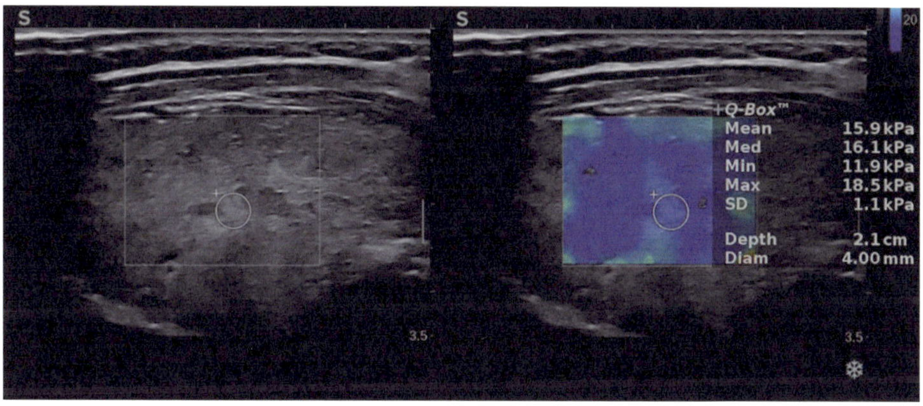

Figure 11.
High-normal mean elasticity index of 15.9 kPa, color map – mostly blue; in a patient with Graves' disease.

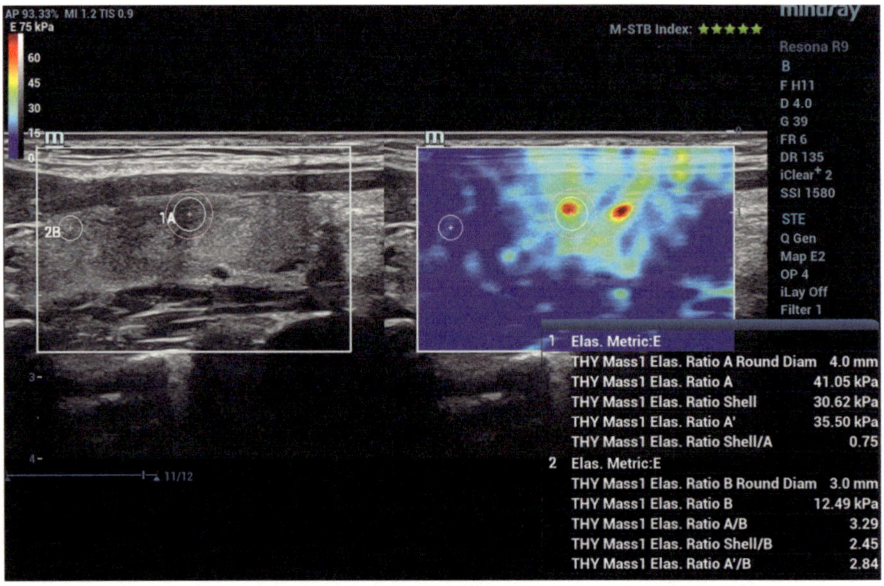

Figure 12.
Stiff areas alternating with normal elasticity areas in a patient with subacute thyroiditis.

Elastography can be of great help in differentiating Graves' from SAT (mean elasticity <24 kPa, AUC 0.953), but may not be able to differentiate Graves' from normal thyroid and, in some cases, from HT [36].

Elastography is instrumental in differentiating SAT from other forms of thyroiditis. It showed markedly higher elasticity measurements, over 100 kPa, an obvious contrast to the mean elasticity values for autoimmune diseases of all forms (mean < 25 kPa). This significant difference is reflected in the area under the curve (AUC) values, where SWE had an AUC of 0.989 for distinguishing SAT from GD, but 0.549 for HT from GD [36]. **Figure 12** displays one SAT case in resolution, euthyroid phase.

6. Advancements in thyroid ultrasound

6.1 Viscosity estimation

Similarly to elasticity estimation, the dispersion slope measurements can be made as potential markers of inflammation, so that viscosity evaluation may be able to differentiate between inflammation and fibrosis, as elastography presents increased values for both and is not able to differentiate between them. Developed by Canon and Supersonic Imagine (Vi PLUS) so far, these techniques utilize algorithmic analyses of tissue viscosity. The significant limitation of the viscosity module is that so far it is exclusively compatible with a curvilinear transducer.

For normal thyroid viscosity, specific values have been determined: In the first study involving 121 healthy subjects, it was found to be 2.42 ± 0.41 Pa·s [34, 37], while a second study with 85 healthy volunteers reported it similarly, as 2.63 ± 0.47 Pa·s [37]. Subsequently, a study assessing thyroid viscosity in adults with HT reported notably higher values in HT patients compared to those with normal thyroid function, with a significant difference between the two groups ($p < 0.0001$). The Vi PLUS demonstrated effective diagnostic capability in identifying chronic autoimmune thyroiditis (**Figures 13** and **14**). An optimal cut-off for diagnosis was identified at above 2.5 Pa·s, (AUC = 0.69; sensitivity = 68.6%; specificity = 64.52%) [38].

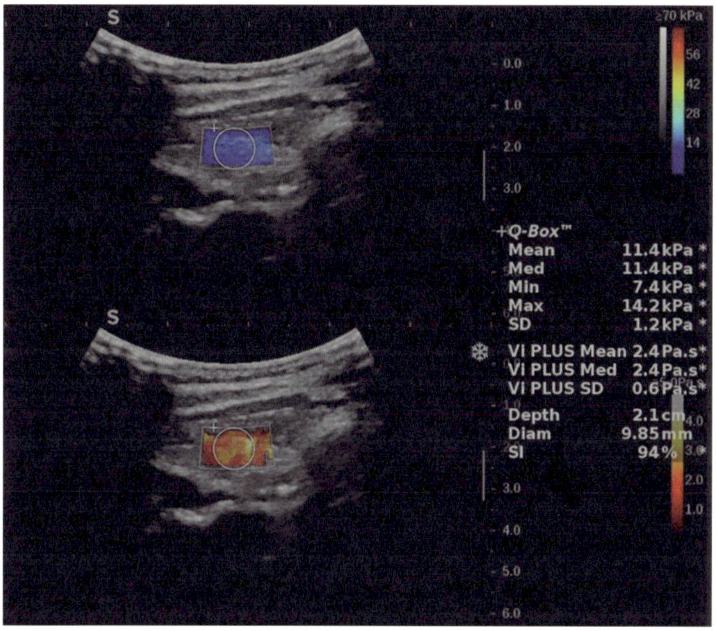

Figure 13.
ViPLUS assessment of thyroid parenchyma in a patient with normal thyroid evaluated with convex probe: Normal mean elasticity index – 11.4 kPa, color map – entirely blue; normal mean viscosity index – 2.4 Pa·s, color map – mostly red.

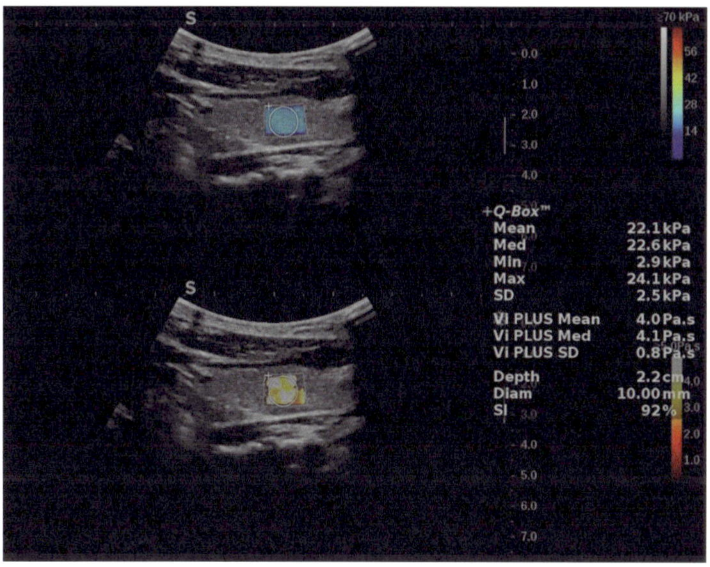

Figure 14.
ViPLUS assessment of thyroid parenchyma in a patient with autoimmune thyroiditis: Mean elasticity index – 22.1 kPa, color map – mostly green; increased mean viscosity index – 4 Pa·s, color map – mostly yellow.

6.2 CEUS

There is no standardized approach in terms of CEUS utilization in DTD [39]. Our team described certain patterns also in qualitative CEUS evaluation for DTD versus normal thyroid, but also between different subtypes of hyperthyroid DTD due to follicular destruction (delayed wash-in; early washout; inhomogeneous contrast enhancement – **Figure 15**) and hyperproduction (early wash-in; prolonged enhancement with late washout; usually homogeneous hyperenhancement – **Figure 16**).

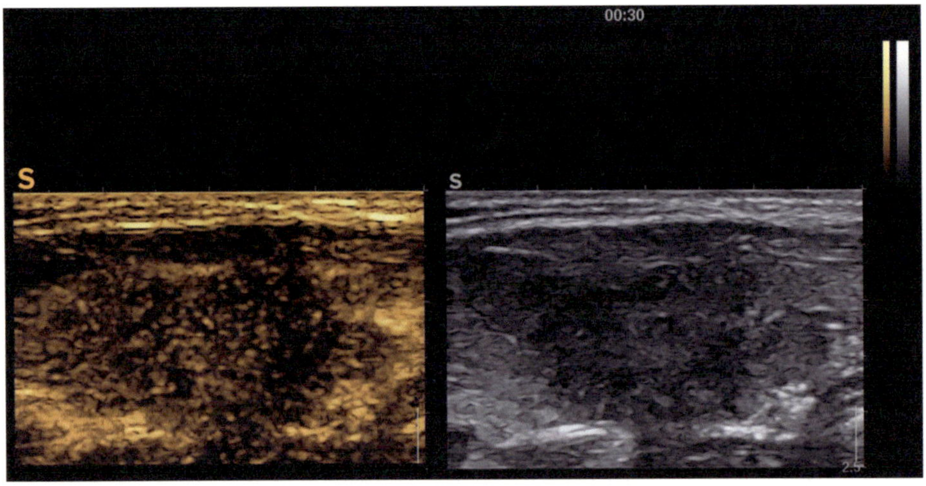

Figure 15.
Inhomogeneous enhancement and early washout in a patient with subacute thyroiditis (destruction).

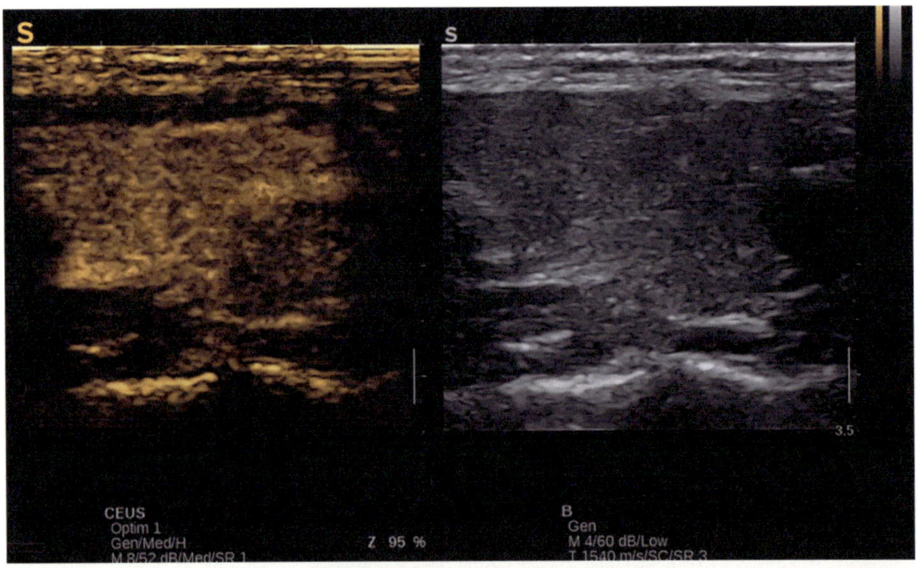

Figure 16.
Homogeneous uptake and prolonged enhancement of the thyroid parenchyma, late washout in a patient with Graves' disease (hyperproduction), and a hypoenhanced area in the posterior part corresponding to a benign thyroid nodule.

Disease	B-mode	Color Doppler	Elastography	CEUS	Biochemical markers
HT	Hypoechoic, heterogeneous	Normal/increased/decreased	Stiff	Not needed	↑TPOAb, ↑/N TSH
GD	Hypoechoic, enlarged	Markedly increased	Normal/slightly stiff	Intense, homogeneous	↑TRAb, ↓/N TSH
DT	Patchy hypoechogenicity	Low/absent	Very stiff (acute phase)	Low or absent	↓TSH, N TRAb, ↑ESR

HT – Hashimoto's thyroiditis; GD – Graves' disease; DT – destructive thyroiditis; N – normal; CEUS – contrast-enhanced ultrasound.

Table 1.
MPUS step-by-step diagnosis.

6.3 Limitations

While MPUS enhances diagnostic accuracy in diffuse thyroid diseases, several limitations remain. Elastography and viscosity values are highly operator- and equipment-dependent, *with varying cut-offs across platforms; they also vary across stages of the disease*. CEUS lacks standardized protocols for DTDs, *and its availability is limited. In addition*, overlapping imaging features *between different DTDs may still require biochemical or nuclear confirmation. Thus, MPUS should still be interpreted in conjunction with clinical and laboratory data*.

7. Conclusion and future directions: Why MPUS approach?

This book chapter highlights the necessity of a systematic, multiphase diagnostic imaging approach for diffuse thyroid diseases (DTDs). The workflow begins with preliminary B-mode and color Doppler ultrasound evaluations, crucial for initial structural and vascular assessment of the thyroid gland. Subsequent laboratory tests are essential for determining thyroid function, thereby deepening the understanding of the thyroid's condition. Spectral Doppler ultrasound is particularly useful in thyrotoxicosis, with peak systolic velocity (PSV) values *above 40–50 cm/s* strongly suggesting Graves' disease. Elastography follows as a key diagnostic step, providing stiffness quantification: *high elasticity (>100 kPa)* indicates subacute thyroiditis (SAT) and important follicular damage, while *moderate elevations (20–35 kPa)* support a diagnosis of Hashimoto's thyroiditis (HT), and *low-normal values (11–17 kPa)* are more typical for Graves' disease (GD). Newer tools like viscosity estimation further help differentiate chronic autoimmune inflammation (*>2.5 Pa·s in HT*) from normal thyroid or GD. CEUS adds perfusion detail—*early, homogeneous enhancement with delayed washout* favors GD, while *delayed, patchy enhancement with early washout* points toward destructive thyroiditis. **Table 1** summarizes this step-by-step diagnostic synergy:

This multiparametric approach allows accurate, real-time differentiation between major DTDs, reducing reliance on nuclear imaging and minimizing treatment errors. For example, differentiating GD from SAT prevents inappropriate antithyroid drug use, while early detection of HT aids monitoring and timely intervention.

The MPUS strategy is therefore essential for precise, personalized thyroid care—integrating structural, vascular, mechanical, and functional insights into a comprehensive diagnostic pathway. This evolving, imaging-led approach represents a promising direction in the future management of thyroid diseases.

Author details

Dana Liana Stoian and Andreea Bena*
"Victor Babes" University of Medicine and Pharmacy, Timisoara, Romania

*Address all correspondence to: borlea.andreea@umft.ro

References

[1] Tomer Y, Ban Y, Conception E, Barbesino G, Villanueva R, Greenberg DA, et al. Common and unique susceptibility loci in Graves and Hashimoto diseases: Results of whole-genome screening in a data set of 102 multiplex families. The American Journal of Human Genetics. 2003;**73**:736-747. DOI: 10.1086/378588

[2] Rizzo M, Rossi RT, Bonaffini O, Scisca C, Altavilla G, Calbo L, et al. Increased annual frequency of Hashimoto's thyroiditis between years 1988 and 2007 at a cytological unit of Sicily. Annales d'endocrinologie. 2010;**71**:525-534. DOI: 10.1016/J.ANDO.2010.06.006

[3] Alexander LF, Patel NJ, Caserta MP, Robbin ML. Thyroid ultrasound: Diffuse and nodular disease. Radiologic Clinics of North America. 2020;**58**:1041-1057. DOI: 10.1016/J.RCL.2020.07.003

[4] Cui Z, Wang Z, Liu X, Cai Y, Xu X, Yang T. Establishment of clinical diagnosis model of Graves' disease and Hashimoto's thyroiditis. Journal of Translational Medicine. 2019;**17**:11. DOI: 10.1186/S12967-018-1765-3

[5] Antonelli A, Ferrari SM, Corrado A, Di Domenicantonio A, Fallahi P. Autoimmune thyroid disorders. Autoimmunity Reviews. 2015;**14**:174-180. DOI: 10.1016/J.AUTREV.2014.10.016

[6] Moini J, Samsam M, Pereira K. Epidemiology of Thyroid Disorders. 1st ed. Elsevier/Academic Press; 2020. pp. 1-336. ISBN: 978-0-12-818500-1. DOI: 10.1007/978-3-319-72102-6_6

[7] Weetman A. Recommended management of thyroid disorders. Prescriber. 2016;**27**:31-38. DOI: 10.1002/PSB.1522

[8] Mahmoud R, Azeem KM, Sayed ASA, Ali FM. Role of ultrasound and Doppler findings as a predictor of thyroid hormonal levels in cases of Hashimoto thyroiditis. Beni-Suef University Journal of Basic and Applied Sciences. 2022;**11**:1-8. DOI: 10.1186/S43088-022-00197-0/TABLES/3

[9] Şahin M, Çakal E, Özbek M, Güngünes A, Arslan MS, Akkaymak ET, et al. Elastography in the differential diagnosis of thyroid nodules in Hashimoto thyroiditis. Medical Oncology. 2014;**31**:97. DOI: 10.1007/s12032-014-0097-2

[10] Vanderpump MPJ. The epidemiology of thyroid disease. British Medical Bulletin. 2011;**99**:39-51. DOI: 10.1093/bmb/ldr030

[11] Waliszewska-Prosół M, Ejma M. Hashimoto encephalopathy—Still more questions than answers. Cells. 2022;**11**:2873. DOI: 10.3390/CELLS11182873

[12] Surks MI, Boucai L. Age- and race-based serum thyrotropin reference limits. The Journal of Clinical Endocrinology and Metabolism. 2010;**95**:496-502. DOI: 10.1210/JC.2009-1845

[13] Stoian D, Pantea S, Margan M, Timar B, Borcan F, Craina M, et al. Individualized follow-up of pregnant women with asymptomatic autoimmune thyroid disease. International Journal of Molecular Sciences. 2016;**17**:88. DOI: 10.3390/ijms17010088

[14] Ruchała M, Szmyt K, Sławek S, Zybek A, Szczepanek-Parulska E. Ultrasound sonoelastography in

the evaluation of thyroiditis and autoimmune thyroid disease. Endokrynologia Polska. 2014;**65**:520-531. DOI: 10.5603/EP.2014.0071

[15] Feldkamp J. Autoimmunthyreoiditis: Diagnostik und Therapie. DMW - Deutsche Medizinische Wochenschrift. 2009;**134**:2504-2509. DOI: 10.1055/S-0029-1243053

[16] Bladowska J, Waliszewska-Prosół M, Ejma M, Sąsiadek M. The metabolic alterations within the normal appearing brain in patients with Hashimoto's thyroiditis are correlated with hormonal changes. Metabolic Brain Disease. 2019;**34**:53-60. DOI: 10.1007/S11011-018-0318-Z/FIGURES/7

[17] Antonelli A, Fallahi P, Elia G, Ragusa F, Paparo SR, Ruffilli I, et al. Graves' disease: Clinical manifestations, immune pathogenesis (cytokines and chemokines) and therapy. Best Practice & Research. Clinical Endocrinology & Metabolism. 2020;**34**:101388. DOI: 10.1016/J.BEEM.2020.101388

[18] Fariduddin MM, Singh G. Thyroiditis. In: StatPearls [Internet]. Treasure Island (FL): StatPearls Publishing; Jan 2025. Available from: https://www.ncbi.nlm.nih.gov/books/NBK555975/ [Updated 2023 Aug 8]

[19] Pearce EN, Farwell AP, Braverman LE. Thyroiditis. The New England Journal of Medicine. 2003;**348**:2646-2655. DOI: 10.1056/NEJMRA021194

[20] Garon-Czmil J, Petitpain N, Rouby F, Sassier M, Babai S, Yelehe-Okouma M, et al. Thyroiditis and immune check point inhibitors: The post-marketing experience using the French National Pharmacovigilance database. Fundamental & Clinical Pharmacology. 2019;**33**:241-249. DOI: 10.1111/FCP.12423

[21] Miller KK, Daniels GH. Association between lithium use and thyrotoxicosis caused by silent thyroiditis. Clinical Endocrinology. 2001;**55**:501-508. DOI: 10.1046/J.1365-2265.2001.01381.X

[22] Patel BN, Kamaya A, Desser TS. Pitfalls in sonographic evaluation of thyroid abnormalities. Seminars in Ultrasound, CT and MRI. 2013;**34**:226-235. DOI: 10.1053/J.SULT.2012.11.001

[23] Solbiati L, Volterrani L, Rizzatto G, Bazzocchi M, Busilacci P, Candiani F, et al. The thyroid gland with low uptake lesions: Evaluation by ultrasound. Radiology. 1985;**155**(1):187-191. DOI: 10.1148/radiology.155.1.3883413

[24] Harris RD, Langer JE, Levine RA, Sheth S, Abramson SJ, Gabriel H, et al. AIUM thyroid and parathyroid ultrasound examination. Journal of Ultrasound in Medicine. 2013;**32**:1319-1329. DOI: 10.7863/ultra.32.7.1319

[25] Hefeda MM. Value of the new elastography technique using acoustic radiation force impulse in differentiation between Hashimoto's thyroiditis and Graves' disease. Journal of Clinical Imaging Science. 2019;**9**:1-8. DOI: 10.25259/JCIS-22-2019

[26] Staniforth JUL, Erdirimanne S, Eslick GD. Thyroid carcinoma in Graves' disease: A meta-analysis. International Journal of Surgery. 2016;**27**:118-125. DOI: 10.1016/j.ijsu.2015.11.027

[27] Ruchala M, Szczepanek-Parulska E, Zybek A, Moczko J, Czarnywojtek A, Kaminski G, et al. The role of sonoelastography in acute, subacute and chronic thyroiditis: A novel application of the method. European Journal of Endocrinology. 2012;**166**:425-432. DOI: 10.1530/EJE-11-0736

[28] Zhao X, Chen L, Liu H, Wang Y, Li L, Lu B, et al. Mean peak systolic

velocity of the superior thyroid artery is correlated with radioactive iodine uptake in untreated thyrotoxicosis. The Journal of International Medical Research. 2012;**40**:640-647. DOI: 10.1177/147323001204000226

[29] Erdoğan MF, Anil C, Cesur M, Başkal N, Erdoğan G. Color flow Doppler sonography for the etiologic diagnosis of hyperthyroidism. Thyroid. 2007;**17**(3):223-228. DOI: 10.1089/thy.2006.0104

[30] Zhou Y, Chen H, Qiang J, Wang D. Systematic review and meta-analysis of ultrasonic elastography in the diagnosis of benign and malignant thyroid nodules. Gland Surgery. 2021;**10**:2734744-2732744. DOI: 10.21037/GS-21-492

[31] Cepeha CM, Paul C, Borlea A, Borcan F, Fofiu R, Dehelean CA, et al. The value of strain elastography in predicting autoimmune thyroiditis. Diagnostics (Basel). 2020;**10**(11):874. DOI: 10.3390/diagnostics10110874

[32] Sigrist RMS, Liau J, El KA, Chammas MC, Willmann JK. Ultrasound elastography: Review of techniques and clinical applications. Theranostics. 2017;**7**:1303-1329. DOI: 10.7150/thno.18650

[33] Kara T, Ateş F, Durmaz MS, Akyürek N, Durmaz FG, et al. Assessment of thyroid gland elasticity with shear-wave elastography in Hashimoto's thyroiditis patients. Ultrasound International Open. 2020;**23**(5):543-551. DOI: 10.1007/s40477-020-00437-y

[34] Stoian D, Moisa L, Taban L, Sporea I, Popa A, Bende F, et al. Quantification of thyroid viscosity in healthy subjects using ultrasound shear wave dispersion (Viscosity PLUS). Diagnostics. 2022;**12**:2194. DOI: 10.3390/DIAGNOSTICS12092194

[35] Wu G, Zou D, Cai H, Liu Y. Ultrasonography in the diagnosis of Hashimoto's thyroiditis. FBL. 2016;**21**:1006-1012

[36] Stoian D, Borlea A, Moisa-Luca L, Paul C. Multiparametric ultrasound-based assessment of overt hyperthyroid diffuse thyroid disease. Frontiers in Endocrinology (Lausanne). 2023;**14**:1300447. DOI: 10.3389/FENDO.2023.1300447/BIBTEX

[37] Petea-Balea DR, Solomon C, Muntean DD, Dulgheriu IT, Silaghi CA, Dudea SM. Viscosity plane-wave ultrasound (Vi PLUS) in the evaluation of thyroid gland in healthy volunteers—A preliminary study. Diagnostics. 2022;**12**:2474. DOI: 10.3390/DIAGNOSTICS12102474

[38] Stoian D, Borlea A, Sporea I, Popa A, Moisa-Luca L, Popescu A. Assessment of thyroid stiffness and viscosity in autoimmune thyroiditis using novel ultrasound-based techniques. Biomedicine. 2023;**11**:938. DOI: 10.3390/BIOMEDICINES11030938

[39] Sidhu PS, Cantisani V, Dietrich CF, Gilja OH, Saftoiu A, Bartels E, et al. The EFSUMB guidelines and recommendations for the clinical practice of contrast-enhanced ultrasound (CEUS) in non-hepatic applications: Update 2017 (long version). Ultraschall in der Medizin. 2018;**39**: e2-e44. DOI: 10.1055/A-0586-1107/ID/JR513-18/BIB

Chapter 2

Thyroid Elastography: A Window to Hashimoto's Thyroiditis in Children

Cristina Mihaela Roi, Andreea Bena, Simina Mihuta, Corina Paul and Dana Liana Stoian

Abstract

This chapter offers a spotlight on the complex field of thyroid elastography, an innovative diagnostic tool performed on children with Hashimoto's thyroiditis (HT). Navigating the intersection of technology and pediatric endocrinology, this chapter explores how elastography provides important information about thyroid tissue elasticity, offering a nuanced understanding of the disease's progression. From unraveling the complexities of Hashimoto's in the pediatric population to elucidating the diagnostic potential of elastography, this chapter serves as a beacon for clinicians and researchers alike. With a focus on precision and innovation, it promises to reshape our approach to diagnosing and managing thyroid disorders in the youngest patients, paving the way for enhanced pediatric thyroid care.

Keywords: thyroid, elastography, strain elastography, shear-wave elastography, children

1. Introduction

Among medical conditions, thyroid diseases rank as some of the most widespread. The diverse manifestations of these conditions significantly differ from one region to another and are primarily influenced by the dietary supply of iodine. Iodine serves as a crucial component of the thyroid hormones thyroxine (T4) and triiodothyronine (T3), both synthesized by the thyroid gland [1].

This chapter will explore Hashimoto's thyroiditis (HT), commonly known as chronic autoimmune thyroiditis (CAT), autoimmune thyroiditis, or chronic lymphocytic thyroiditis, representing an autoimmune thyroid condition encompassing thyroid enlargement, lymphocyte infiltration, and the detection of specific antibodies [2, 3]. Many factors, including the geographical region and time period, affect the incidence and prevalence of thyroiditis. Longitudinal, long-term follow-ups are not enough, even with the abundance of research on the frequency of autoimmune disorders. Over the previous 30 years, there has been a significant increase in both incidence and prevalence [4]. The frequency of HT

IntechOpen

varies from 4.8 to 25.8% in women and from 0.9 to 7.8% in males, depending on the area and socioeconomic class [5]. HT stands as the primary cause of hypothyroidism [6, 7]. Additionally, HT represents the most widespread autoimmune disease among the pediatric population. Approximately 4–10% of children are estimated to be affected by CAT [8, 9]. The diagnosis of CAT involves clinical examination, antithyroid antibodies, and imaging assays. Among these, serum antithyroid peroxidase antibodies (TPOAb) are considered the most crucial indicator of HT, with approximately 95% of patients exhibiting their presence [10, 11]. In contrast to TPOAb, antibodies against thyroglobulin (TgAb) exhibit lower sensitivity (se), being positive in only 60–80% of patients with HT. Additionally, these antibodies are less specific, with a higher percentage of positive results observed in healthy controls [12]. There are rarely any clinical symptoms or indicators. When symptoms do occur, they are usually associated with hypothyroidism (dry skin, weight gain, sensitivity to cold, constipation, etc.), but they may also result from the thyroid gland compressing surrounding tissues (dyspnea, dysphonia, dysphagia, etc.) [10].

Thyroid ultrasound (US) has been extensively used to diagnose thyroid lesions and has also proved to be helpful in CAT detection. The US examination of a patient with HT usually reveals either focal or diffuse enlargement of the thyroid, accompanied by a coarse, heterogeneous, and hypoechoic pattern in the parenchyma. Although echogenicity is often reduced because of the inflammatory cells infiltrating the thyroid tissue, it can be normal in certain circumstances [13]. Diminished brightness, or echogenicity, in comparison to normal thyroid tissues is known as diffuse hypoechogenicity. In CAT, a heterogeneous echotexture is among the most frequently observed US findings (**Figure 1**) [14–17].

The thyroid gland's texture may appear irregular or uneven, but it might also appear macro- or micronodular. Thyroid pseudonodules are regions of the gland that show up as distinct nodules on ultrasonography; however, they are not actual thyroid nodules. There are two types of pseudonodules: micronodules and macronodules. Micro-pseudonodules are utterly small, sometimes less than

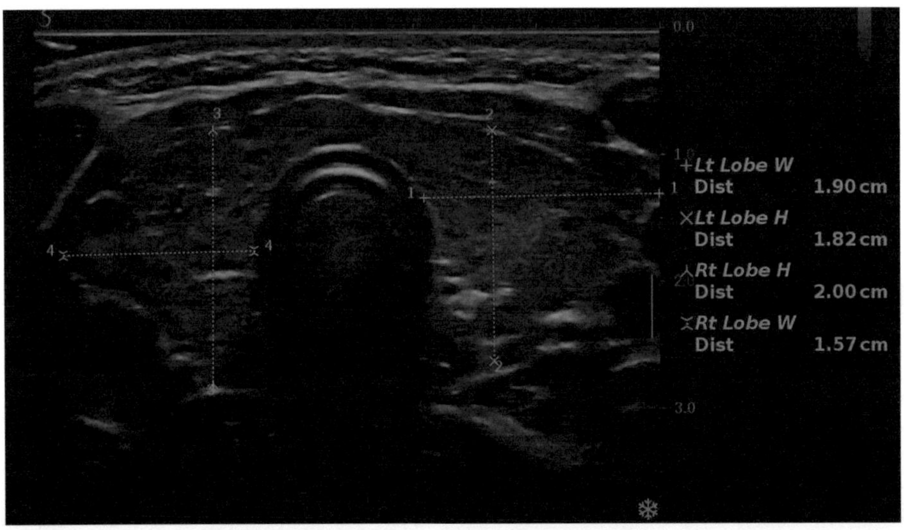

Figure 1.
B-mode US of a thyroid affected by HT; heterogeneous echotexture, hypoechogenicity; transverse plane.

one centimeter in diameter. These small pseudonodules usually do not need to be treated because they do not have any clinical significance. Usually, macro-pseudonodules are more than one centimeter in size. Several hypoechoic micronodules clearly suggest the presence of chronic thyroiditis. The external contour becomes more nodular as inflammation and fibrosis progress, and hyperechoic linear and curvilinear lines can appear with an uneven appearance. Fibrous septae can give the appearance that the parenchyma is pseudolobulated [18–21]. There are various thyroid volume ranges: extremely small (atrophic gland), normal, or significantly increased (goiter) (**Figure 2**).

The thyroid tissue impacted by CAT may exhibit a moderate to considerable increase in vascularity, or it may exhibit normal vascularity, as revealed by Color Doppler Imaging (CDI). Increased vascularity appears to be associated with hypothyroidism, most likely as a result of thyroid-stimulating hormone's (TSH) trophic stimulation [22]. Reduced or absent vascularization is frequently linked to the gland's small size and atrophic state [23, 24].

Modern technologies, like elastography, have the potential to provide important information for the diagnostic methodology, hence increasing its quality and accuracy. Tissue strain is measured using elastography, a noninvasive US technique. Both shear-wave elastography (SWE) and strain elastography (SE) can accurately predict the probability of malignancies linked to increasing stiffness [25–31]. Less research has been done on diffuse thyroid pathology, with most studies centered on nodular thyroid pathology. However, there is evidence that suggests that HT-affected thyroid tissue is stiffer than normal thyroid tissue. Unfortunately, limited data is available regarding the pediatric population. In the next chapters, this subject will be covered in more detail.

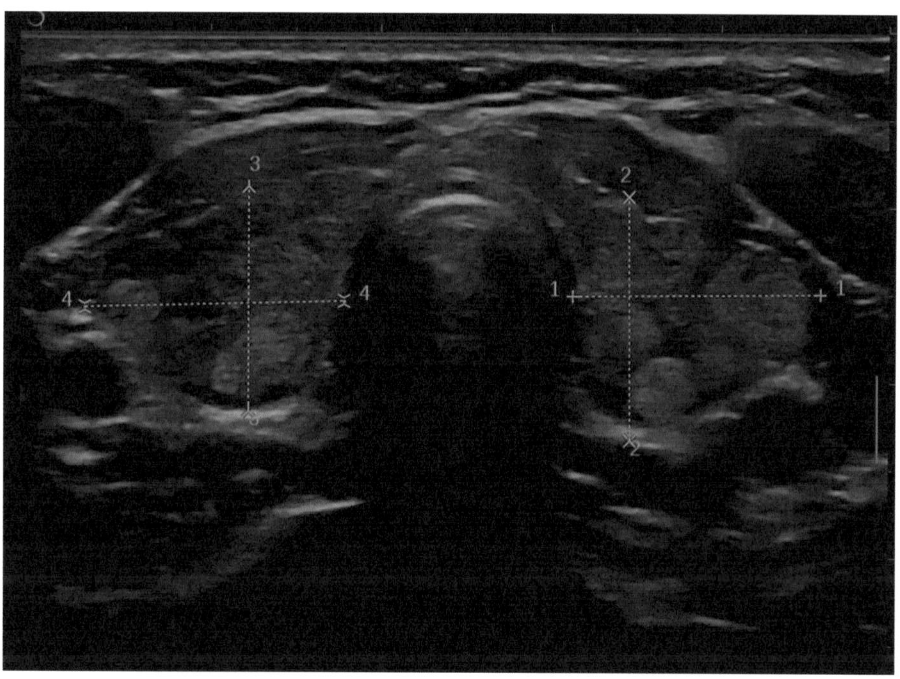

Figure 2.
Hyperechoic regenerative nodules in a hypoechoic thyroid parenchyma in a patient with HT - transverse view.

2. Ultrasound features in pediatric patients

Thyroid US procedures for children are essentially quite similar to those for adults, with the exception of a few requirements on volume measuring accuracy. A change in gland volume is a common feature of almost all pediatric thyroid disorders. Regarding the normal size of the pediatric thyroid gland, opinions vary. Both the alternative thyroid formula, height x width x length x 0.47, and the ellipsoid formula, height x width x length x 0.523, have been used [32–35]. A group of researchers compared various correction methods, including height, weight, a combination of height and weight, body surface area, and body mass index. Their study concluded that body surface area-corrected volume was the most reliable method for assessing thyroid volume in children aged 8–10 years [36]. Ozdikici conducted a study aimed at establishing normative reference values for thyroid volume in children, stratified by age and gender. This comprehensive investigation defined normal ranges of thyroid volume within a 95% confidence interval [37].

Pediatric thyroid size has been linked to somatometric characteristics, ethnicity, and local iodine intake [35, 38]. The World Health Organization (WHO) reference values for total thyroid volume, established in 2004, are limited to children aged 6–12 years from regions with long-standing iodine sufficiency, which does not accurately represent most European countries. For example, in German boys and girls, the 97th percentile thyroid volumes exceed the WHO standards by 33.4 and 28.5%, respectively—findings consistent with other contemporary European studies. These results suggest that the WHO reference values may be overly conservative and could be revised for use in other European countries with similar iodine histories [39]. Also, there may be variations in reported normal values as a result of these factors and variations in operator technique [34, 40]. Depending on gestational age, newborn thyroid volumes can range from 0.84 ± 0.38 mL to 1.62 ± 0.44 mL [41, 42]. Although highly important, research indicates that neither subjective nor objective assessments reliably predict whether congenital hypothyroidism (CH) is permanent or transient. Changes in gland shape may interfere with both methods and reduce the accuracy of standard formulas used to calculate lobe volume. Until more precise techniques for evaluating thyroid size are developed, the use of both subjective and objective assessments is advised in cases of CH [43]. The tracheal index is used in a simplified manner, and the usual range for the thyroid/trachea ratio is 1.7–2.4 [44]. The depth of the isthmus is typically not taken into account in situations where there is a noticeable rise in the overall volume of the thyroid lobes. The size of the isthmus can be estimated indirectly if the thyroid volume is close to the highest limit. In children under the age of 10 years, an isthmus thicker than 3 mm, and in adolescents, more than 5 mm, is considered an enlarged thyroid. The thyroid tissue's echo density is measured in relation to the salivary gland in both children and adults. Normal thyroid tissue has a homogeneous echo structure [45].

Children with the diffuse sclerosing type of papillary carcinoma might present with an enlarged heterogeneous thyroid with echogenic regions that indicate microcalcifications, with the background of thyroiditis; this has to be diagnosed as such and requires a biopsy. It is important to distinguish this uneven look from thyroiditis's micronodular pattern [46–48].

The intrathyroidal thymus, an embryological remnant, is a specific US finding in infants. It appears as a well-defined hypovascular lesion, often measuring less than 1 cm, and sometimes has angulated borders with a starry-sky pattern. These lesions can occasionally show extrathyroidal extension, characterized by a thymic tissue protrusion toward the mediastinum or a thymus-lesion link. It is crucial to distinguish ectopic thymus from other nodular thyroid tumors [49–51].

3. Ultrasound-based elastography

3.1 General principles

Elastography, a noninvasive technique based on ultrasound, measures tissue strain. Its increasing use aims to enhance the differentiation of thyroid nodules. Both shear-wave elastography (SWE) and strain elastography (SE) have demonstrated effectiveness in predicting the risk of malignancy by identifying increased rigidity as a suspicion criterion [52–54]. US elastography evaluates tissue stiffness noninvasively by assessing the displacement of the tissue in response to internal or external mechanical pressure. Ultrasound elastography methods are categorized as quasi-static, or strain-based, and dynamic, or shear-wave-based [55–57]. A deformation occurs when the tissue is exposed to an external pressure, as in strain scanning, or to the shear-waves emitted by the US probe, as in SWE [58]. The capacity of a tissue to resist deformation in the presence of an external force and to return to its initial form upon removal of the force is known as its elasticity. Clinically observed loss of elasticity with palpation or elastography (virtual palpation) increases the possibility of a disease [59, 60]. A recent study compared two types of elastography—SWE and strain elastography—in evaluating children with Hashimoto's thyroiditis, concluding that there were no significant differences between the methods. The authors recommend using either technique, depending on availability [61].

3.2 Shear-wave elastography

The SWE method relies on the generation and detection of shear-waves (SW), which are transverse components of particle displacement. Shear indicates a shape change, but volume does not change [25, 27]. The velocity of wave propagation is contingent on tissue elasticity, and shear-waves move through the tissue at a considerably slower speed than longitudinal waves [62]. Deformation of the tissue induced by wave generation leads to changes in the US pattern. The movement of tissue is monitored by using multiple locations of the ultrasound probe. Shear waves typically have a speed ranging from 1 to 50 m/s and are generated at frequencies between 10 and 2000 Hz [63, 64]. Because shear-wave elastography is less operator-dependent, it may be reproduced more precisely. Tissue elasticity may be evaluated both quantitatively and qualitatively by measuring the SW velocity [25, 65].

1-D monoplane: A common method for evaluating liver fibrosis is transient elastography, such as Echosens and Fibroscan. It is not accessible on normal US devices using standard US transducers. This device has a vibrating instrument in addition to a specialized ultrasonic transducer that uses an external vibrating "punch" to create shear-waves that penetrate the tissues [60].

Using push pulses that induce local tissue displacement perpendicular to the surface, the ARFI (acoustic radiation force impulse) physically stimulates the ROI's (region of interest) tissue in monoplane SWE (point-SWE, pSWE). The operator can select the suitable acoustic window for assessments with the use of visual assistance in point shear-wave elastography. SW velocity (m/s) estimations may be achieved up to a maximum of 8 cm depth [60].

Using biplane SWE (2D SWE) and 3D SWE, a quantitative color elastogram is superimposed over 2B images in real time, and SW speed is determined. Supersonic shear-wave technology uses focused ultrasonic beams. These beams spread out over the imaging region and show the elasticity index (EI), which is measured in kilopascals (kPa), for each pixel of the ROI. This indicates the speed (m/s) of the SW. The mean, minimum, and maximum stiffness values, as well as the standard deviation (SD), may all be measured inside the ROI [25, 60].

Compared to SE, image acquisition is acknowledged as being easier to get accustomed to and more rapid. 2D SWE equipment provides results that are both quantitative and qualitative. Images are stored and assessed once the SWE map has stabilized, usually following an undisturbed exposure of five to seven seconds. Color-coded maps are supplied for each US machine, with different codes displayed on scales denoting soft-to-hard lesions.

Some drawbacks of the ARFI method will be briefly highlighted. The first one has to do with the ROI's predetermined fixed dimension. Additionally, nodules larger than 20 mm cause instability in SW speed. Lesions with liquid areas and intralesional calcifications cannot be examined since the ROI is hard to identify within the nodule. When utilizing point- and 2D-SWE, deep localization presents a major challenge; nodular structures deeper than 40–50 mm are inaccessible to the ARFI. Lesions on the thyroid isthmus are a challenge because of their position between the surface of the skin and the stiff trachea (**Figures 3** and **4**) [66, 67].

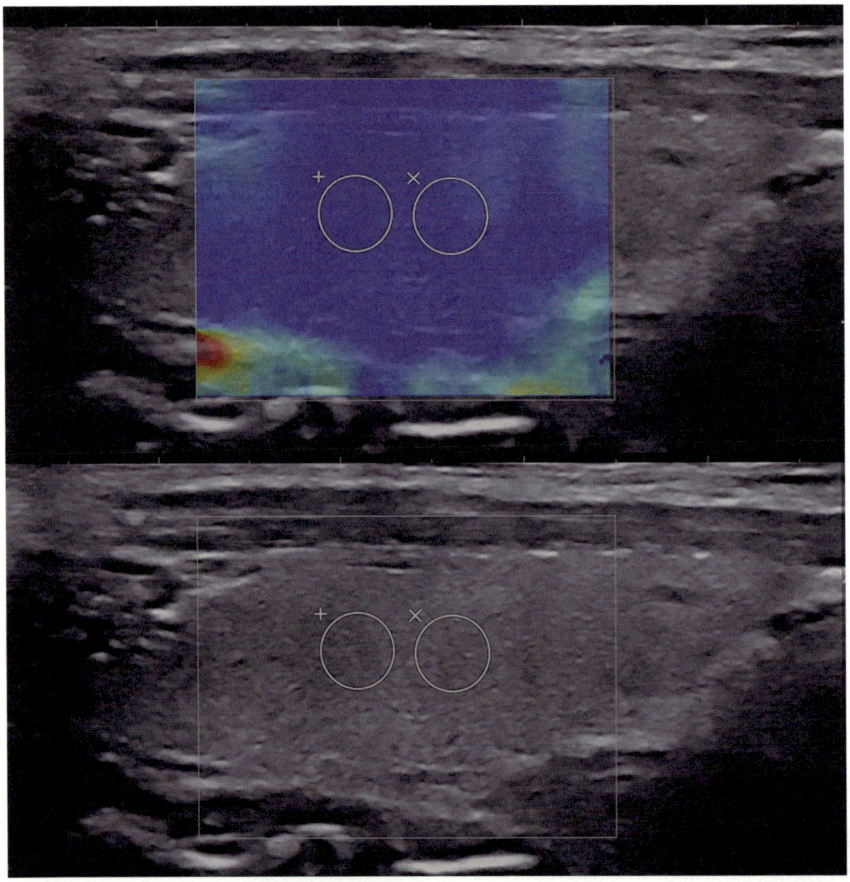

Figure 3.
2D-SWE of a healthy thyroid; homogeneous blue appearance; longitudinal view.

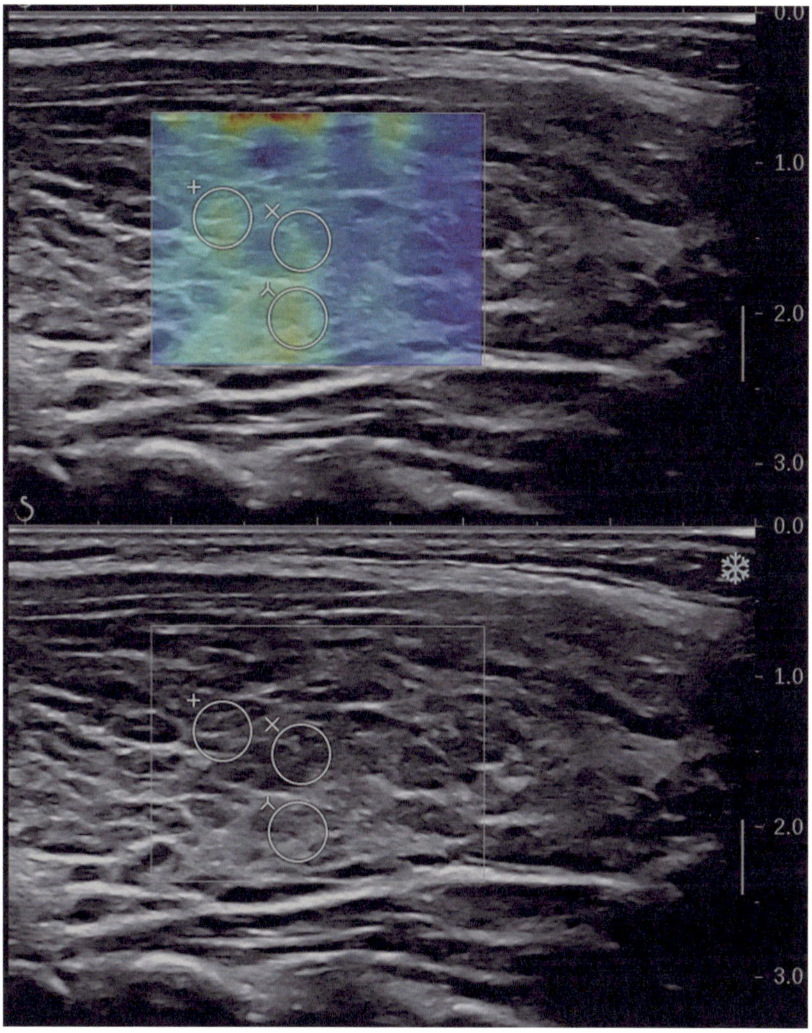

Figure 4.
2D-SWE - Thyroid affected by HT, stiffer thyroid tissue, heterogeneously blue and green appearance; longitudinal view.

3.3 Strain elastography

Initially, and most commonly, strain elastography is the technique employed. The external pressure is either created by an ARFI or the operator typically applies a minimally controlled external pressure. In recent years, the equipment has acquired the ability to identify even the smallest internal physiological motions, such as muscle contraction and vascular pulse [52, 59].

Devices equipped with strain elastography are unable to measure stress directly. Elastograms, which are based on signal differences before and after compression, show relative stiffness together with B-mode pictures on a dual-screen system or overlaid on the grayscale image. Usually, a continuous color map that ranges from red (soft) to green (equal strain or intermediate) to blue (hard) is used to depict the tissue stiffness. Several systems use an inverted color scale [60, 68, 69].

With the use of special software, strain elastography equipment generates an objective, semiquantitative assessment that yields a numerical value known as the strain ratio (SR). The measure used to evaluate stiffness is the parenchyma-to-nodule ratio (PTNR), which is the ratio of the strain in the thyroid parenchyma to the strain in the nodule, or the strain in the proximal strap muscle to the thyroid tissue. SR is thought to be more precise than evaluating qualitative elasticity (**Table 1**).

The average of the three consecutive measurements determines the final result. A number of recommendations need to be considered when determining where the ROI will be located. It should include the whole nodule and surrounding parenchyma as close to the transducer as possible. Strain depreciation with distance can be avoided by positioning the elastographic ROI as close to the transducer as is practical [66]. To increase the contrast between nodules and parenchyma in SE, it is imperative to include as much "normal" reference parenchyma as possible in the picture. Furthermore, the blood vessels (particularly the carotid), the esophagus, the trachea, the bones, and the muscles must all be removed from the ROI as much as possible. There is an important relevance to holding one's breath and not speaking or swallowing. A large amount of gel and minimal skin contact are necessary. For this application, a probe stabilizer is inappropriate because of the neck's anatomical particulars [70, 71]. Longitudinal sections are favored over transverse ones in the SE assessment. To improve reproducibility regarding the external, operator-dependent manual compression, each system offers suggestions on the ideal displacement quantity and frequency [66, 67].

The approach has several limitations, including subjectivity, operator dependence, and compressibility. It is believed that the size of the nodule has little impact on the accuracy of SE assessment, even though certain studies show that nodules less than 3 cm or greater than 3 cm perform differently. The World Federation for Ultrasound in Medicine and Biology (WFUMB) standards state that because of their deeper regions and absence of healthy surrounding tissue, nodules bigger than three centimeters cannot be examined appropriately. When coalescent nodules are present, the SE assessment is not accurate. Increased stiffness in benign lesions with calcifications or fibrosis can be detected, leading to false-positive findings. Identifying anterior lesions that extend to the capsule as soft may be an error due to the reference tissue being the strap muscles rather than the thyroid parenchyma. Isthmic lesions are challenging to assess because they are limited between two firm planes (the probe and the trachea) and lack reference tissue [72]. When external pressure is

Modality	Strengths	Limitations
B-mode US	Structural detail, widely available	Operator-dependent, does not provide information about elasticity
Color Doppler	Evaluates vascularity	Nonspecific for thyroiditis
Strain elastography	Qualitative, semiquantitative	Operator-dependent, less reproducible
Shear-wave elastography	Quantitative, reproducible	Equipment variability, deep lesions are problematic

Table 1.
Comparison of ultrasound modes.

applied, carotid pulsations may interfere, especially in transverse sections. Real-time elastography (RTE) with external force is less suitable for transverse thyroid scans because it is more susceptible to carotid pulse interference. However, they have the benefit of internal force. Longitudinal scans offer greater thyroid reference tissue and are less affected by carotid pulsations. The surrounding reference parenchyma inside the ROI must exhibit at least 50% green color to determine an appropriate strain ratio. Lesions that are smaller than 5 mm, significant cystic components (only the solid part should be measured), nodules with peripheral rim calcification (which might inaccurately increase stiffness), and overweight individuals are some further limitations of SE (**Figures 5** and **6**) [27, 68].

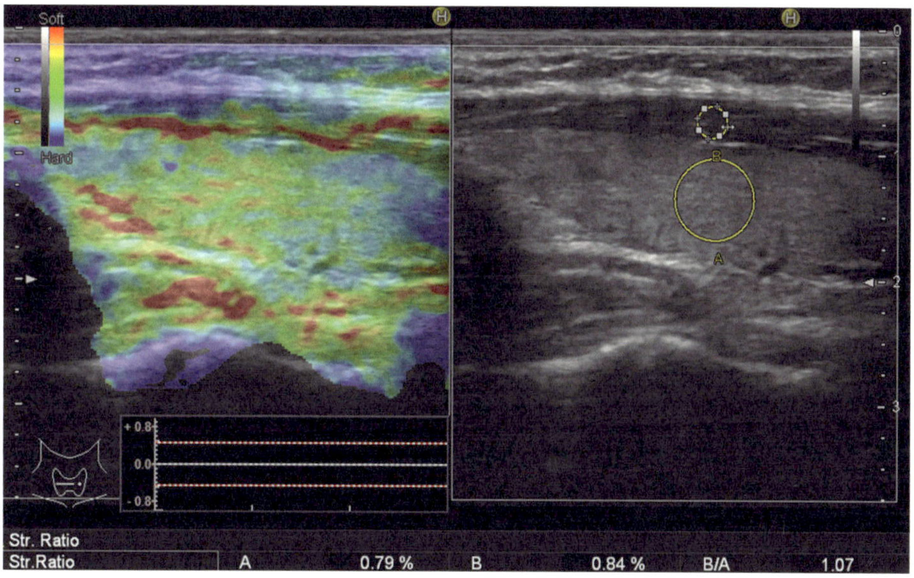

Figure 5.
SE (left) and B-mode US (right) of a normal thyroid; SR = 1.07; longitudinal view.

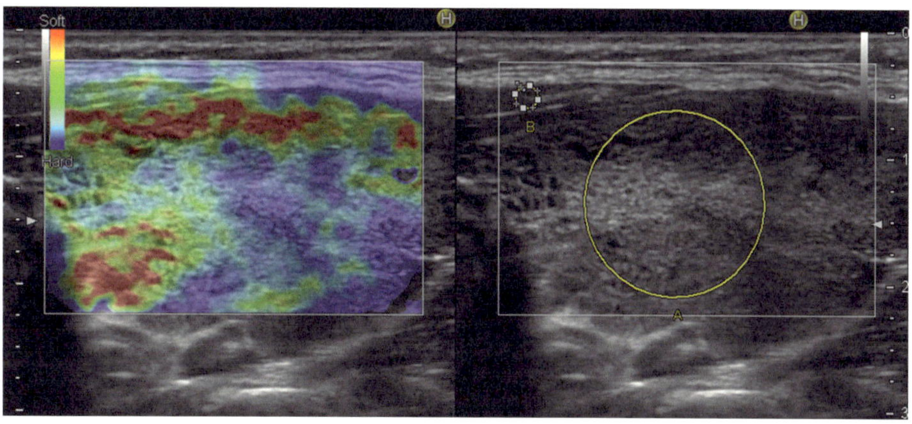

Figure 6.
SE (left) and B-mode US (right) of a thyroid affected by HT; longitudinal view.

3.4 Thyroid elastography in children with HT – current perspective

3.4.1 Shear-wave elastography

There has been limited research on the pediatric population. Elasticity scores were measured in 107 healthy children, and a median value of 6.38 ± 1.97 kPa was suggested as the norm for a healthy thyroid [73]. Additional studies on children with healthy thyroids have revealed similar findings, with thyroid stiffness (TS) values ranging from 8.2 ± 2.82 kPa [74] to 11.24 ± 1.99 kPa [75]. Normal elasticity scores were reported as 10.9 ± 1.78 kPa [76], 9.36 ± 1.63 kPa [77], 10.41 ± 2.01 kPa [78], or 10.6 kPa [79] in several articles. Given the wide range of variability, more expansive cohorts of children must be investigated. The evaluation should also consider the ROI's depth and size.

The cut-off value with the best diagnostic accuracy for elasticity values was 12.3 kPa (sensitivity 86.4%, specificity 96.3%) in research with 59 pediatric patients with CAT diagnoses and 26 healthy controls [79]. Twenty healthy volunteers and 74 patients with diffuse thyroid diseases (DTD) participated in another study on children with graves' disease (GD), HT, and simple goiter. It was discovered that 12.8 kPa was the optimal SWE cut-off value for distinguishing between DTD and a normal thyroid [76]. Another research that showed a se of 82% and a sp of 88% determined a cut-off value of 12.2 kPa for the mean SWE value in predicting CAT in children. A cut-off value of 13.13 kPa for the highest SWE value obtained a sensitivity of 80% and a specificity of 92% in accurately differentiating between children with CAT and healthy participants [78]. A group of Egyptian researchers found similar results after studying 64 children. The elasticity values of the CAT patients were significantly higher than those of the control group (9.35 kPa vs. 35.6 kPa). In addition to having a sensitivity of 96.9% and a specificity of 100%, the test was found to have a threshold value for elasticity of 12.317 kPa [77]. Koca et al. assessed 46 children who were recently given a diagnosis of CAT and 46 healthy individuals. Mean SWE values of 12.5 ± 5.1 kilopascals (kPa) were observed in children with euthyroid CAT, whereas healthy controls exhibited mean SWE values of 8.2 ± 2.82 kPa ($p < 0.001$). With a sensitivity of 68%, a specificity of 72%, a positive predictive value of 70%, and a negative predictive value of 69%, they determined a cut-off value of 9.68 kPa for diagnosing HT [74]. In a different study, the thyroid glands of 18 children (5 boys and 13 girls) with newly diagnosed HT and 27 healthy controls (21 boys and 6 girls) were assessed using grayscale ultrasound followed by SWE. The median SWE value in the HT group was 20.6 kPa, compared to 10.7 kPa in the control group. This difference was statistically significant ($W = 438.5$, $P < .001$) [80]. Another study concluded that SWE can not only aid in the diagnosis of Hashimoto's thyroiditis but also assist in grading its severity, as SWE values were found to increase with advancing stages of the disease. However, no significant differences were observed between stages 2 and 3 [81].

There was no association observed between thyroid elasticity levels and TSH levels [78, 82, 83]. However, one study reported a mild negative correlation between the two parameters [80]. Furthermore, two studies reported a weak to mildly positive correlation between thyroid elasticity level and TPOAb [78, 79] but no link between TS and TGAb [79]. A weak positive correlation was seen in another analysis between TS and TGAb, but no link was discovered between TS and TPOAb [84].

Additionally, it was verified if children with CAT diagnoses who were getting levothyroxine hormone replacement therapy had different TS than those who were not. Nevertheless, no noticeable differences in elasticity were seen between these two youth patient categories [78]. However, research by Magri found that there were significant differences in thyroid elasticity between individuals receiving medication and those who were not, although it is important to highlight that Magri's study included adult participants [85].

A recent meta-analysis was conducted to evaluate the utility of two-dimensional shear-wave elastography (2D-SWE) in children with Hashimoto's thyroiditis. Although the analysis included only five studies, all reported that the method is useful for diagnosing children with Hashimoto's thyroiditis. However, larger studies are needed to reach a consensus on standardized cut-off values [86].

3.4.2 Strain elastography

It was found that the stiffness of several thyroid diseases in adults may be ranked in ascending order using a list as follows: control group < hyperthyroidism< HT < subacute thyroiditis (SAT) [87]. SE can be a useful tool in distinguishing cases of SAT from healthy individuals as well as between several autoimmune diseases, including GD and HT [88]. Real-time elastography is a viable technique for differential diagnosis when thyroid nodules and CAT coexist, and SR evaluation could be a helpful predictor [89, 90].

Until this point, there has been limited research conducted on thyroid elastography specifically focused on pediatric individuals diagnosed with thyroiditis. The existing body of literature concerning this subject is currently scarce.

In a study including 54 healthy children, Yurttutan et al. evaluated the SR of normal thyroid parenchyma. Their suggested mean value is 0.54 +/– 0.38. Their analysis found no evidence of a significant association between SR and gender ($r = 0.007$; $p = 0.96$) or age ($r = 0.22$; $p = 0.15$) [91].

A study that included 47 children without thyroid conditions and 63 children with HT revealed differences between the two groups (1.75 ± 1.46 vs. 0.26 ± 0.77; $p < 0.001$). For CAT presence, the cut-off value was 0.31 (92.1% sensitivity (se), 66% sp, and AUROC of 0.828) [92]. A different study with 76 teenagers with HT and 46 without thyroid disease suggested using SR >0.98 (se of 83%, sp of 93%, AUROC 0.929) as the cut-off value for CAT diagnosis. The children with CAT had mean SR values of 1.2 ± 0.2, which were considerably higher than the control participants' mean SR values of 0.77 ± 0.18 ($p < 0.01$) [93].

In another study, 22 children without thyroid pathology and 52 children with CAT diagnoses were included. When comparing the control group to the CAT group, the mean SR values were considerably lower (0.68 ± 0.2 vs. 1.19 ± 0.25; $p < 0.0001$). For CAT, a mean value greater than 0.9 was determined to be predictive, with AUROC 0.9, 84.62% se, 95.45% sp, 97.8% PPV, and 72.4% NPV [94].

Regarding the relationships between different variables and tissue elasticity level, there is no consensus in the literature. Positive correlations between SR and TPOAb ($r = 6.85$) were noted by Ozturk et al., but no evaluation was done into the possible association between SR and TGAb [92]. Similar findings were made by Çekiç et al.; they found no association between SR and TGAb but a correlation between SR and TPOAb ($r = 0.439$, $p < 0.01$) [93]. Additionally, Cepeha et al. found a mildly positive association ($r = 0.29$) between SR and TGAb levels and a strong correlation ($r = 0.65$) between SR and TPOAb values [94].

Only one study addressed the differences between patients receiving treatment and those who did not need it. There were no significant differences noticed between children receiving levothyroxine therapy and those who were not [94]. Given the disparities between treated and untreated patients seen in previous adult population studies [69], this line of inquiry deserves more examination.

4. Conclusions

Elastography has emerged as a promising tool in the evaluation and follow-up of children with HT. Although the number of studies in pediatric populations is still relatively limited, the existing research shows encouraging results regarding the accuracy and usefulness of this technique. Both SWE and strain elastography have demonstrated the ability to noninvasively measure thyroid stiffness, offering additional information that complements conventional ultrasound. Some studies even suggest that elastography may help in grading disease severity, although clear differences between all stages have not been consistently observed.

Despite these promising results, some limitations remain. The small number of large studies, differences in examination methods, and the lack of clear reference values mean that elastography is not yet fully standardized for routine use in clinical practice.

In clinical settings, elastography provides a unique benefit by reducing the need for invasive procedures and allowing for easy, repeatable monitoring over time, an important consideration when dealing with children. Its role should be viewed as complementary to conventional ultrasound techniques, including grayscale and Doppler imaging, to provide a more complete picture of thyroid health.

Looking ahead, further research is essential to define normal reference ranges for children, establish standard protocols, and clarify the potential of elastography in tracking disease progression and treatment response. With continued advances in ultrasound technology and growing experience among clinicians, elastography may become an even more reliable and routine part of thyroid imaging in pediatric patients.

Conflict of interest

The authors declare no conflict of interest.

Author details

Cristina Mihaela Roi[1*], Andreea Bena[2], Simina Mihuta[3], Corina Paul[3] and Dana Liana Stoian[2]

1 Victor Babes University of Medicine and Pharmacy, Timisoara, Romania

2 Department of Internal Medicine II, Victor Babes University of Medicine and Pharmacy, Timisoara, Romania

3 Department of Pediatrics, Victor Babes University of Medicine and Pharmacy, Timisoara, Romania

*Address all correspondence to: cristina.cepeha@umft.ro

References

[1] Vanderpump MPJ. Epidemiology of thyroid disorders. In: The Thyroid and its Diseases. Cham: Springer International Publishing; 2019. pp. 75-85. DOI: 10.1007/978-3-319-72102-6_6

[2] Ralli M, Angeletti D, Fiore M, D'Aguanno V, Lambiase A, Artico M, et al. Hashimoto's thyroiditis: An update on pathogenic mechanisms, diagnostic protocols, therapeutic strategies, and potential malignant transformation. Autoimmunity Reviews. 2020;**19**:102649. DOI: 10.1016/j.autrev.2020.102649

[3] Ajjan RA, Weetman AP. The pathogenesis of Hashimoto's thyroiditis: Further developments in our understanding. Hormone and Metabolic Research. 2015;**47**:702-710. DOI: 10.1055/s-0035-1548832

[4] Lerner A, Jeremias P, Matthias T. The world incidence and prevalence of autoimmune diseases is increasing. International Journal of Celiac Disease. 2015;**3**:151-155. DOI: 10.12691/ijcd-3-4-8

[5] Hu X, Chen Y, Shen Y, Tian R, Sheng Y, Que H. Global prevalence and epidemiological trends of Hashimoto's thyroiditis in adults: A systematic review and meta-analysis. Frontiers in Public Health. 2022;**10**:1020709. DOI: 10.3389/fpubh.2022.1020709

[6] Ragusa F, Fallahi P, Elia G, Gonnella D, Rosaria S, Giusti C, et al. Hashimotos' thyroiditis: Epidemiology, pathogenesis, clinic and therapy. Best Practice & Research Clinical Endocrinology & Metabolism. 2019;**33**:101367. DOI: 10.1016/j.beem.2019.101367

[7] Delemer B, Aubert J, Nys P. An observational study of the initial management of hypothyroidism in France: The ORCHIDÉE study. European Journal of Endocrinology. 2012;**167**:817-823. DOI: 10.1530/EJE-11-1041

[8] Brown RS. Autoimmune thyroiditis in childhood. JCRPE Journal of Clinical Research in Pediatric Endocrinology. 2013;**5**:45-49. DOI: 10.4274/Jcrpe.855

[9] Skarpa V, Kousta E, Tertipi A, Anyfandakis K, Vakaki M, Dolianiti M, et al. Epidemiological characteristics of children with autoimmune thyroid disease. Hormones. 2011;**10**:207-214. DOI: 10.14310/horm.2002.1310

[10] Caturegli P, De Remigis A, Rose NR. Hashimoto thyroiditis: Clinical and diagnostic criteria. Autoimmunity Reviews. 2014;**13**:391-397. DOI: 10.1016/j.autrev.2014.01.007

[11] Radetti G. Clinical aspects of Hashimoto's thyroiditis. Endocrine Development. 2014;**26**:158-170. DOI: 10.1159/000363162. Epub 2014 Aug 29

[12] McLachlan SM, Rapoport B. Why measure thyroglobulin autoantibodies rather than thyroid peroxidase autoantibodies? Thyroid. 2004;**14**:510-520. DOI: 10.1089/1050725041517057

[13] Mazziotti G, Sorvillo F, Iorio S, Carbone A, Romeo A, Piscopo M, et al. Grey-scale analysis allows a quantitative evaluation of thyroid echogenicity in the patients with Hashimoto's thyroiditis. Clinical Endocrinology. 2003;**59**:223-229. DOI: 10.1046/j.1365-2265.2003.01829.x

[14] Schiemann U, Avenhaus W, Konturek JW, Gellner R, Hengst K, Gross M. Relationship of clinical features and laboratory parameters to thyroid

echogenicity measured by standardized grey scale ultrasonography in patients with Hashimoto's thyroiditis. Medical Science Monitor. 2003;**9**:MT13-MTI7

[15] Kim DW, Eun CK, In HS, Kim MH, Jung SJ, Bae SK. Sonographic differentiation of asymptomatic diffuse thyroid disease from normal thyroid: A prospective study. American Journal of Neuroradiology. 2010;**31**:1956-1960. DOI: 10.3174/ajnr.A2164

[16] Lai SM, Chang TC, Chang CC, Kuo SH, Chen FW. Sonographic presentation in autoimmune thyroiditis. Journal of the Formosan Medical Association. 1990;**89**:1057-1062

[17] Baek HJ, Kim DW, Lee YJ, Ahn HS, Ryu JH. Comparison of real-time and static ultrasonography diagnoses for detecting incidental diffuse thyroid disease: A multicenter study. Ultrasound Quarterly. 2019;**35**:233-239. DOI: 10.1097/RUQ.0000000000000391

[18] Alexander LF, Patel NJ, Caserta MP, Robbin ML. Thyroid ultrasound: Diffuse and nodular disease. Radiologic Clinics of North America. 2020;**58**:1041-1057. DOI: 10.1016/j.rcl.2020.07.003

[19] Kharchenko VP, Kotlyarov PM, Mogutov MS, Alexandrov YK, Sencha AN, Patrunov YN, et al. Diffuse changes of the thyroid gland. In: Ultrasound Diagnostics of Thyroid Diseases. Berlin, Heidelberg: Springer Berlin Heidelberg; 2010. pp. 57-83. DOI: 10.1007/978-3-642-12387-0_5

[20] Koprowski R, Zieleźnik W, Wróbel Z, Małyszek J, Stępień B, Wójcik W. Assessment of significance of features acquired from thyroid ultrasonograms in Hashimoto's disease. Biomedical Engineering Online. 2012;**11**:48. DOI: 10.1186/1475-925X-11-48

[21] Chaudhary V, Bano S. Thyroid ultrasound. Indian Journal of Endocrinology and Metabolism. 2013;**17**:219. DOI: 10.4103/2230-8210.109667

[22] Chung J, Lee YJ, Choi YJ, Ha EJ, Suh CH, Choi M, et al. Clinical applications of Doppler ultrasonography for thyroid disease: Consensus statement by the Korean Society of Thyroid Radiology. Ultrasonography. 2020;**39**:315-330. DOI: 10.14366/usg.20072

[23] Dighe M, Barr R, Bojunga J, Cantisani V, Chammas MC, Cosgrove D, et al. Thyroid ultrasound: State of the art part 1 – Thyroid ultrasound reporting and diffuse thyroid diseases. Medical Ultrasonography. 2017;**19**:79. DOI: 10.11152/mu-980

[24] Schulz SL, Seeberger U, Hengstmann JH. Color Doppler sonography in hypothyroidism. European Journal of Ultrasound. 2003;**16**:183-189. DOI: 10.1016/S0929-8266(02)00072-1

[25] Kwak JY, Kim E-K. Ultrasound elastography for thyroid nodules: Recent advances. Ultrasonography. 2014;**33**:75-82. DOI: 10.14366/usg.13025

[26] Cantisani V, De Silvestri A, Scotti V, Fresilli D, Tarsitano MG, Polti G, et al. US-elastography with different techniques for thyroid nodule characterization: Systematic review and meta-analysis. Frontiers in Oncology. 2022;**12**:845549. DOI: 10.3389/fonc.2022.845549

[27] Cantisani V, Grazhdani H, Drakonaki E, D'Andrea V, Di Segni M, Kaleshi E, et al. Strain US elastography for the characterization of thyroid nodules: Advantages and limitation. International Journal of Endocrinology. 2015;**2015**:1-8. DOI: 10.1155/2015/908575

[28] Bojunga J, Herrmann E, Meyer G, Weber S, Zeuzem S, Friedrich-Rust M. Real-time elastography for the differentiation of benign and malignant thyroid nodules: A meta-analysis. Thyroid. 2010;**20**:1145-1150. DOI: 10.1089/thy.2010.0079

[29] Borlea A, Stoian D, Cotoi L, Sporea I, Lazar F, Mozos I. Thyroid multimodal ultrasound evaluation—Impact on presurgical diagnosis of intermediate cytology cases. Applied Sciences. 2020;**10**:3439. DOI: 10.3390/app10103439

[30] Borlea A, Cotoi L, Mozos I, Stoian D. Advanced ultrasound techniques in preoperative diagnostic of thyroid cancers. In: Knowledges on Thyroid Cancer. London: IntechOpen; 2019. DOI: 10.5772/intechopen.83032

[31] Hazem M, Zakaria OM, Daoud MYI, Al Jabr IK, AlYahya AA, Hassanein AG, et al. Accuracy of shear-wave elastography in characterization of thyroid nodules in children and adolescents. Insights into Imaging. 2021;**12**:128. DOI: 10.1186/s13244-021-01074-7

[32] Aydıner Ö, Karakoç Aydıner E, Akpınar İ, Turan S, Bereket A. Normative data of thyroid volume-ultrasonographic evaluation of 422 subjects aged 0-55 years. Journal of Clinical Research in Pediatric Endocrinology. 2015;7:98-101. DOI: 10.4274/jcrpe.1818

[33] Ng SM, Turner MA, Avula S. Ultrasound measurements of thyroid gland volume at 36 weeks' corrected gestational age in extremely preterm infants born before 28 weeks' gestation. European Thyroid Journal. 2018;7:21-26. DOI: 10.1159/000481857

[34] Taş F, Bulut S, Eğilmez H, Öztoprak İ, Ergür AT, Candann F. Normal thyroid volume by ultrasonography in healthy children. Annals of Tropical Paediatrics. 2002;**22**:375-379. DOI: 10.1179/027249302125002047

[35] Zimmermann MB, Hess SY, Molinari L, de Benoist B, Delange F, Braverman LE, et al. New reference values for thyroid volume by ultrasound in iodine-sufficient schoolchildren: a World Health Organization/Nutrition for Health and Development Iodine Deficiency Study Group Report. The American Journal of Clinical Nutrition. 2004;**79**:231-237. DOI: 10.1093/ajcn/79.2.231

[36] Liu L, Qian T, Sun R, Du Y, Li M, Liu L, et al. Comparative analysis of five correction methods for thyroid volume by ultrasound and their recommended reference values in Chinese children aged 8-10 years. British Journal of Nutrition. 2023;**129**:301-311. DOI: 10.1017/S0007114522001003

[37] Özdikici M. Ultrasound measurement of thyroid volume in healthy children. Ultrasound Quarterly. 2025;**41**(1):e00711. DOI: 10.1097/RUQ.0000000000000711

[38] Moradi M, Hashemipour M, Akbari S, Kor Z, Mirbod S, Kooshanmehr M. Ultrasonographic evaluation of the thyroid gland volume among 8-15-year-old children in Isfahan, Iran. Advanced Biomedical Research. 2014;**3**:9. DOI: 10.4103/2277-9175.124637

[39] Hirtz R, Thamm R, Kuhnert R, Liesenkötter K-P, Thamm M, Grasemann C. New reference values for thyroid volume by ultrasound in German children and adolescents from a population-based study. The Journal of Clinical Endocrinology and Metabolism. 2025;**110**:e382-e390. DOI: 10.1210/clinem/dgae194

[40] Zygmunt A. Are the normal values of thyroid gland in children fulfilling the role attributed to them? Thyroid Research. 2015;**8**:A27. DOI: 10.1186/1756-6614-8-S1-A27

[41] Goldis M, Waldman L, Marginean O, Rosenberg HK, Rapaport R. Thyroid imaging in infants. Endocrinology and Metabolism Clinics of North America. 2016;**45**:255-266. DOI: 10.1016/j.ecl.2016.02.005

[42] Delange F, Benker G, Caron P, Eber O, Ott W, Peter F, et al. Thyroid volume and urinary iodine in European schoolchildren: Standardization of values for assessment of iodine deficiency. European Journal of Endocrinology. 1997;**136**:180-187. DOI: 10.1530/eje.0.1360180

[43] Mansour C, Ouarezki Y, Jones JH, Green M, Stenhouse EJ, Irwin G, et al. Determination of thyroid volume in infants with suspected congenital hypothyroidism—the limitations of both subjective and objective evaluation. BJR|Open. 2020;**2**:20200001. DOI: 10.1259/bjro.20200001

[44] Yasumoto M, Inoue H, Ohashi I, Shibuya H, Onishi T. Simple new technique for sonographic measurement of the thyroid in neonates and small children. Journal of Clinical Ultrasound. 2004;**32**:82-85. DOI: 10.1002/jcu.10234

[45] Kharchenko VP, Kotlyarov PM, Mogutov MS, Alexandrov YK, Sencha AN, Patrunov YN, et al. Ultrasound examination of the thyroid gland in children. In: Ultrasound Diagnostics of Thyroid Diseases. Berlin, Heidelberg: Springer Berlin Heidelberg; 2010. pp. 35-45. DOI: 10.1007/978-3-642-12387-0_3

[46] Koo JS, Hong S, Park CS. Diffuse sclerosing variant is a major subtype of papillary thyroid carcinoma in the young. Thyroid. 2009;**19**:1225-1231. DOI: 10.1089/thy.2009.0073

[47] Vlachopapadopoulou E, Thomas D, Karachaliou F, Chatzimarkou F, Memalai L, Vakaki M, et al. Evolution of sonographic appearance of the thyroid gland in children with Hashimoto's thyroiditis. Journal of Pediatric Endocrinology and Metabolism. 2009;**22**(4):339-344. DOI: 10.1515/JPEM.2009.22.4.339

[48] Wang X, Xu F, Gao J, Agyekum EA, Sun H, Zhang G, et al. Differential diagnosis of diffuse sclerotic thyroid papillary carcinoma and Hashimoto's thyroiditis using fine-needle aspiration cytology, $BRAF^{V600E}$, and ultrasound elastography. Journal of Clinical Ultrasound. 2022;**50**:942-950. DOI: 10.1002/jcu.23260

[49] Raissaki M, Tritou I, Smirnaki P. Sonographic appearances of intrathyroid thymus: Emphasis on details. Hellenic Journal of Radiology. 2018;**3**:42-51

[50] Hong HS, Lee EH, Jeong SH, Park J, Lee H. Ultrasonography of various thyroid diseases in children and adolescents: A pictorial essay. Korean Journal of Radiology. 2015;**16**:419. DOI: 10.3348/kjr.2015.16.2.419

[51] Tritou I, Vakaki M, Sfakiotaki R, Kalaitzaki K, Raissaki M. Pediatric thyroid ultrasound: A radiologist's checklist. Pediatric Radiology. 2020;**50**:563-574. DOI: 10.1007/s00247-019-04602-2

[52] Bamber J, Cosgrove D, Dietrich C, Fromageau J, Bojunga J, Calliada F, et al. EFSUMB guidelines and recommendations on the clinical use of ultrasound elastography. Part 1: Basic principles and technology. Ultraschall in Der Medizin-European

Journal of Ultrasound. 2013;**34**:169-184. DOI: 10.1055/s-0033-1335205

[53] Tian W, Hao S, Gao B, Jiang Y, Zhang X, Zhang S, et al. Comparing the diagnostic accuracy of RTE and SWE in differentiating malignant thyroid nodules from benign ones: A meta-analysis. Cellular Physiology and Biochemistry. 2016;**39**:2451-2463. DOI: 10.1159/000452513

[54] Hu X, Liu Y, Qian L. Diagnostic potential of real-time elastography (RTE) and shear-wave elastography (SWE) to differentiate benign and malignant thyroid nodules. Medicine. 2017;**96**:e8282. DOI: 10.1097/MD.0000000000008282

[55] Zhao C-K, Xu H-X. Ultrasound elastography of the thyroid: Principles and current status. Ultrasonography. 2019;**38**:106-124. DOI: 10.14366/usg.18037

[56] Andrioli M, Persani L. Elastographic techniques of thyroid gland: Current status. Endocrine. 2014;**46**:455-461. DOI: 10.1007/s12020-014-0178-1

[57] Ozturk A, Grajo JR, Dhyani M, Anthony BW, Samir AE. Principles of ultrasound elastography. Abdominal Radiology. 2018;**43**:773-785. DOI: 10.1007/s00261-018-1475-6

[58] Russ G, Bonnema SJ, Erdogan MF, Durante C, Ngu R, Leenhardt L. European thyroid association guidelines for ultrasound malignancy risk stratification of thyroid nodules in adults: The EU-TIRADS. European Thyroid Journal. 2017;**6**:225-237. DOI: 10.1159/000478927

[59] Monpeyssen H, Tramalloni J, Poirée S, Hélénon O, Correas J-M. Elastography of the thyroid. Diagnostic and Interventional Imaging. 2013;**94**:535-544. DOI: 10.1016/j.diii.2013.01.023

[60] Sigrist RMS, Liau J, El Kaffas A, Chammas MC, Willmann JK. Ultrasound elastography: Review of techniques and clinical applications. Theranostics. 2017;**7**:1303-1329. DOI: 10.7150/thno.18650

[61] Roi CM, Borlea A, Mihuta MS, Paul C, Stoian D. A comparative analysis of strain and 2D shear-wave elastography in the diagnosis of autoimmune thyroiditis in pediatric patients. Biomedicine. 2023;**11**:1970. DOI: 10.3390/biomedicines11071970

[62] Nowicki A, Dobruch-Sobczak K. Wprowadzenie do ultradźwiękowej elastografii. Journal of Ultrasonography. 2016;**16**:113-124. DOI: 10.15557/JoU.2016.0013

[63] Gennisson J-L, Deffieux T, Fink M, Tanter M. Ultrasound elastography: Principles and techniques. Diagnostic and Interventional Imaging. 2013;**94**:487-495. DOI: 10.1016/j.diii.2013.01.022

[64] Hoskins PR. Principles of ultrasound elastography. Ultrasound. 2012;**20**:8-15. DOI: 10.1258/ult.2011.011005

[65] Mihaela Cepeha C, Borlea A, Paul C, Velea I, Stoian D. Shear-wave elastography in diffuse thyroid diseases. In: Elastography - Applications in Clinical Medicine. London: IntechOpen; 2022. DOI: 10.5772/intechopen.102636

[66] Dudea SM, Jid CB. Ultrasound elastography in thyroid disease. Medical Ultrasonography. 2015;**17**:74. DOI: 10.11152/mu.2013.2066.171.smd

[67] Cosgrove D, Barr R, Bojunga J, Cantisani V, Chammas MC, Dighe M, et al. WFUMB guidelines and

recommendations on the clinical use of ultrasound elastography: Part 4. Ultrasound in Medicine & Biology. 2017;**43**:4-26. DOI: 10.1016/j.ultrasmedbio.2016.06.022

[68] Dietrich C, Barr R, Farrokh A, Dighe M, Hocke M, Jenssen C, et al. Strain elastography - How to do it? Ultrasound International Open. 2017;**03**:E137-E149. DOI: 10.1055/s-0043-119412

[69] Cepeha CM, Paul C, Borlea A, Borcan F, Fofiu R, Dehelean CA, et al. The value of strain elastography in predicting autoimmune thyroiditis. Diagnostics. 2020;**10**(11):874. DOI: 10.3390/diagnostics10110874

[70] Xing P, Wu L, Zhang C, Li S, Liu C, Wu C. Differentiation of benign from malignant thyroid lesions. Journal of Ultrasound in Medicine. 2011;**30**:663-669. DOI: 10.7863/jum.2011.30.5.663

[71] Calvete AC, Rodríguez JM, de Dios B-MJ, Ríos A, Abellán-Rivero D, Reus M. Interobserver agreement for thyroid elastography. Journal of Ultrasound in Medicine. 2013;**32**:495-504. DOI: 10.7863/jum.2013.32.3.495

[72] Dhyani M, Li C, Samir AE, Stephen AE. Elastography: Applications and limitations of a new technology. In: Advanced Thyroid and Parathyroid Ultrasound. Cham: Springer International Publishing; 2017. pp. 67-73. DOI: 10.1007/978-3-319-44100-9_8

[73] Uysal E, Öztürk M. Quantitative assessment of thyroid glands in healthy children with shear-wave elastography. Ultrasound Quarterly. 2019;**35**:297-300. DOI: 10.1097/RUQ.0000000000000426

[74] Koca SB, Seber T. Factors affecting thyroid elastography in healthy children and patients with Hashimoto's thyroiditis. Journal of Clinical Research in Pediatric Endocrinology. 2023;**15**:7-15. DOI: 10.4274/jcrpe.galenos.2022.2022-4-5

[75] Li L, Zhang A, Chen D, Taragin BH, Luo X. Preliminary study of sound touch elastography in diffuse thyroid disease in children. Frontiers in Pediatrics. 2022;**10**:964413. DOI: 10.3389/fped.2022.964413

[76] Hazem M, Al Jabr IK, AlYahya AA, Hassanein AG, Algahlan HAE. Reliability of shear-wave elastography in the evaluation of diffuse thyroid diseases in children and adolescents. European Journal of Radiology. 2021;**143**:109942. DOI: 10.1016/j.ejrad.2021.109942

[77] Kamel SM, ElKhashab KM, Bhagat S, Elzayat WA. Shear wave elastography as a quantitative method for thyroid gland elasticity assessment in pediatrics patients with autoimmune-related thyroid disease, diagnostic utility and laboratory correlation. Egyptian Journal of Radiology and Nuclear Medicine. 2022;**53**:189. DOI: 10.1186/s43055-022-00882-1

[78] Cepeha CM, Paul C, Borlea A, Fofiu R, Borcan F, Dehelean CA, et al. Shear-wave elastography—diagnostic value in children with chronic autoimmune thyroiditis. Diagnostics. 2021;**11**(2):248. DOI: 10.3390/diagnostics11020248

[79] Kandemirli SG, Bayramoglu Z, Caliskan E, Sari ZNA, Adaletli I. Quantitative assessment of thyroid gland elasticity with shear-wave elastography in pediatric patients with Hashimoto's thyroiditis. Journal of Medical Ultrasonics. 2018;**45**:417-423. DOI: 10.1007/s10396-018-0859-0

[80] Agarwal D, Bhatia A, Saxena AK, Dayal D, Sodhi KS. Role of shear-wave

elastography of thyroid gland in children with newly diagnosed Hashimoto's thyroiditis: Preliminary study. Journal of Ultrasound in Medicine. 2022;**41**:2217-2225. DOI: 10.1002/jum.15903

[81] Koca SB, Seber T. Can thyroid elastography with ultrasound be used to stage children with Hashimoto's thyroiditis? Journal of Pediatric Endocrinology and Metabolism. 2023;**36**:346-352. DOI: 10.1515/jpem-2022-0573

[82] Yucel S, Ceyhan Bilgici M, Kara C, Can Yilmaz G, Aydin HM, Elmali M, et al. Acoustic radiation force impulse quantification in the evaluation of thyroid elasticity in pediatric patients with Hashimoto thyroiditis. Journal of Ultrasound in Medicine. 2018;**37**:1143-1149. DOI: 10.1002/jum.14459

[83] Bakırtaş Palabıyık F, İnci E, Papatya Çakır ED, Hocaoğlu E. Evaluation of normal thyroid tissue and autoimmune thyroiditis in children using shear-wave elastography. JCRPE Journal of Clinical Research in Pediatric Endocrinology. 2019;**11**:132-139. DOI: 10.4274/jcrpe.galenos.2018.2018.0137

[84] Liu J, Zhang Y, Ji Y, Wan Q, Dun G. The value of shear-wave elastography in diffuse thyroid disease. Clinical Imaging. 2018;**49**:187-192. DOI: 10.1016/j.clinimag.2018.03.019

[85] Magri F, Chytiris S, Capelli V, Alessi S, Nalon E, Rotondi M, et al. Shear wave elastography in the diagnosis of thyroid nodules: Feasibility in the case of coexistent chronic autoimmune Hashimoto's thyroiditis. Clinical Endocrinology (Oxford). 2012;**76**:137-141. DOI: 10.1111/j.1365-2265.2011.04170.x

[86] Decker T, Schnittka E, Stolzenberg L, Yalowitz J. Shear-wave elastography for the diagnosis of pediatric Hashimoto's thyroiditis: A systematic review and meta-analysis. Cureus. 2023;**15**(2):e35490. DOI: 10.7759/cureus.35490

[87] Yang Z, Zhang H, Wang K, Cui G, Fu F. Assessment of diffuse thyroid disease by strain ratio in ultrasound elastography. Ultrasound in Medicine & Biology. 2015;**41**:2884-2889. DOI: 10.1016/j.ultrasmedbio.2015.07.012

[88] Ayca H, Korkmaz A, Baki G, Köse M, Çobanoğlu BY. Value of real-time and strain ratio elastography in differential diagnosis of graves' disease and subacute and hashimoto's thyroiditis. Iranian Journal of Radiology. 2017;**14**(4):e22019. DOI: 10.5812/iranjradiol.22019

[89] Borysewicz-Sańczyk H, Sawicka B, Bossowski F, Dzięcioł J, Bossowski A. Elastographic evaluation of thyroid nodules in children and adolescents with Hashimoto's thyroiditis and nodular goiter with reference to cytological and/or histopathological diagnosis. Journal of Clinical Medicine. 2022;**11**:6339. DOI: 10.3390/jcm11216339

[90] Wang J, Li P, Sun L, Sun Y, Fang S, Liu X. Diagnostic value of strain ratio measurement in differential diagnosis of thyroid nodules coexisted with Hashimoto thyroiditis. International Journal of Clinical and Experimental Medicine. 2015;**8**(4):6420-6426

[91] Yurttutan N, Gungor G, Bilal N, Kizildag B, Baykara M, Sarica MA. Interpretation of thyroid glands in a group of healthy children: Real-time ultrasonography elastography study. Journal of Pediatric Endocrinology and Metabolism. 2016;**29**:933-937. DOI: 10.1515/jpem-2015-0409

[92] Öztürk M, Yildirim R. The usefulness of strain wave elastography in the

diagnosis and grading of Hashimoto's thyroiditis in children. Radiologia Medica. 2017;**122**:960-966. DOI: 10.1007/s11547-017-0801-3

[93] Cekic B et al. Real-time ultrasound elastography evaluation of the thyroid gland in adolescent patients with Hashimoto thyroiditis. Biomedical Research-India. 2017;**28**(17):7534-7539

[94] Cepeha CM, Paul C, Borlea A, Bende R, Mihuta MS, Stoian D. Is strain elastography useful in diagnosing chronic autoimmune thyroiditis in children? Applied Sciences. 2022;**12**(17):8881. DOI: 10.3390/app12178881

Chapter 3

Perspective Chapter: Ultrasound Techniques for Assessment of Thyroid Nodules with Indeterminate Cytology

Luciana Moisa-Luca and Andreea Borlea

Abstract

The Bethesda class III encompasses around 15% of biopsied nodules and has an estimated malignancy risk ranging from 10% to 30%. Managing this category can be challenging in clinical practice, as nearly 50% have undetermined cytology even after repeated fine needle aspiration biopsy. While molecular testing is expensive and is not widely available, lobectomy is associated with increased morbidity, and therefore, additional evaluation is needed. In the context of grayscale ultrasound criteria, such as hypoechogenicity, irregular margins, and microcalcifications, which are associated with the risk of cancer, Doppler applications, including color Doppler, PW Doppler, spectral Doppler, superb microvascular imaging, and contrast-enhanced ultrasound (CEUS), may be employed to predict malignancy in indeterminate cytology nodules. Additionally, the stiffness of the Bethesda III nodules can be evaluated using elastography, which includes strain and shear-wave elastography. It is noteworthy that malignant lesions are generally stiffer than benign nodules.

Keywords: Bethesda III, grayscale ultrasound, Doppler applications, strain elastography, shear-wave elastography

1. Introduction

The detection of thyroid nodules has significantly increased with the advancement and use of high-resolution imaging techniques. As a result, it is estimated that up to 60% of the adult population may have one or more thyroid nodules, depending on factors such as age, sex, and geographical location [1, 2]. Although the majority of thyroid nodules are benign, it is important to note that the risk of malignancy (ROM) is up to 5%.

The ultrasound features allow risk stratification and management of thyroid lesions through a system called the Thyroid Imaging, Reporting, and Data System (TIRADS). The TIRADS score, ranging from 1 to 5, and the maximum diameter of the nodules determine whether monitoring or fine needle aspiration biopsy (FNAB) is recommended [3]. The diagnosis of thyroid cytopathology is classified into one of six categories according to the Bethesda System for Reporting Thyroid Cytopathology (BSRTC): I (nondiagnostic), II (benign), III (atypia of undetermined significance), IV (follicular neoplasm), V (suspicious for malignancy), and VI (malignant). Each category has an associated estimated ROM [4] and cytopathology-based management. It is estimated that approximately 30% of nodules that undergo biopsy cannot be definitively classified as either malignant or benign based solely on cytological criteria [5]. The Bethesda III classification represents the most prominent subset among these indeterminate cases, encompassing atypia of undetermined significance (AUS) or follicular lesion of undetermined significance (FLUS). The malignancy risk associated with this classification ranges from 10% to 30% [1], with a higher risk of carcinoma for AUS than FLUS [6].

Managing indeterminate cytology nodules in clinical practice can prove challenging, as a significant proportion of these nodules, up to 50%, exhibit indeterminate cytology upon repeat FNAB [7]. Another approach for assessing the malignant potential of Bethesda III lesions involves employing molecular diagnostic tests, such as gene sequencing and messenger RNA (mRNA) expression analysis. These tests furnish precise data about the malignant risk of the nodules, thereby aiding in distinguishing between individuals who necessitate surgical intervention and those who can be managed through surveillance [8]. Regrettably, the high expenses and sporadic accessibility of these tests significantly constrain their application in medical practice. Moreover, there are no established guidelines for the management of nodules in light of genetic mutations identified through molecular testing [8]. In cases where patients have indeterminate cytology following repeat FNAB or where molecular testing is not feasible, surgical intervention may be advised based on the ultrasound features of the nodule or the presence of associated risk factors [9]. This strategy must consider the expenses, as well as the potential morbidity that could arise from the surgical procedure such as hemorrhage, airway obstruction, hypocalcemia, and recurrent laryngeal nerve palsy [10]. Additionally, it is important to take into account the requirement for hormone replacement therapy.

Considering all these, it is apparent that additional methods are necessary to assess indeterminate cytology nodules. In addition to the ultrasonographic (US) evaluation of thyroid lesions, the utilization of Doppler ultrasonography and elastography in assessing thyroid lesions is of great significance in the stratification of malignancy risk and will be explored in subsequent sections.

2. Grayscale ultrasound evaluation

High-resolution ultrasound is the preferred imaging modality for evaluating thyroid nodules, as it allows for the assessment of their number, location, size, ultrasound features, vascularity, relationship with surrounding structures, and regional lymph nodes [11]. A high-frequency linear probe, ranging from 7 to 15 MHz, is employed to attain high-resolution images and ensure adequate tissue penetration during the examination of the thyroid gland [12].

According to TIRADS models, thyroid nodules are evaluated based on their dimensions and ultrasound characteristics, including composition (cystic, spongiform, mixed, and solid), echogenicity (hyperechoic, isoechoic, mildly hypoechoic, and markedly hypoechoic), shape (oval, round, taller than wide), margin (smooth, ill-defined, irregular), microcalcification [13]. In light of the primary TIRADS models, which include the American Thyroid Association, the American College of Radiology TI-RADS, and the European Thyroid Association Thyroid Imaging, Reporting, and Data System, the sensitivity was observed to be 87, 74, and 54%, respectively, while the specificity was 31, 64, and 53%, respectively. The ACR TI-RADS system shows higher performance compared to ATA and EU-TIRADS in selecting malignant thyroid nodules for fine-needle aspiration (FNA). The sensitivities and specificities of US risk stratification systems vary widely, with ACR TI-RADS achieving better discriminative power. While the specificity of ACR TI-RADS is notably higher, leading to a greater likelihood ratio and diagnostic odds ratio, its sensitivity, negative predictive values, and positive predictive values are comparable to other systems. Differences in the classification criteria and definitions, such as those for microcalcifications, and variations in FNA cut-offs for intermediate and high-risk nodules, contribute to the performance variations among these systems. ACR TI-RADS tends to categorize fewer nodules as intermediate- or high-risk compared to other systems, which might explain its superior performance. However, challenges such as time-consuming assessments and the potential for missing certain cancer types like follicular thyroid cancer should be considered when adopting ultrasound risk stratification systems [14].

In the Bethesda III category, several high-risk ultrasound characteristics are indicative of thyroid cancer. These features include a solid structure, hypoechogenicity, irregular margins, a taller-than-wide shape, microcalcification, and solitary nodules, which have consistently been associated with malignancy [2, 9, 15, 16]. The diagnostic specificity for malignancy is greater when Bethesda class III nodules exhibit more ultrasonographic features of malignancy [17].

The management of Bethesda III nodules can be improved by integrating ultrasound features according to the EU-TIRADS and conducting repeat FNAB. Ultrasound follow-up is a suitable course of action for Bethesda III category nodules that persist after FNAB repetition and exhibit ultrasound features corresponding to the EU-TIRADS 3 class (**Figure 1**).

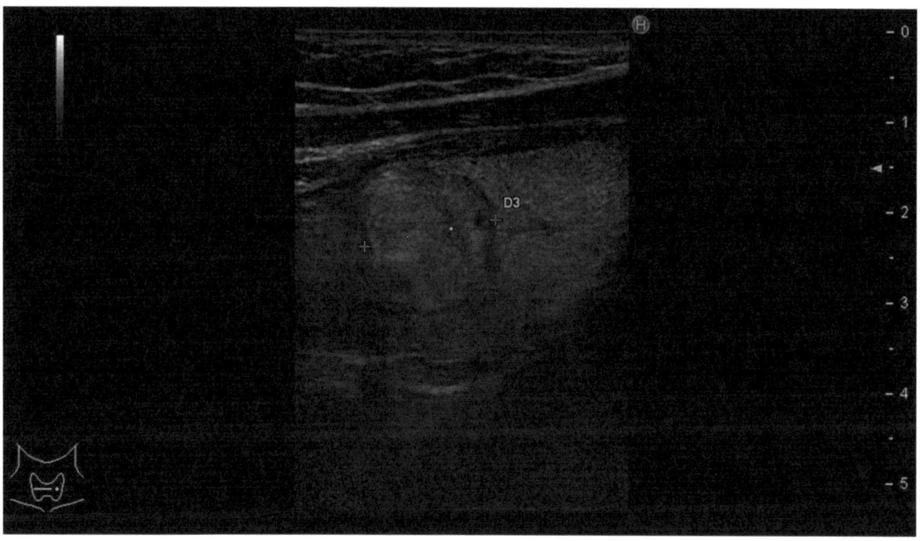

Figure 1.
EU-TIRADS 3 (solid, oval, isoechoic, and smooth margin).

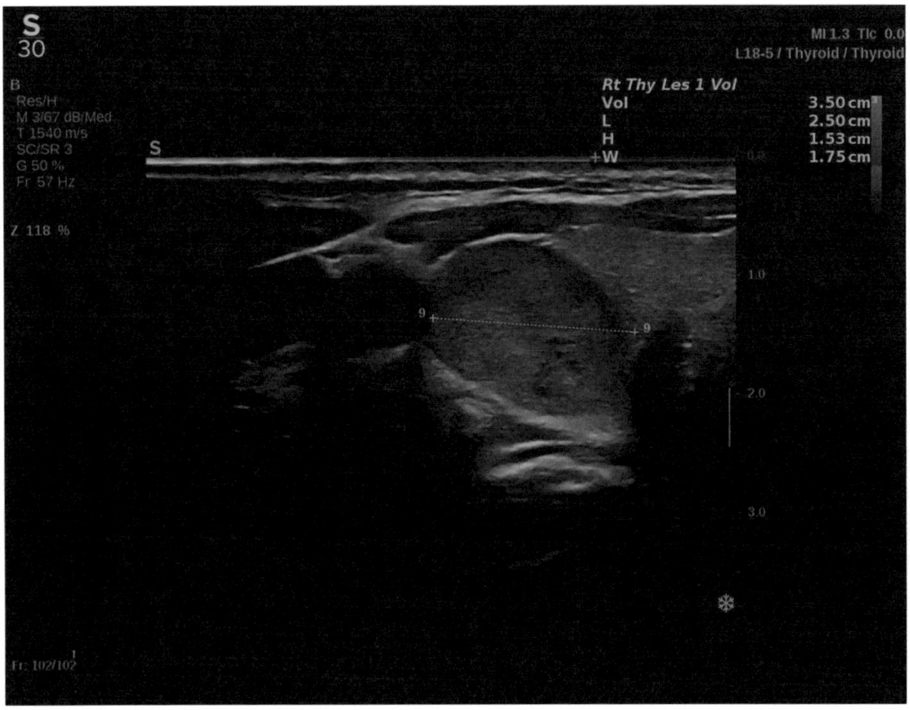

Figure 2.
EU-TIRADS 4 (solid, oval, hypoechoic, and smooth margin).

Conversely, nodules classified as EU-TIRADS 4 are associated with a higher ROM therefore surgical intervention appears to be a more appropriate approach (**Figure 2**) [1, 18].

This underlines the importance of performing a thorough ultrasonographic examination, as it may change the therapeutic management of nodules with indeterminate cytology.

3. Doppler ultrasonography

Doppler ultrasound is a diagnostic tool that provides information on blood flow and is closely related to the vascularization of thyroid nodules. Numerous Doppler applications are used to evaluate thyroid lesions.

3.1 Color Doppler imaging

Color Doppler imaging (CDI) is a US technique that utilizes a color map to register the blood flow direction and velocity superimposed on grayscale images. Blood flow velocity and direction are arbitrarily color-coded. Flow that moves away from the transducer is represented by the color blue, while flow that approaches the transducer is represented by red. Lighter shades of these colors indicate higher velocities. Additionally, a third color, such as green or yellow, is typically used to designate areas of high-flow turbulence [19].

Thyroid nodules may exhibit four types of vascular patterns: type 1 (no blood flow detected-**Figure 3**, left image), type 2 (perinodular—blood flow is registered at the

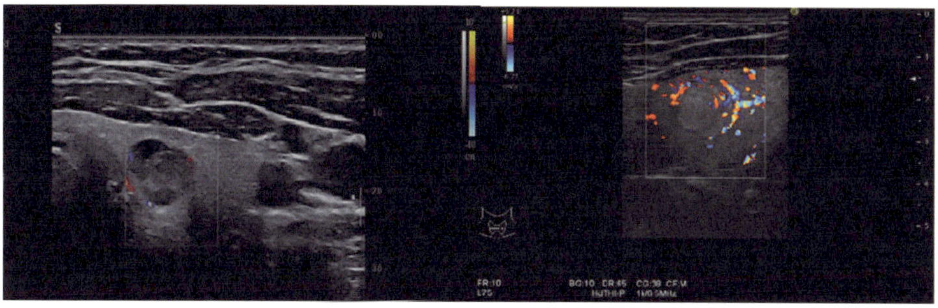

Figure 3.
Left image: Type 1 vascularity (no blood vessels), Right image: Type 2 vascularity (blood vessel at the periphery of the nodule).

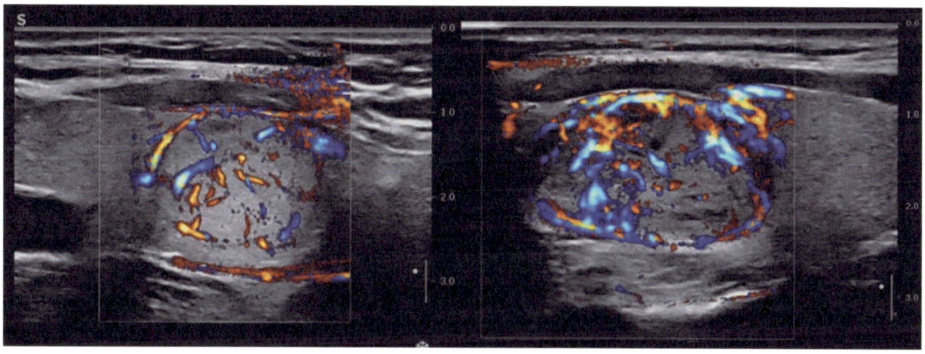

Figure 4.
Left image: Type 3 vascularity (some blood vessels inside and at the periphery of the nodule), Right image: Type 4 vascularity (multiple blood vessels inside and at the periphery of the nodule).

periphery of the nodule—**Figure 3**, right image), type 3 (mild intranodular vascularity with or without peripheral flow—**Figure 4**, left image), and type 4 (marked intranodular-multiple vessels within the lesion with or without perinodular flow—**Figure 4**, right image) [20].

Although there is no definitive consensus regarding the value of CDI in distinguishing between benign and malignant lesions, the presence of marked intranodular vascularity may be a significant predictor of cancer, particularly in larger nodules [20–23]. It is also applicable to Bethesda III nodules, where the CDI evaluation and volumetric (3D) color Doppler assessment demonstrated significant vascularity in both the intranodular and peripheral regions [24, 25].

3.2 Power Doppler and spectral Doppler imaging

Power Doppler Imaging (PDI) is more sensitive than CDI in detecting the slow flow and distribution of small vessels (**Figure 5**) and can be employed in the assessment of thyroid nodules for risk stratification as marked intranodular blood flow is an important feature that is correlated with malignancy [1, 25, 26].

Spectral Doppler imaging (SDI) is an ultrasound method that involves computer analysis to transform frequency into velocity and plot it as a function of time. This analysis facilitates the determination of various parameters, such as peak systolic velocity (PSV), mean systolic velocity (MSV), end-diastolic velocity (ESV),

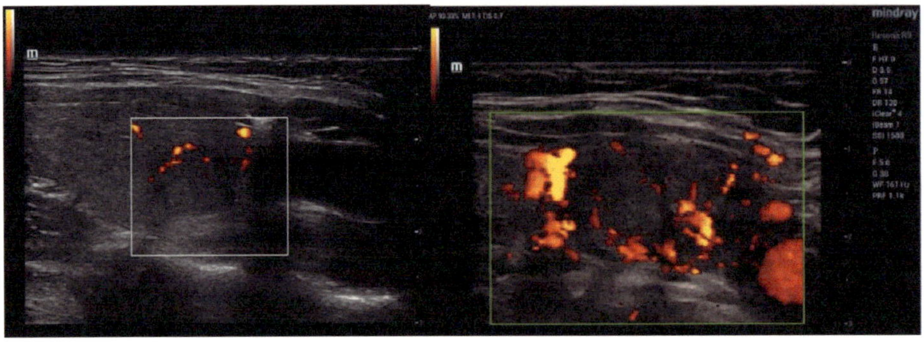

Figure 5.
Power Doppler: Left image: low intranodular vascularity, Right image: marked intranodular vascularity.

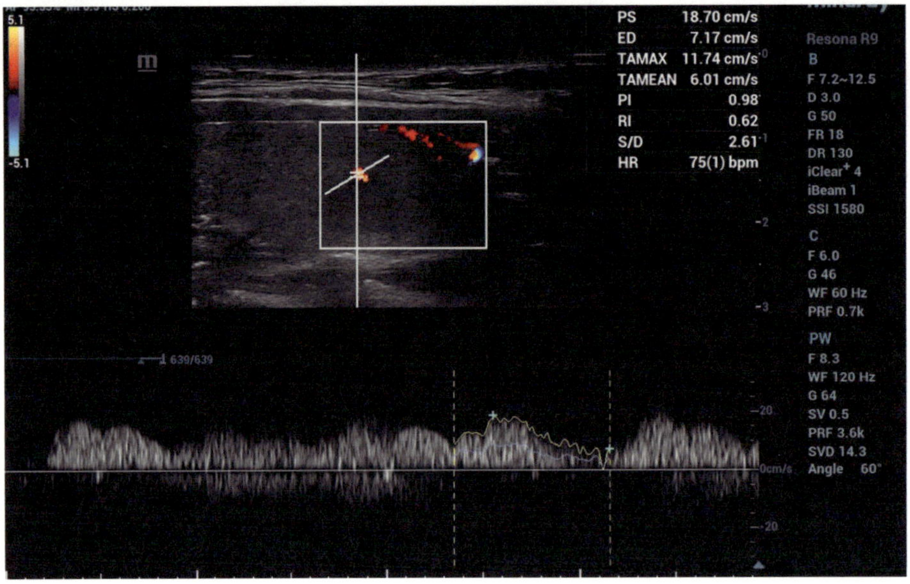

Figure 6.
SDI nodule with low RI and PI.

resistance index (RI), and pulsatility index (PI) (**Figure 6**). Malignant nodules are typically characterized by a significantly higher RI and PI compared to benign nodules, with a cutoff of 0,73 for RI and 1,3 for PI [26, 27], making them valuable tools for predicting the likelihood of malignancy even in AUS/FLUS class.

3.3 Superb microvascular imaging

The recently developed ultrasound imaging technique known as Superb microvascular imaging (SMI) or microvascular flow imaging is designed to visualize the low velocity and small diameter blood vessel flow by suppressing noise caused by motion artifacts, without eliminating the weak signal originating from small vessel blood flow. The utilization of SMI offers the advantage of affording more comprehensive information concerning the microvascular circulation within thyroid nodules than CDI or PDI [28].

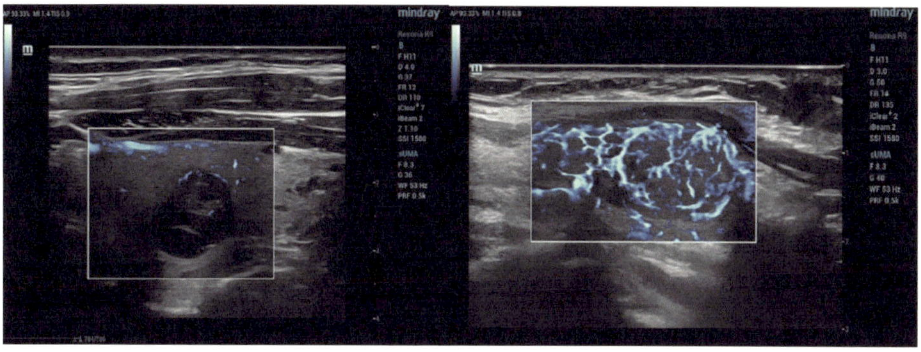

Figure 7.
Left image: minimal peripheral vascularity, Right image: marked peripheral vascularity.

The assessment of vascularity through SMI can be categorized based on its pattern, which includes absence, peripheral, or intranodular. Among these, intranodular vascularity demonstrates high sensitivity and specificity for malignancy (**Figure 7**). The explanation for this phenomenon lies in the fact that many peripheral vessels identified through PDI are, in fact, numerous small vessels of neoformation that infiltrate the nodules [29, 30]. Another method of classifying vascularity on SMI is to determine the number of vessels within the nodule. A score of 1 is attributed to thyroid nodules exhibiting a maximum of two blood vessels, while a score of 2 is assigned to nodules containing three or more vessels. Thyroid lesions with a score of 2 are associated with a higher ROM, particularly when accompanied by suspicious ultrasonographic features [29–31].

3.4 Contrast-enhanced ultrasound

Contrast-enhanced ultrasound (CEUS) is a technology that uses intravenously contrast agents to assess vascular perfusion and hemodynamics in thyroid lesions. The procedure for performing CEUS on thyroid nodules involves placing the focal zone at the base of the nodule and utilizing a low mechanical index (less than 0.10). The CEUS mode is initiated and a microbubble contrast agent is administered intravenously as a bolus, followed by a saline infusion. The CEUS timer is started upon the contrast administration, and images are captured during the subsequent 2–3 minutes [28, 32].

After the images are acquired, the nodule is assessed based on qualitative analysis that includes contrast agent arrival time (synchronous, earlier or later than adjacent thyroid tissue) and peak intensity (iso-, hyper-, hypo-, or non-enhancement), enhancement direction (scattered, centripetal or centrifugal), enhancement pattern (homogeneous or heterogeneous), ring enhancement (present or absent), nodule borders (clearly or unclear), contrast wash-out (fast wash-out, wash-out similar to thyroid parenchyma, slow wash-out). Malignant thyroid nodules exhibit heterogeneous patterns and hypoenhancement, which is attributed to fibrosis, calcification, and focal necrosis within the tumor (**Figure 8**). Additionally, these nodules tend to display irregular ring enhancement, while peripheral ring enhancement is considered highly specific for benign nodules (**Figure 9**) [32–34]. The utilization of quantitative analysis through the use of processing software is characterized by a greater degree of objectivity, resulting in the provision of more reliable data. The presence of a slow wash-in, low peak intensity, and hypoenhancement are commonly associated with malignancy [28, 32].

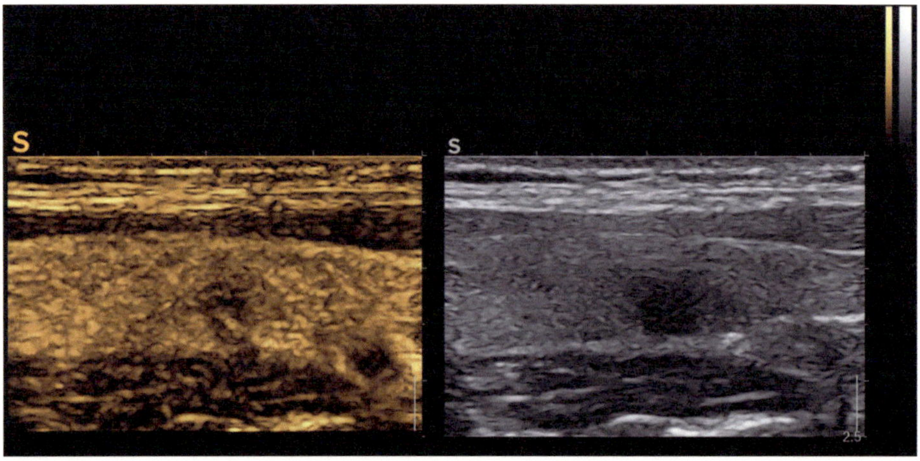

Figure 8.
High-risk nodule: on the left on CEUS (heterogeneous, hypoenhancement, unclear border, absent ring enhancement) and on the right on US (solid, marked hypoechoic, heterogeneous, irregular margins).

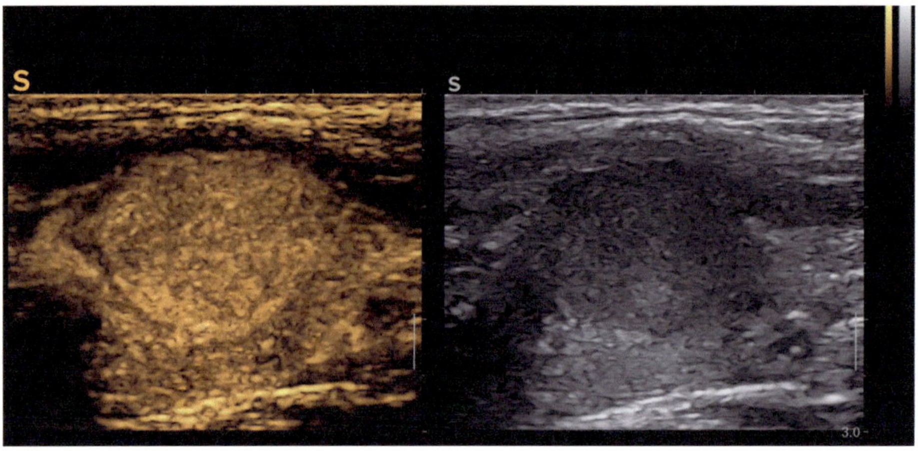

Figure 9.
Low-risk nodule: on the left on CEUS (homogeneous, isoenhancement, clear border, peripheral ring enhancement) and on the right on US (solid, mild hypoechoic, oval, regular margins, posterior enhancement).

Although CEUS is not yet universally standardized, it presents a promising diagnostic method due to its capacity to distinguish malignant from benign thyroid lesions by identifying pathological modifications in microvascularization, even in cases where cytology is indeterminate [34]. Furthermore, addition of CEUS to TIRADS results in increased sensitivity and specificity, reaching 89 and 87%, respectively, as opposed to individual TIRADS models. This enhances the identification of nodules that are suitable for FNAB [33].

4. Elastography

Elastography is an ultrasound method for evaluating the elastic properties of tissues (stiffness), surpassing the reliability of clinical palpation in detecting hard tumors. Two primary elastographic techniques can be employed for assessing thyroid nodules: strain elastography (SE) and shear-wave elastography (SWE).

4.1 Strain elastography

Strain elastography uses an external force (stress) to calculate strain from the axial gradient of the displacements. To obtain images, repetitive, uniform compression, and decompression movements are applied with the transducer perpendicular to the skin over the thyroid lesion or using physiological pulsations from cardiac, respiratory, or muscle contractions to calculate the displacement gradient before and after compression. Visible blood vessels should be excluded from the region of interest (ROI) to prevent the artificial appearance of significant displacement or "softness" caused by blood movement. Strain elastography is a method that provides a qualitative assessment of tissue elasticity, as it is unable to measure the applied stress directly. Therefore, only relative stiffness can be depicted. The tissue stiffness is represented using either a grayscale or a color map superimposed over a grayscale image, with various systems assigning different colors to different levels of stiffness. For instance, some systems use red to signify high stiffness, green for intermediate stiffness, and blue for low stiffness, while others adopt an inverse color scale [35, 36].

The evaluation of lesion stiffness can be accomplished through the utilization of a visual 5-point scoring system. A score of 1 signifies complete elasticity within the nodule, while a score of 2 denotes elasticity present in a substantial portion of the nodule. A score of 3 is attributed to elasticity only at the peripheral region of the nodule, a score of 4 indicates the absence of elasticity within the nodule, and a score of 5 indicates the absence of elasticity both within the nodule and its surrounding tissue. Thyroid nodules that have a score between 1 and 3 are considered benign, while those with a score of 4 or 5 are considered malignant. Another classification system employs a 4-point color scale, wherein a score of 1 signifies elasticity present throughout the assessed area, a score of 2 denotes elasticity present in a significant portion of the assessed area, a score of 3 indicates stiffness in a substantial portion of the assessed area, and a score of 4 indicates the presence of a nodule devoid of elasticity. Thyroid nodules that have a score between 1 and 3 on a 5-point color map, or 1 and 2 on a 4-point color system are considered benign, while those with a score of 4 or 5 using a 5-point color map, and 3 and 4 using a 4-point color map are considered malignant [36–38].

A more accurate assessment of nodule stiffness can be made by using the strain ratio (SR) between the nodule and the surrounding thyroid parenchyma (**Figure 10**) at the same depth or strain ratio between the nodule and strap muscles (**Figure 11**) with no difference between them. The ROI should be placed to cover the entire nodule. A consensus regarding the cutoff point to differentiate malignant nodules from benign ones has not been reached, but a value of around 4 has good sensitivity and specificity [36].

SE holds significant value in the assessment of the Bethesda III category. Nodules with indeterminate cytology and high stiffness on strain elastography, with a score of 3 or 4 on the color map, are more likely to be malignant (**Figure 12**) than those with a score of 1 or 2. Additionally, a strain ratio greater than 4 is a reliable predictor for malignancy [24, 36, 39].

The strain elastography, in conjunction with ultrasound features, plays an important role in the risk stratification and management of Bethesda Category III nodules.

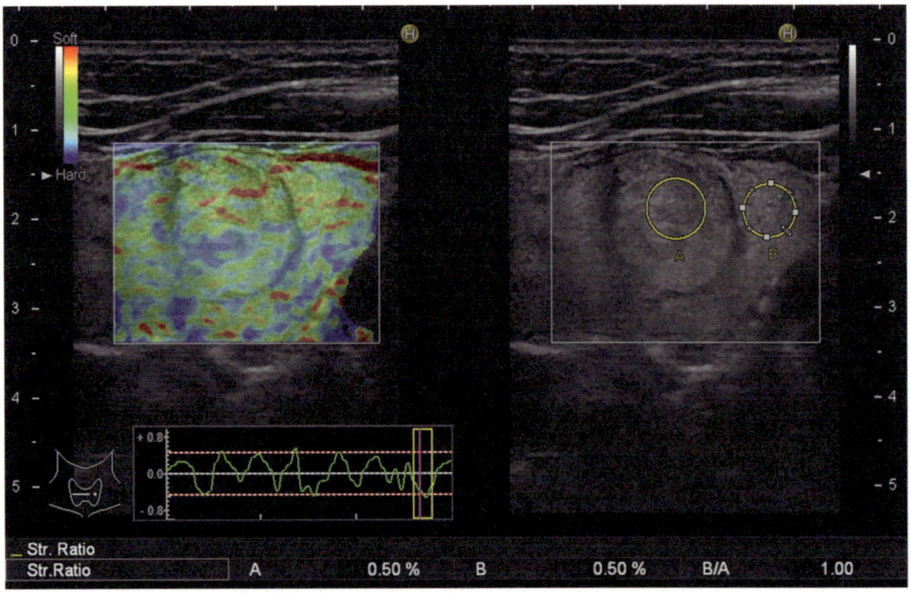

Figure 10.
SE score 1, SR = 1.0 (SR between nodule and surrounding thyroid parenchyma).

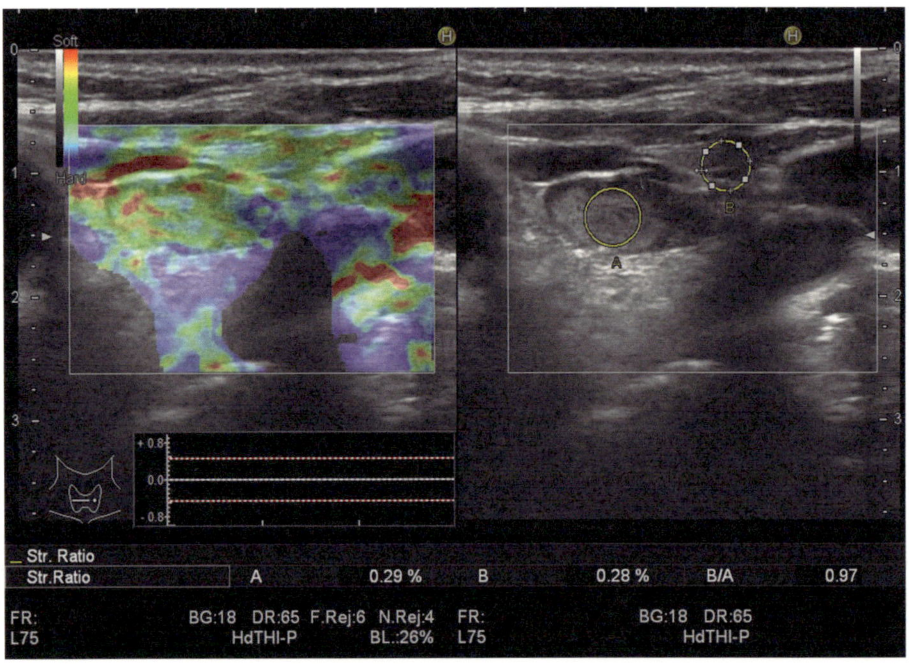

Figure 11.
SE score 1, SR = 0.97 (SR between nodule and strap muscle).

Consequently, low-risk lesions can be closely monitored, while high-risk lesions may require repeated fine needle aspiration or surgical intervention for diagnostic purposes [24, 36, 39, 40].

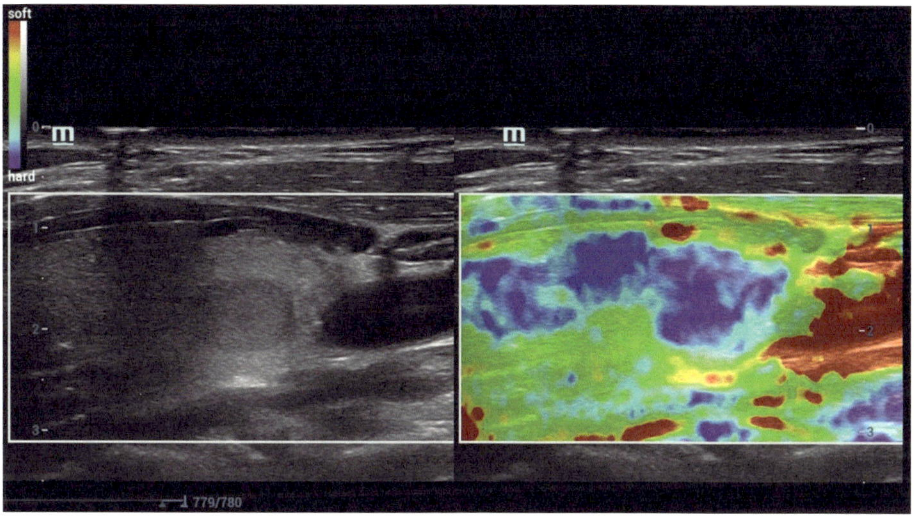

Figure 12.
SE score 3.

4.2 Shear-wave elastography

Shear-wave elastography (SWE) uses high-energy ultrasound impulses that are sent from the probe into the tissue and generate shear waves that propagate in a direction orthogonal to the direction of tissue displacement, being less operator-dependent. The method is a quantitative one, in which the assessment of tissue stiffness may be accomplished through the measurement of shear-wave speed by the ultrasound machine, as shear waves are propagated more rapidly in stiffer tissues [36]. Two techniques are available for the clinical assessment of thyroid nodules: the point shear-wave elastography and the 2-dimensional shear-wave elastography (2D SWE).

2D SWE utilizes a color-coded map that is superimposed on a gray-scale image, allowing the assessment of nodule stiffness. Soft tissue is typically depicted in blue, while hard tissue appears in red. By placing an ROI within the field of view, the mean stiffness (Emean), maximal stiffness (Emax), and standard deviation (SD) can be determined and expressed in terms of shear-wave speed (m/sec) or elasticity (kPa) [41].

SWE has demonstrated significant potential in distinguishing malignant from benign thyroid nodules, with promising outcomes. While there is no universally accepted threshold for SWE, various values ranging from 30 kPa [42] to 65 kPa [43, 44] or from 2.4–4.7 m/s [36] have been proposed to differentiate between these two types of nodules. Additionally, the elasticity ratio between the nodule and the thyroid parenchyma can be calculated by placing ROIs: one in the stiffer part of the nodule and another in the thyroid parenchyma at the same depth. Different values have been reported for the stiffness ratio, ranging from 2.8 [42] to 3.7 [45].

The role of SWE in indeterminate cytology nodules remains controversial. To assess its utility in risk stratification for malignancy, several studies have been conducted to determine the optimal cutoff for SWE parameters. Regarding the value of Emean, the cutoff values ranged from 24 kPa to 39,2 kPa (**Figure 13**), depending on the SWE ultrasound system used. Meanwhile, Emax values ranged from 41,2 kPa to

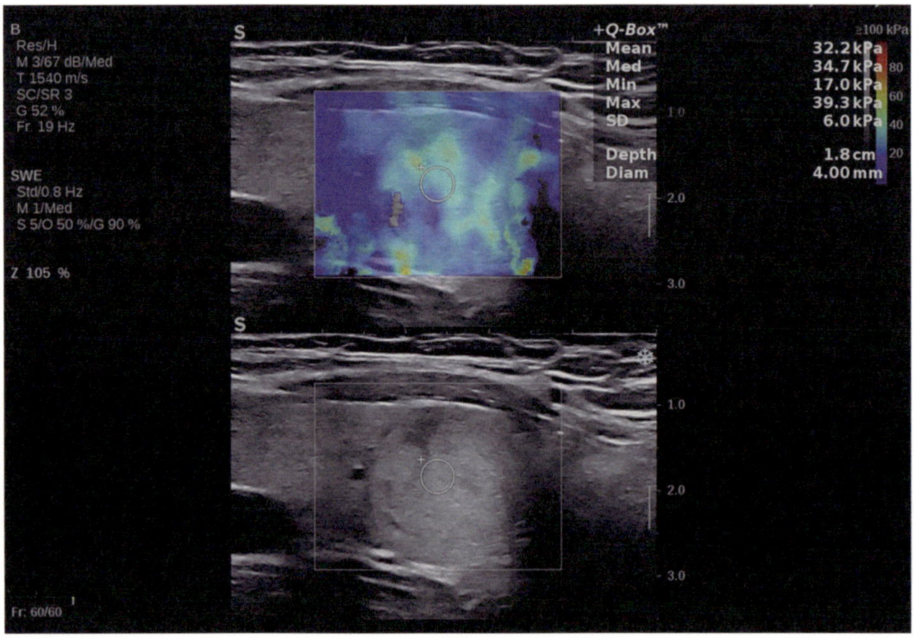

Figure 13.
SWE: low stiffness nodule (Emean = 32.2 kPa, Emax = 39.3 kPa).

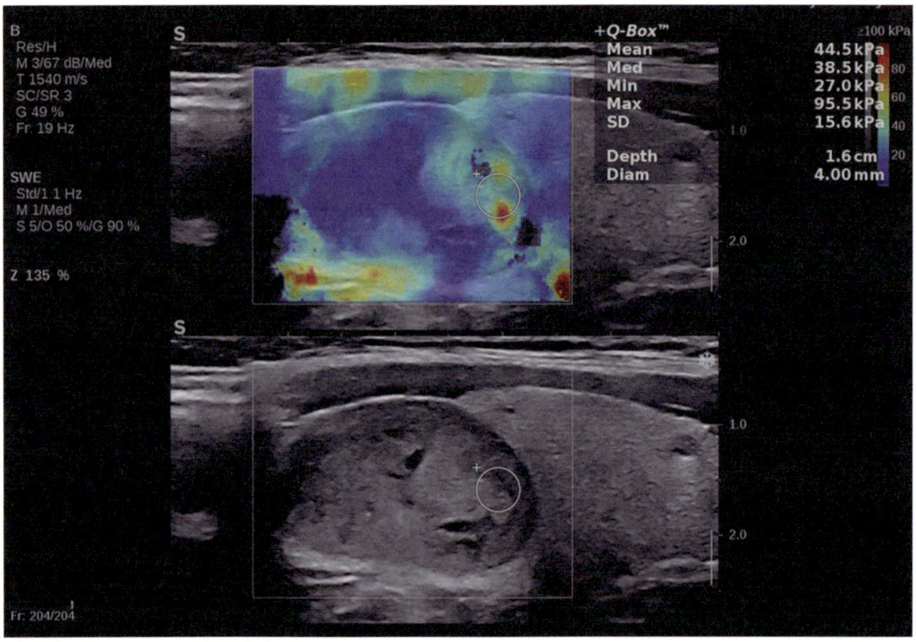

Figure 14.
SWE: high stiffness nodule (Emean = 60.7 kPa, Emax = 83.6 kPa).

65 kPa (**Figure 14**) [46]. Interestingly, a low value of 22.3 kPa was found to be sufficient for differentiating between malignant and benign follicular thyroid lesions [35, 46]. Therefore, the utilization of Emean instead of Emax in the evaluation of

indeterminate cytology could be more reliable, given the common occurrence of follicular carcinoma within this category [47].

Elastography, when used in conjunction with TIRADS, can be a useful tool for classifying thyroid nodules as either high or low risk based on their degree of stiffness. Therefore, lesions that are stiff on SWE can be upgraded to a higher risk class, while those that are soft can be downgraded to a lower risk classification. Emean proves to be the best parameter, exhibiting a sensitivity and a specificity of 98% for upgrading or downgrading the nodules category [48].

SWE can be a valuable auxiliary tool in conjunction with grayscale ultrasound for evaluating thyroid nodules with indeterminate cytology. The integration of SWE and the ACR TIRADS system enhances diagnostic precision and accuracy and can be used in selecting the nodules that are eligible for FNAB [36, 49].

5. Discussion

In the context of assessing thyroid nodules with indeterminate cytology, advanced ultrasound techniques play a crucial role in risk stratification and management. High-resolution ultrasound, employing high-frequency linear probes, allows for detailed visualization of nodule characteristics such as size, shape, and echogenicity, integral to TIRADS classification. The distinctiveness of each TIRADS model (American Thyroid Association, American College of Radiology, and European Thyroid Association) highlights variable sensitivities and specificities, underscoring the importance of selecting an appropriate model based on clinical context.

For Bethesda III category nodules, ultrasound features such as solid composition, hypoechogenicity, and irregular margins are strong predictors of malignancy. These nodules benefit from a tailored approach—repeated fine needle aspirations or surgical interventions for those exhibiting high-risk ultrasound features and careful monitoring for others showing features consistent with lower risk.

Incorporating Doppler ultrasound into the evaluation process enhances the characterization of thyroid nodules further. Color Doppler imaging (CDI) and spectral Doppler imaging (SDI) assess vascularity and blood flow within the nodules, providing critical insights, particularly in nodules with indeterminate cytology. Significant intranodular vascularity, assessed through parameters like resistance index (RI) and pulsatility index (PI), is notably higher in malignant nodules.

The integration of novel modalities like contrast-enhanced ultrasound (CEUS) and elastography further refines diagnostic accuracy. CEUS, although not universally standardized, enhances the detection of malignant features within nodules through detailed assessment of microvascularization. Elastography, particularly strain elastography and shear-wave elastography (SWE), adds valuable information regarding nodule stiffness, correlating stiffness with potential malignancy. Here, parameters like strain ratio and Emean provide quantitative data that significantly influence the management decisions for nodules categorized as Bethesda III.

6. Conclusions

The management of nodules with indeterminate cytology is proving to be difficult, as no single imaging method has sufficient accuracy in differentiating malignant from benign nodules. Thorough ultrasound examination, combined with Doppler and elastographic techniques, helps to identify high-risk nodules, reduce fine needle aspiration, and avoid unnecessary surgery.

Acknowledgements

We would like to acknowledge Victor Babes University of Medicine and Pharmacy Timisoara for their support in covering the costs of publication for this research paper.

Conflict of interest

The authors declare no conflict of interest.

Appendices and nomenclature

2D SWE	2-Dimensional shear-wave elastography
ACR TIRADS	American College of Radiology Thyroid Imaging, Reporting, and Data System
AUS	atypia of undetermined significance
BSRTC	Bethesda System for Reporting Thyroid Cytopathology
CDI	Color Doppler Imaging
CEUS	Contrast-enhanced ultrasound
Emax	maximal stiffness
Emean	mean stiffness
ESV	end-diastolic velocity
EU-TIRADS	European Thyroid Association Thyroid Imaging, Reporting and Data System
FLUS	follicular lesion of undetermined significance
FNAB	fine needle aspiration biopsy
mRNA	messenger RNA
MSV	mean systolic velocity
PDI	Power Doppler Imaging
PI	pulsatility index
PSV	peak systolic velocity
RI	resistance index
ROI	region of interest
ROM	risk of malignancy
SD	standard deviation
SDI	Spectral Doppler Imaging
SE	Strain elastography
SMI	Superb microvascular imaging
SR	strain ratio
SWE	shear-wave elastography
TIRADS	Thyroid Imaging, Reporting, and Data System
US	ultrasonographic

Author details

Luciana Moisa-Luca[1] and Andreea Borlea[2*]

1 Department of Doctoral Studies, "Victor Babes" University of Medicine and Pharmacy, Timisoara, Romania

2 2nd Department of Internal Medicine, "Victor Babes" University of Medicine and Pharmacy, Timisoara, Romania

*Address all correspondence to: borlea.andreea@umft.ro

References

[1] Durante C, Hegedüs L, Czarniecka A, Paschke R, Russ G, Schmitt F, et al. European thyroid association clinical practice guidelines for thyroid nodule management. European Thyroid Journal. 2023;**12**:5. DOI: 10.1530/ETJ-23-0067

[2] Hacim N, Akbaş A, Ulgen Y, et al. Impact of ultrasonographic features for thyroid malignancy in patients with Bethesda categories III, IV, and V: A retrospective observational study in a tertiary center. Cureus. 2021;**13**(7):e16708. DOI: 10.7759/cureus.16708

[3] Tessler F, Middleton W, Grant E. Thyroid imaging reporting and data system (TI-RADS): A user's guide. Radiology. 2018;**287**(1):29-36. DOI: 10.1148/radiol.2017171240

[4] Ali SZ, Baloch ZW, Cochand-Priollet B, Schmitt FC, Vielh P, VanderLaan PA. The 2023 Bethesda system for reporting thyroid cytopathology. Thyroid. 2023;**33**(9):1039-1044. DOI: 10.1089/thy.2023.0141. Epub 2023 Jul 8

[5] Wong LQ, Baloch ZW. Analysis of the Bethesda system for reporting thyroid cytopathology and similar precursor thyroid cytopathology reporting schemes. Advances in Anatomic Pathology. 2012;**19**(5):313-319. DOI: 10.1097/PAP.0b013e3182666398

[6] Mosca L, Silva LFFD, Carneiro PC, Chacon DA, Araujo-Neto VJF, Araujo-Filho VJF, et al. Malignancy rates for Bethesda III subcategories in thyroid fine needle aspiration biopsy (FNAB). Clinics (São Paulo, Brazil). 2018;**73**:e370. DOI: 10.6061/clinics/2018/e370. Epub 2018 May 28

[7] Rosario PW. Thyroid nodules with atypia or follicular lesions of undetermined significance (Bethesda category III): Importance of ultrasonography and cytological subcategory. Thyroid. 2014;**24**(7):1115-1120. DOI: 10.1089/thy.2013.0650. Epub 2014 May 9

[8] Patel J, Klopper J, Cottrill EE. Molecular diagnostics in the evaluation of thyroid nodules: Current use and prospective opportunities. Frontiers in Endocrinology (Lausanne). 2023;**14**:1101410. DOI: 10.3389/fendo.2023.1101410

[9] Haugen BR, Alexander EK, Bible KC, Doherty GM, Mandel SJ, Nikiforov YE, et al. 2015 American Thyroid Association management guidelines for adult patients with thyroid nodules and differentiated thyroid cancer: The American Thyroid Association guidelines task force on thyroid nodules and differentiated thyroid cancer. Thyroid. 2016;**26**(1):1-133. DOI: 10.1089/thy.2015.0020

[10] Hassan-Smith ZK, Gopinath P, Mihaimeed F. A UK-wide survey of life-threatening thyroidectomy complications. Journal of Thyroid Research. 2011;**2011**:329620. DOI: 10.4061/2011/329620

[11] Morgan M, Atkinson H, Jones J, et al. Assessment of Thyroid Lesions (Ultrasound). Reference article, Radiopaedia.org. 2015. DOI: 10.53347/rID-35024 [Accessed: December 27, 2023]

[12] Beck-Razi N, Gaitini D, Evans R, Ivanac G, Dietrich C. Ultrasound of the thyroid. In: Dietrich C, editor. EFSUMB Course Book. 2nd ed. London, United Kingdom: EFSUM (European Federation of Societies for Ultrasound in Medicine and Biology); 2019. pp. 1-84. DOI: 10.37713/ECB18

[13] Russ G, Bonnema SJ, Erdogan MF, Durante C, Ngu R, Leenhardt L. European thyroid association guidelines for ultrasound malignancy risk stratification of thyroid nodules in adults: The EU-TIRADS. European Thyroid Journal. 2017;**6**(5):225-237. DOI: 10.1159/000478927. Epub 2017 Aug 8

[14] Castellana M, Castellana C, Treglia G, Giorgino F, Giovanella L, Russ G, et al. Performance of five ultrasound risk stratification systems in selecting thyroid nodules for FNA. The Journal of Clinical Endocrinology & Metabolism. 2020;**105**(5):1659-1669. DOI: 10.1210/clinem/dgz170

[15] Jeong SH, Hong HS, Lee EH, Cha JG, Park JS, Kwak JJ. Outcome of thyroid nodules characterized as atypia of undetermined significance or follicular lesion of undetermined significance and correlation with ultrasound features and BRAF(V600E) mutation analysis. AJR. American Journal of Roentgenology. 2013;**201**(6):W854-W860. DOI: 10.2214/AJR.12.9901

[16] Orlando G, Graceffa G, Mazzola S, Vassallo F, Proclamà MP, Richiusa P, et al. The role of "critical" ultrasound reassessment in the decision-making of Bethesda III thyroid nodules. Medicina (Kaunas, Lithuania). 2023;**59**(8):1484. DOI: 10.3390/medicina59081484

[17] Kımıloğlou E, Özdemir M, Çobanoğlu P, Kavuncu B, Gönüllü D. Evaluation of risk factors for malignancy obtained by means of fine needle aspiration biopsies in thyroid nodules and surgical outcomes of patients with Bethesda category III (AUS/FLUS). Chirurgia (Bucharest). 2023, 1990;**118**:137-145. DOI: 10.21614/chirurgia.2812

[18] Gao LY, Wang Y, Jiang YX, Yang X, Liu RY, Xi XH, et al. Ultrasound is helpful to differentiate Bethesda class III thyroid nodules: A PRISMA-compliant systematic review and meta-analysis. Medicine (Baltimore). 2017;**96**(16):e6564. DOI: 10.1097/MD.0000000000006564

[19] Carroll D, Bickle I, Chieng R, et al. Color Flow Doppler (Ultrasound). Reference article, Radiopaedia.org. 2019. DOI: 10.53347/rID-67339 [Accessed: December 28, 2023]

[20] Shin JH, Baek JH, Chung J, Ha EJ, Kim JH, Lee YH, et al. Ultrasonography diagnosis and imaging-based management of thyroid nodules: Revised Korean society of thyroid radiology consensus statement and recommendations. Korean Journal of Radiology. 2016;**17**(3):370-395. DOI: 10.3348/kjr.2016.17.3.370. Epub 2016 Apr 14

[21] Papini E, Guglielmi R, Bianchini A, Crescenzi A, Taccogna S, Nardi F, et al. Risk of malignancy in nonpalpable thyroid nodules: Predictive value of ultrasound and color-doppler features. The Journal of Clinical Endocrinology and Metabolism. 2002;**87**(5):1941-1946. DOI: 10.1210/jcem.87.5.8504

[22] Russ G. Risk stratification of thyroid nodules on ultrasonography with the French TI-RADS: Description and reflections. Ultrasonography. 2016;**35**(1):25-38. DOI: 10.14366/usg.15027. Epub 2015 Jul 13

[23] Slapa RZ, Jakubowski WS, Slowinska-Srzednicka J, Szopinski KT. Advantages and disadvantages of 3D ultrasound of thyroid nodules including thin slice volume rendering. Thyroid Research. 2011;**4**(1):1. DOI: 10.1186/1756-6614-4-1

[24] Borlea A, Stoian D, Cotoi L, Sporea I, Lazar F, Mozos I. Thyroid multimodal ultrasound evaluation—Impact on

presurgical diagnosis of intermediate cytology cases. Applied Sciences. 2020;**10**:3439. DOI: 10.3390/app10103439

[25] Cerbone G, Spiezia S, Colao A, Di Sarno A, Assanti AP, Lucci R, et al. Power doppler improves the diagnostic accuracy of color doppler ultrasonography in cold thyroid nodules: Follow-up results. Hormone Research. 1999;**52**(1):19-24. DOI: 10.1159/000023427

[26] Palaniappan MK, Aiyappan SK, Ranga U. Role of gray scale, color doppler and spectral doppler in differentiation between malignant and benign thyroid nodules. Journal of Clinical and Diagnostic Research. 2016;**10**(8):TC01-TC06. DOI: 10.7860/JCDR/2016/18459.8227. Epub 2016 Aug 1

[27] Algin O, Algin E, Gokalp G, Ocakoğlu G, Erdoğan C, Saraydaroglu O, et al. Role of duplex power Doppler ultrasound in differentiation between malignant and benign thyroid nodules. Korean Journal of Radiology. 2010;**11**(6):594-602. DOI: 10.3348/kjr.2010.11.6.594. Epub 2010 Oct 29

[28] Chung J, Lee YJ, Choi YJ, Ha EJ, Suh CH, Choi M, et al. Clinical applications of doppler ultrasonography for thyroid disease: Consensus statement by the Korean Society of Thyroid Radiology. Ultrasonography. 2020 Oct;**39**(4):315-330. DOI: 10.14366/usg.20072. Epub 2020 Aug 25

[29] Kong J, Zhang Y, Jin J. Role of superb micro-vascular imaging in the preoperative evaluation of thyroid nodules: Comparison with power Doppler flow imaging. Journal of Ultrasound in Medicine. 2017;**36**(7):1329-1337. DOI: 10.7863/ultra.16.07004

[30] Zhu YC, Zhang Y, Deng SH, Jiang Q. A prospective study to compare superb microvascular imaging with grayscale ultrasound and color doppler flow imaging of vascular distribution and morphology in thyroid nodules. Medical Science Monitor. 2018;**24**:9223-9231. DOI: 10.12659/MSM.911695

[31] Cappelli C, Pirola I, Gandossi E, Marini F, Cristiano A, Casella C, et al. Ultrasound microvascular blood flow evaluation: A new tool for the management of thyroid nodule? International Journal of Endocrinology. 2019;**2019**:7874890. DOI: 10.1155/2019/7874890

[32] Radzina M, Ratniece M, Putrins DS, Saule L, Cantisani V. Performance of contrast-enhanced ultrasound in thyroid nodules: Review of current state and future perspectives. Cancers (Basel). 2021;**13**(21):5469. DOI: 10.3390/cancers13215469

[33] Ruan J, Xu X, Cai Y, Zeng H, Luo M, Zhang W, et al. A practical CEUS thyroid reporting system for thyroid nodules. Radiology. 2022;**305**(1):149-159. DOI: 10.1148/radiol.212319. Epub 2022 Jun 14

[34] Sorrenti S, Dolcetti V, Fresilli D, Del Gaudio G, Pacini P, Huang P, et al. The role of CEUS in the evaluation of thyroid cancer: From diagnosis to local staging. Journal of Clinical Medicine. 2021;**10**(19):4559. DOI: 10.3390/jcm10194559

[35] Dietrich CF, Barr RG, Farrokh A, Dighe M, Hocke M, Jenssen C, et al. Strain elastography—How to do it? Ultrasound International Open. 2017;**3**(4):E137-E149. DOI: 10.1055/s-0043-119412. Epub 2017 Dec 7

[36] Cosgrove D, Barr R, Bojunga J, Cantisani V, Chammas MC, Dighe M, et al. WFUMB guidelines and recommendations on the clinical use of ultrasound Elastography: Part 4. Thyroid.

Ultrasound Med Biology. 2017;**43**(1):4-26. DOI: 10.1016/j.ultrasmedbio.2016.06.022. Epub 2016 Aug 25

[37] Rago T, Santini F, Scutari M, Pinchera A, Vitti P. Elastography: New developments in ultrasound for predicting malignancy in thyroid nodules. The Journal of Clinical Endocrinology and Metabolism. 2007;**92**(8):2917-2922. DOI: 10.1210/jc.2007-0641. Epub 2007 May 29

[38] Kwak JY, Kim EK. Ultrasound elastography for thyroid nodules: Recent advances. Ultrasonography. Apr 2014;**33**(2, 82):75. DOI: 10.14366/usg.13025. Epub 2014 Feb 26

[39] Stoian D, Borcan F, Petre I, Mozos I, Varcus F, Ivan V, et al. Strain elastography as a valuable diagnosis tool in intermediate cytology (Bethesda III) thyroid nodules. Diagnostics (Basel). 2019;**9**(3):119. DOI: 10.3390/diagnostics9030119

[40] Cantisani V, Ulisse S, Guaitoli E, De Vito C, Caruso R, Mocini R, et al. Q-elastography in the presurgical diagnosis of thyroid nodules with indeterminate cytology. PLoS One. 2012;**7**(11):e50725. DOI: 10.1371/journal.pone.0050725. Epub 2012 Nov 29

[41] Zhao CK, Xu HX. Ultrasound elastography of the thyroid: Principles and current status. Ultrasonography. Apr 2019;**38**(2):106-124. DOI: 10.14366/usg.18037. Epub 2018 Oct 1

[42] Borlea A, Sporea I, Popa A, Derban M, Taban L, Stoian D. Strain versus 2D shear-wave elastography parameters—Which score better in predicting thyroid cancer? Applied Sciences. 2022;**12**(21):11147. DOI: 10.3390/app122111147

[43] Sebag F, Vaillant-Lombard J, Berbis J, Griset V, Henry JF, Petit P, et al. Shear wave elastography: A new ultrasound imaging mode for the differential diagnosis of benign and malignant thyroid nodules. The Journal of Clinical Endocrinology & Metabolism. 2010;**95**(12):5281-5288. DOI: 10.1210/jc.2010-0766

[44] Kim H, Kim JA, Son EJ, Youk JH. Quantitative assessment of shear-wave ultrasound elastography in thyroid nodules: Diagnostic performance for predicting malignancy. European Radiology. 2013;**23**(9):2532-2537. DOI: 10.1007/s00330-013-2847-5. Epub 2013 Apr 19

[45] Monpeyssen H, Tramalloni J, Poirée S, Hélénon O, Correas J-M. Elastography of the thyroid. Diagnostic and Interventional Imaging. 2013;**94**(5):535-544. ISSN 2211-5684. DOI: 10.1016/j.diii.2013.01.023

[46] Qiu Y, Xing Z, Yang Q, Luo Y, Ma B. Diagnostic performance of shear wave elastography in thyroid nodules with indeterminate cytology: A systematic review and meta-analysis. Heliyon. 2023;**9**(10):e20654. DOI: 10.1016/j.heliyon.2023.e20654

[47] Samir AE, Dhyani M, Anvari A, Prescott J, Halpern EF, Faquin WC, et al. Shear-wave Elastography for the preoperative risk stratification of follicular-patterned lesions of the thyroid: Diagnostic accuracy and optimal measurement plane. Radiology. 2015;**277**(2):565-573. DOI: 10.1148/radiol.2015141627. Epub 2015 May 7

[48] Luo J, Chen J, Sun Y, Xu F, Wu L, Huang P. A retrospective study of reducing unnecessary thyroid biopsy for American College of Radiology Thyroid Imaging Reporting and Data Systems 4 assessment through applying shear wave

elastography. Archives of Endocrinology and Metabolism. 2020;**64**(4):349-355. DOI: 10.20945/2359-3997000000267. Epub 2020 Jul 24

[49] Zhang WB, Li JJ, Chen XY, He BL, Shen RH, Liu H, et al. SWE combined with ACR TI-RADS categories for malignancy risk stratification of thyroid nodules with indeterminate FNA cytology. Clinical Hemorheology and Microcirculation. 2020;**76**(3):381-390. DOI: 10.3233/CH-200893

Chapter 4

Contrast-Enhanced Thyroid Ultrasound in Detecting Thyroid Cancer

Andreea Bena, Luciana Moisa Luca and Dana Liana Stoian

Abstract

Thyroid nodules pose a diagnostic challenge, with some displaying suspicious features that may be present both in benign and malignant entities. While ultrasound evaluation is the frontline imaging method, it sometimes falls short in distinguishing between the two. This chapter explores the innovative approach of Contrast-Enhanced Ultrasound (CEUS) as a complementary tool in thyroid nodule assessment. CEUS provides invaluable insights into nodular microvascular perfusion, offering a safe and easily accessible method with minimal adverse reactions or contraindications. Numerous studies suggest that CEUS features such as early washout, heterogeneous or hypo-enhancement, and areas of no enhancement in solid thyroid nodules, improve the predictive value for malignancy. In this chapter, we explore the role of CEUS as a potential game-changer in improving ultrasound diagnostic accuracy for thyroid nodules, particularly in cases with unclear results or indeterminate fine-needle aspiration cytology.

Keywords: microvascular perfusion, CEUS, thyroid nodules, thyroid cancer, MPUS

1. Introduction

Over the past few decades, there has been a considerable increase in the prevalence of thyroid cancer, a serious public health concern [1]. This increase is partly attributed to the enhanced detection of thyroid nodules, often discovered incidentally during imaging for unrelated conditions [2]. Despite being widespread, thyroid nodules can be difficult to diagnose; while the majority of them are benign, a small but significant percentage do harbor malignancy. However, despite the increasing incidence, mortality rates have remained consistently low [1, 3]. This trend in epidemiology is largely attributed to an overdiagnosis effect. Accurately diagnosing the malignant nodules that need further attention is a crucial challenge for clinicians in order to prevent needless interventions while ensuring prompt medical interventions.

Conventionally, ultrasound imaging has been the preferred imaging in the evaluation of thyroid nodules. Given its non-invasive nature, widespread availability, and cost-effectiveness, it is currently considered the first-line imaging modality in thyroid nodule assessment [4–6]. However, despite its many advantages, B-mode ultrasound also has limitations, being able to make a correct diagnosis in about 51.25–59.93% of cases [7]. The typical features suggestive of malignancy are: hypoechogenicity, solid composition, the presence of calcifications, spiculated or irregular borders, "taller than wide" or vertical shape, and the absence of a complete, thick perinodular "halo" [4, 5, 8]. This diagnostic uncertainty often leads to further procedures like fine-needle aspiration (FNA) cytology, or even thyroid surgery. While FNA is in most cases helpful, it can return indeterminate results in a notable number of cases, its sensitivity and specificity being about 60–98% and 54–90%, respectively [9, 10].

In this context, Contrast-Enhanced Ultrasound (CEUS) emerges as a promising complementary tool. CEUS evaluation consists of the use of ultrasound contrast agents—microbubbles that enhance vascular patterns within the thyroid nodule during imaging [11]. This technique allows for a more detailed evaluation of nodular vascularity and perfusion, characteristics that are crucial in differentiating between benign and malignant nodules. CEUS has been gaining attention for its potential to provide additional diagnostic information that could refine the assessment of thyroid nodules, especially in cases where conventional ultrasound findings are inconclusive [12]. It is important to note that only the solid component of a nodule is relevant to be assessed in a nodule.

The adoption of CEUS in thyroid nodule evaluation signifies a paradigm shift in thyroid imaging. The primary diagnostic use of this technology in this specific field is the identification and analysis of various microvascular patterns, which has a higher level of diagnostic precision compared to using Color-Doppler alone [12]. Its ability to provide real-time, dynamic assessment of nodule vascularity provides a unique and highly valuable perspective, which has the ability to enhance the precision of diagnosis and decrease the need for invasive diagnostic procedures [13]. This chapter aims to explore the innovative role of CEUS in thyroid nodule evaluation, highlighting its utility, the nuances of its interpretation, and how it might improve the overall diagnostic pathway for thyroid cancer.

In the following sections, we will explore the underlying principles of CEUS, its application in thyroid nodule assessment, the interpretation of its findings in the context of thyroid cancer, and the potential impact this advanced imaging technique could have on clinical practice.

2. How to perform thyroid CEUS

2.1 Contrast agent

Microbubbles contain a high molecular weight gas core surrounded by a lipid or albumin shell and have evolved to be more permanent in circulation, allowing longer imaging periods, which may help evaluate differences between perfusion patterns in malignant and benign settings. Microbubble contrast agents (MCA) are currently safer than CT and MRI contrast agents, especially for patients with kidney, liver and thyroid disease. No kidney problems have been linked to the use of microbubble agents. The medicine is well-tolerated, with most side effects being brief and not requiring medical care. True allergic reactions to microbubble gas have been observed in 0.006–0.009% of patients [14, 15].

Currently available contrast agents for ultrasound evaluation include:

- Sonovue®/lumason® (Bracco Imaging)—a sulfur hexafluoride microbubble contrast agent, widely used in echocardiography, liver imaging, and other vascular applications; available in North America, New Zealand, Europe, Brazil, Asia;
- Definity®/luminity® (Lantheus medical imaging)—composed of lipid-coated microbubbles filled with octafluoropropane gas; widely used in echocardiography in North America, Europe, Australia, Asia;
- Optison (GE Healthcare)—made of human albumin microspheres filled with octafluoropropane, also commonly used in cardiac ultrasound, in North America, Europe.
- Sonazoid (GE Healthcare)—a perfluorobutane microbubble contrast agent, used in liver imaging and also for investigating other organs, available in Japan, South Korea and Norway.

The optimum imaging protocol (contrast agent, delivery method, and imaging modality) depends on the individual experience of each center, radiology team and clinical circumstances [16]. For thyroid evaluation, which is a superficial structure, a dose of 1.0–2.0 mL of contrast agent is administered as an intravenous bolus, followed by 5–10 mL of saline. In some instances, more than one administration may be needed for evaluating multiple nodules.

The catheter for administration of the MCA should be placed, if possible, into the left arm, specifically the antecubital vein, to prevent any interference between the injector and the examiner on the right side. For optimal preservation of microbubbles while passing through the cannula, it is preferable to have a venous line with a diameter of 20 gauge or greater, and to keep its length as minimal as feasible [17, 18].

2.2 Ultrasound system and image acquisition

An ultrasound machine with CEUS application available for a linear probe is required in order to perform the evaluation. The mechanical index (MI) should be set <0.1 in order to obtain. If the mode is reverted to non-contrast B-mode, the contrast agent will be destroyed due to an immediate increase in the MI. In order to avoid this, the low MI contrast mode should be kept activated during the examination [17, 19].

Immediately after the MCA bolus and the saline flush are injected in the bloodstream, the timer is started on the machine and, optionally, the dynamic images can be saved as a clip. The focus area should always be positioned in the bottom region of the field of view [17].

3. CEUS characteristics used in thyroid nodule evaluation

There are certain characteristics that we follow specifically when evaluating thyroid nodules, that significantly differ from liver, breast or cardiac evaluation, given the specific vascularization in each organ and the dynamics in the development of thyroid neoplasia.

3.1 Qualitative evaluation

The first and most easily available type of evaluation refers to the qualitative type of assessment, or real-time CEUS, which is analyzed for up to 3 minutes after MCA injection. The fundamental components of qualitative analysis involve assessing the timing of contrast medium entry into the nodule and the highest level of enhancement, which can be higher, lower, or roughly the same as the surrounding tissue (referred to as hyper-, hypo-, or iso-enhancement, respectively), or the absence of enhancement [20].

3.1.1 Contrast wash-in

The contrast wash-in is regarded as centripetal, when the MCA first arrives in the peripheral part towards the center of the nodule; centrifugal, with opposite direction of enhancement, first arrival in the center; and non-concentric, or a diffuse, eccentric enhancement [21].

3.1.2 Type of enhancement

In terms of the pattern of enhancement after the MCA injection, thyroid nodules are divided as follows: no enhancement - when no MCA is detected in the nodule; low enhancement—when the intensity of the nodule after enhancement is lower compared to the surrounding thyroid parenchyma; iso-enhancement—when the intensity of the nodule after MCA administration is similar to the surrounding thyroid; hyper-enhancement—when the intensity of the nodule after MCA arrival is higher compared to the surrounding thyroid parenchyma [22]. **Figure 1** displays enhancement patterns for all variants.

3.1.3 Homogeneity of enhancement

As the previously mentioned characteristics, the homogeneity of enhancement is also compared to the adjacent parenchyma, considered healthy. The homogeneity of nodule enhancement can be inhomogeneous (**Figure 2a**) or homogeneous (**Figure 2b**).

3.1.4 Enhancement completeness

There are two types of enhancement, incomplete and complete. Complete enhancement means that the entire lesion is filled with contrast medium, with no defects of arrival of the MCA, whereas incomplete enhancement means that there are regions inside the lesion where the contrast agent is not present, or defects of enhancement are present inside the nodule. **Figure 3** displays these two enhancement variants. These defects should not be confounded with cystic areas of a mixed nodule or a spongiform consistency.

3.1.5 Peripheral ring

The outer rings described in the periphery of the nodules were categorized into four types: a consistently intense ring of enhanced tissue, an inconsistently intense ring of enhanced tissue, a consistently unenhanced ring, and an inconsistently

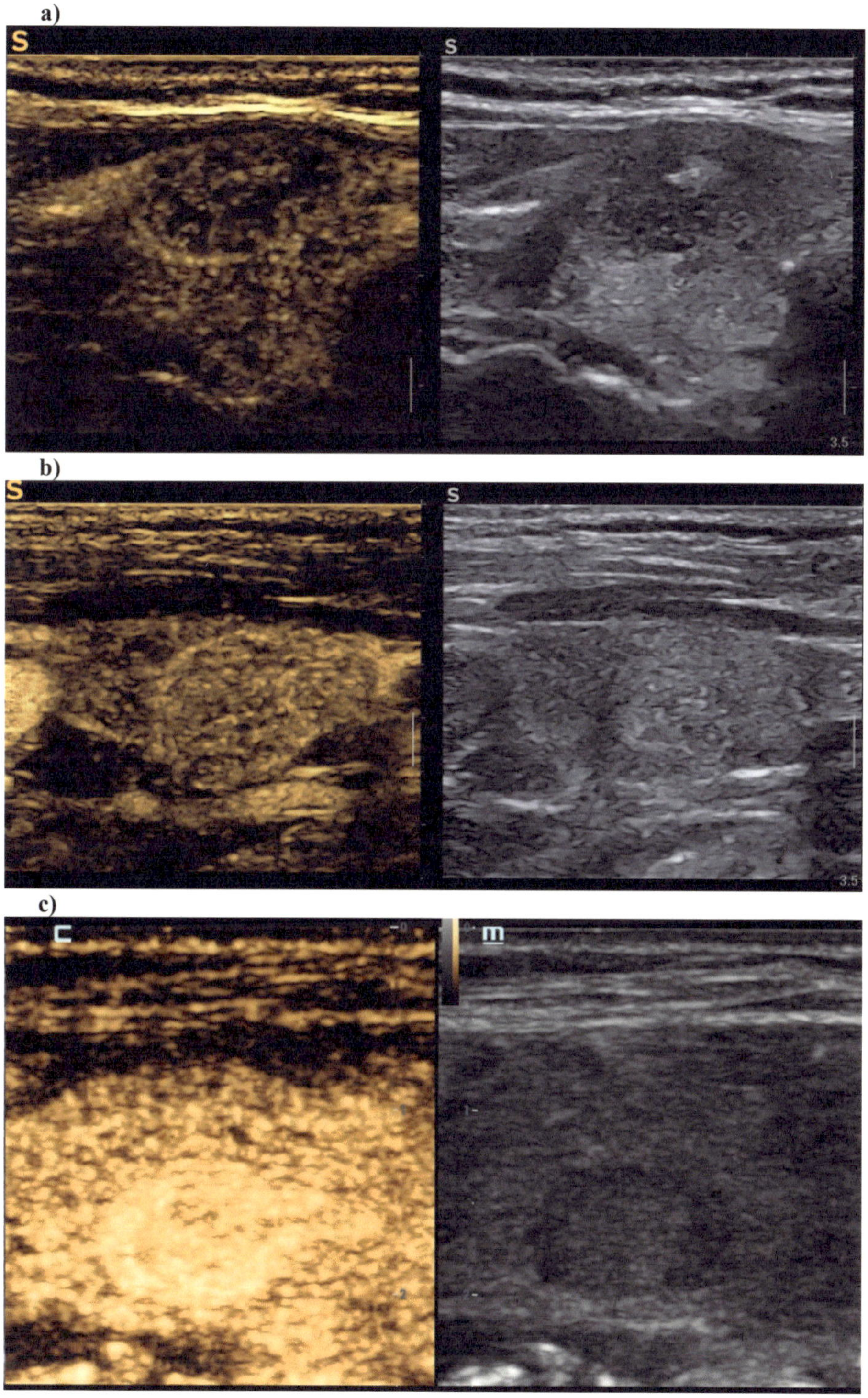

Figure 1.
Types of enhancement for thyroid nodules: (a) left figure—CEUS: low enhancement in a solid nodule (Hologic SuperSonic Mach30), right figure—B mode; (b) left figure—CEUS: iso-enhancement in a solid nodule, right figure—B mode; (c) left figure—B mode, right figure—CEUS: hyper-enhancement in a solid thyroid nodule (Mindray Resona 9).

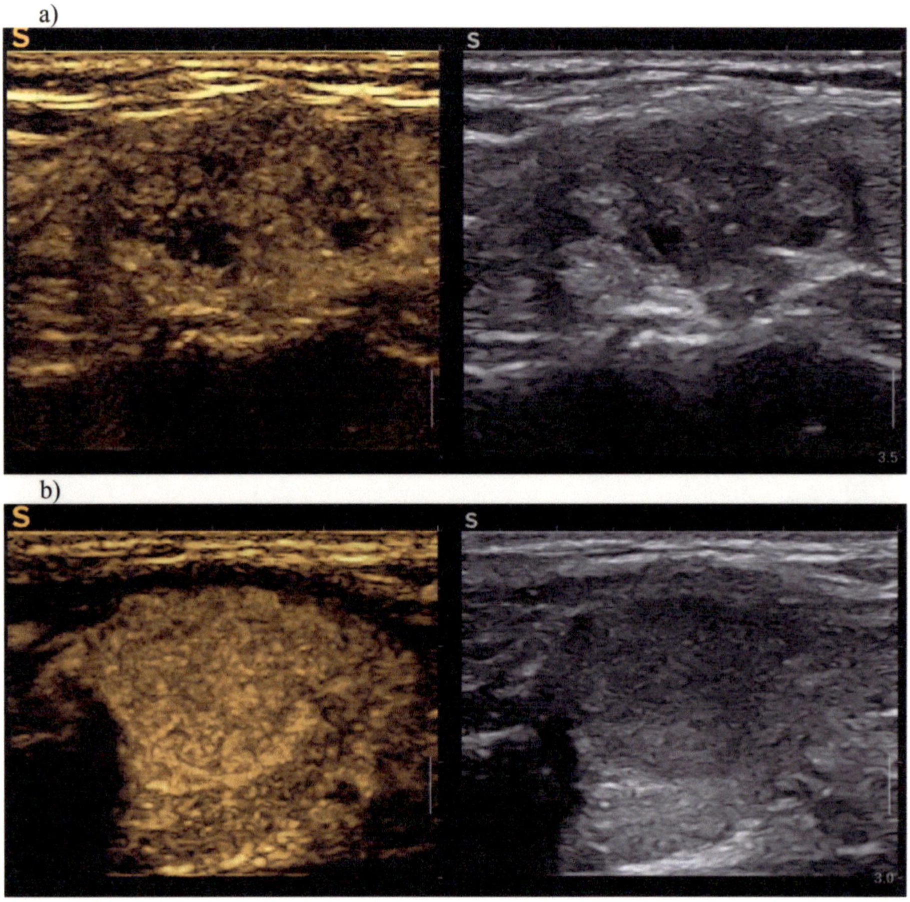

Figure 2.
Homogeneity of enhancement in thyroid nodules: (a) left figure—CEUS: inhomogeneous enhancement, right figure—B mode; (b) left figure—CEUS: homogeneous enhancement, right figure—B mode.

unenhanced ring. Conventional rings follow the oval or circular shape of the nodule, and their thickness remains consistent throughout. In contrast, irregular rings exhibited deformities and had uneven thicknesses along the margins of the nodule. A fifth type is the complete absence of a peripheral ring [22]. A complete peripheral enhanced ring and an absent ring are presented in **Figure 4**.

3.1.6 Washout of MCA

An early wash-out comparative to the neighboring parenchyma has also been presented as a typically malignant feature. This feature is evaluated in the washout phase, after the peak enhancement and is interpreted qualitatively by the operator [20].

3.2 Quantitative evaluation

Several quantitative parameters can be assessed using CEUS, providing valuable diagnostic information in the evaluation of thyroid nodules. These parameters are very different, for every manufacturer. Some ultrasound machines (e.g. Mindray, GE)

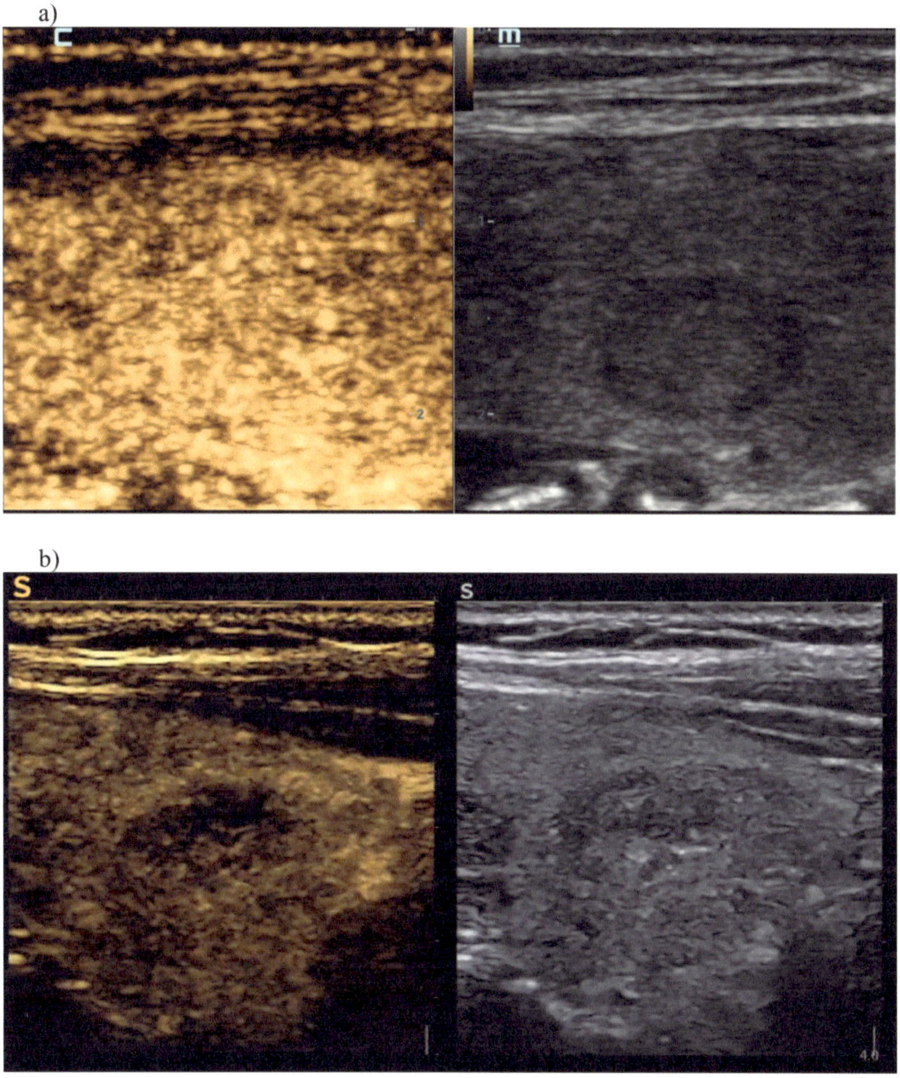

Figure 3.
Completeness of enhancement: (a) left figure—CEUS: complete enhancement in a solid thyroid nodule, right figure—B mode (Mindray Resona 9); (b) left figure—CEUS: enhancement defects inside a solid thyroid nodule, right figure—B mode (Hologic SuperSonic Mach30).

provide specific software which are machine-integrated and can be used after the evaluation for image post-processing, while others do not and a computer application (e.g. VueBox, Bracco, Italy; QLab, Philips, Netherlands) can also be used for compatible machines [23, 24]. The quantitative parameters include:

- Time Intensity Curves (TIC) are graphical representations that show the changes in contrast enhancement within a specific region of interest (ROI) over time.

- Peak Enhancement (PE) measures the maximum intensity of contrast enhancement in ROI selected by the operator, reflecting the blood volume via the uptake of contrast agents in the tissues.

a)
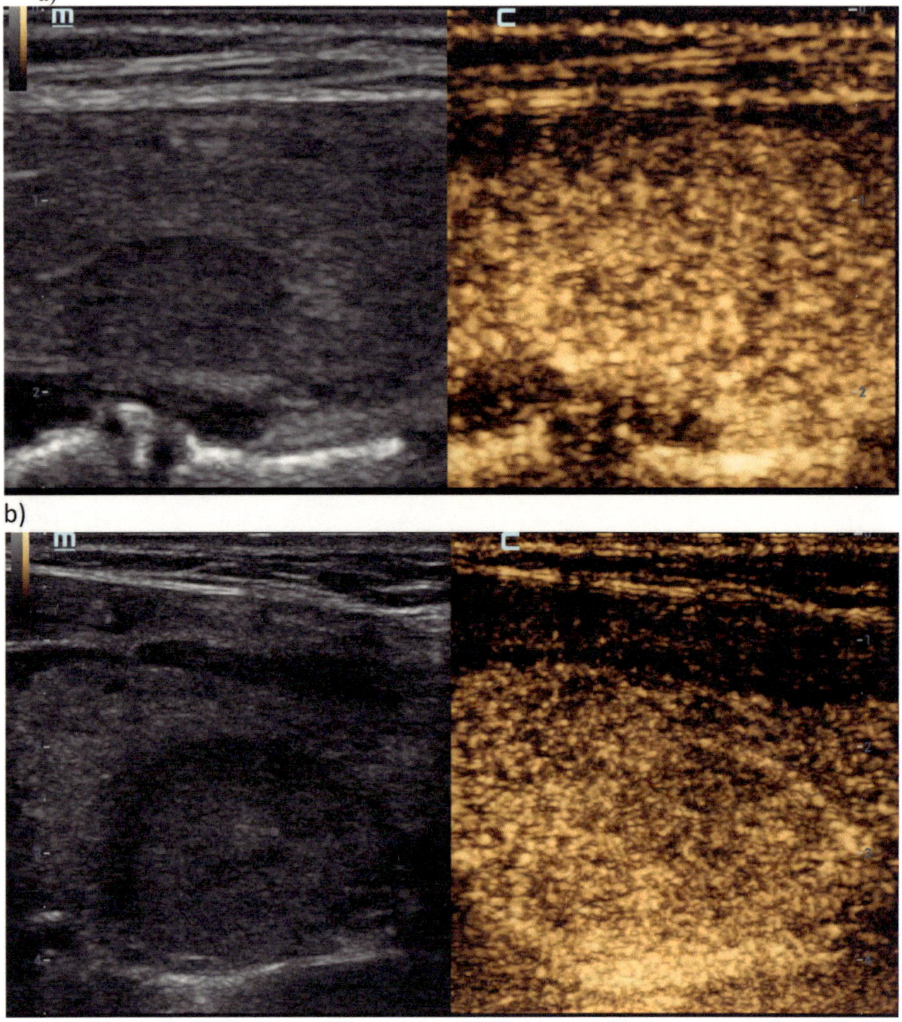
b)

Figure 4.
Peripheral ring in thyroid CEUS: (a) left figure—CEUS: absence of an enhanced peripheral ring and, right figure—B mode; (b) left figure—CEUS: complete peripheral hyperenhancement (Mindray Resona 9), right figure—B mode.

- Time to Peak (TTP) is the time interval between the injection of the contrast agent and the moment of peak enhancement and it can indicate the speed of blood flow which may vary in different substrates.

- Wash-in Rate (WiR) measures how quickly the contrast agent flows into the ROI: a faster wash-in rate might indicate higher blood flow, which can be significant in assessing tumors or inflammation.

- Wash-out Rate (WoR) assesses how quickly the contrast agent leaves the ROI. Different patterns of wash-out can help differentiate between benign and malignant lesions.

- Mean Transit Time (MTT) is the average time taken by the contrast agent to pass through the vascular bed of the ROI. It can provide information about blood flow efficiency and vascular permeability.

- Area Under the Curve (AUC) is a measure of the total contrast enhancement over time within the ROI, which integrates both the intensity and duration of enhancement and can be useful in quantifying blood volume and flow per global per evaluation/nodule.

- Rise Time (RT) represents the time taken for the contrast enhancement to go from baseline to a certain threshold level. It can help in assessing the speed of blood flow to the ROI.

- Fall Time (FT) measures the time it takes for the contrast enhancement to decrease from its peak to a certain lower threshold and provides insights into wash-out characteristics of the evaluated tissue.

- Heterogeneity Value (HV) is an advanced CEUS parameter calculated using the formula: standard deviation/mean intensity × 100. This calculation is performed at the time of peak PE of the thyroid nodule and its surrounding parenchyma; HV quantifies the variation in contrast enhancement within a region of interest (ROI). A higher HV indicates greater heterogeneity in blood flow and perfusion, which can be characteristic of certain types of lesions or abnormalities.

- Heterogeneity Ratio (HR): HR is the ratio of the HV of the nodule to that of the surrounding parenchyma and is calculated for the peak time. This ratio helps to compare the heterogeneity of the nodule against the background tissue, providing a relative measure that can be useful in differentiating between benign and malignant nodules. The parameter may be calculated using Adobe Photoshop.

- Additionally, various perfusion indices can be calculated, which reflect the blood flow per unit tissue volume; these parameters can be particularly useful in tumor assessment and in monitoring the tissue response to therapy [15, 17, 20, 23, 25].

4. Diagnostic accuracy of CEUS in thyroid cancer detection

To date, the thyroid CEUS procedure has not yet been completely standardized and is not included in any diagnostic guideline for routine assessment [15]. There are no established references for measuring the quantity or quality of the assessment. Furthermore, as in conventional ultrasound of thyroid nodules, no single parameter in CEUS appears to be sufficiently sensitive and specific for diagnosing malignancy [24]. Although the thyroid gland contains many small blood vessels and shows quick and consistent enhancement of its tissue after contrast agent injection, the vascular structures of nodules exhibit a contrasting enhancement compared to the normal tissue [26].

The most consistent malignancy-related finding in qualitative CEUS is an *inhomogeneous enhancement* of the nodule [20, 21, 27]. In papillary cancers, microcalcifications are often present and their detection on B-mode ultrasound may be sometimes misinterpreted with colloid deposit displaying micro-linear artifacts. However, in CEUS this could lead to inhomogeneous appearance and MCA uptake, due to the presence of psammoma bodies, which are calcified structures commonly found in papillary carcinoma that influence tumor angiogenesis. This results in a reduced microvessel density within the tumor, leading to a diminished blood supply [28]. Another reason for inhomogeneous uptake may be the presence of newly formed but abnormally structured vessels in the tumor tissue, coupled with the malignant growth; this tends to disrupt and even destroy existing vascular and tissue structures. Consequently, the rate of vascular necrosis in these tumors may surpass the rate of angiogenesis, leading to a notably decreased enhancement in malignant nodules, observable as inhomogeneous hypo-enhancement in CEUS. Furthermore, the development of interstitial fibrosis, often occurring in thyroid papillary carcinoma, exacerbates this effect by reducing the vascular content within the nodule even further [29, 30].

Benign thyroid nodules are typically characterized by important blood supply, which is reflected in their imaging features during CEUS evaluations. These nodules usually exhibit enhanced and homogeneous enhancement, and they generally lack perfusion defects or unenhanced areas. The uniform enhancement and absence of perfusion deficits are indicative of the consistent and abundant vascular supply that is often associated with benign thyroid conditions as opposed to the heterogeneous enhancement patterns described in thyroid cancers [31]. An example of typical benign (**Figure 5**) and malignant (**Figure 6**) thyroid nodules are displayed below.

The quantitative analysis of CEUS is also operator-dependent: The ROI is manually adjusted in the post-processing period and placed within the nodule and surrounding parenchyma. This generates variable color-coded curves, and automatically calculated parameters. Typical quantitative parameters suggesting malignancy are the subject of current research and scientific discussion. One study by Wang et al. found that slow wash-in, heterogeneous enhancement, ill-defined enhancement border, and fast wash-out rate were suggestive of malignancy. Furthermore, quantitative features include polyphasic washout curves, early arrival time, and shorter TTP [20, 32]. One study proposed an algorithm for assessing nodule heterogeneity, their

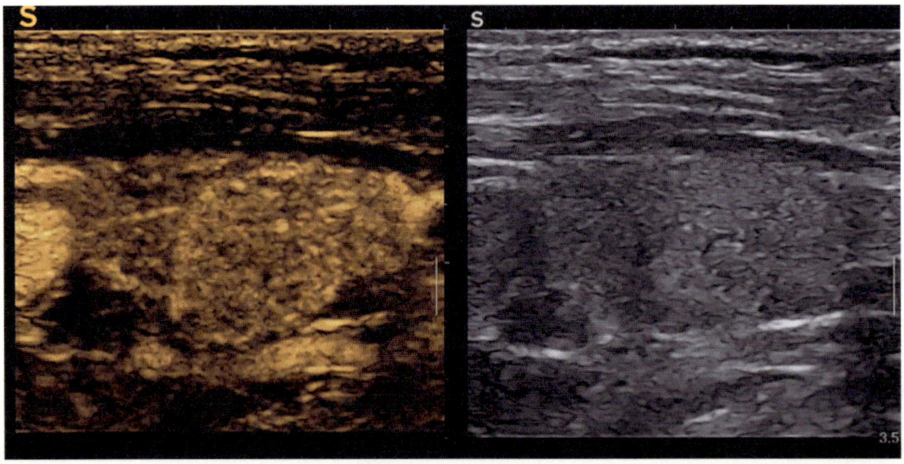

Figure 5.
Typical benign thyroid nodule: homogeneous enhancement, iso-enhancement, hyperenhanced, fine, peripheral ring.

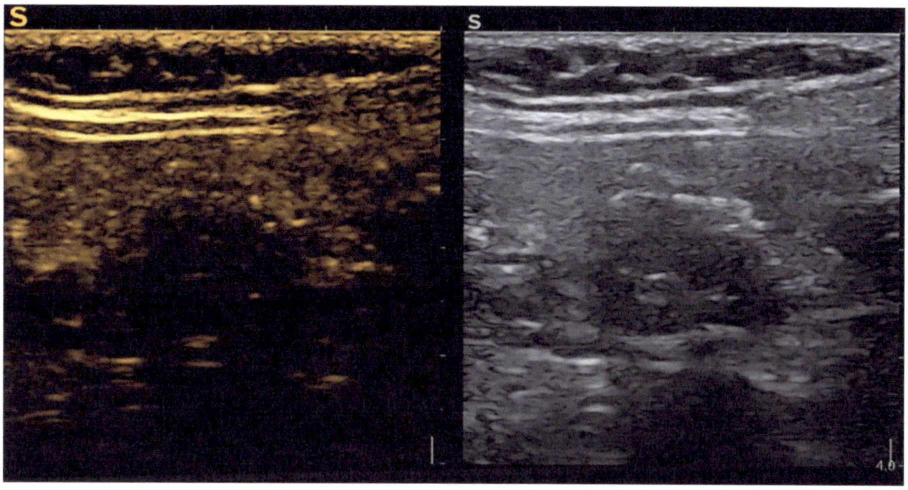

Figure 6.
Typical malignant thyroid nodule: left figure—CEUS; unclear margins, inhomogeneous enhancement with an important unenhanced area, absent peripheral ring; right figure—B mode.

findings indicating that the heterogeneity ratio HR, particularly during the ascending phase, is markedly elevated in malignant thyroid nodules as compared to benign ones (95.57 ± 43.87 vs. 73.06 ± 44.04, p = 0.009) [25].

There is currently a significant body of published data that validates the efficacy of CEUS in diagnosing thyroid cancer, including several meta-analyses [27, 33]. One meta-analysis that included only studies with histology reference standard for enhanced accuracy—revealed that thyroid nodules CEUS has a pooled sensitivity of 85% and specificity of 82%, with the sensitivity showing consistency and specificity demonstrating only mild inconsistency [34]. The Positive Predictive Value (PPV) and Negative Predictive Value (NPV) were found to be 83% and 85%, respectively. Interestingly, these findings align with previous meta-analyses which used non-histological references [35, 36]. Notably, this study stands out as the first meta-analysis in this area that employs histological diagnosis as the sole reference standard.

Overall, the performance of CEUS seems to improve conventional ultrasound diagnosis in thyroid nodule evaluation. The combination of CEUS with Thyroid Imaging Reporting and Data System (TIRADS) categories based on conventional US significantly increased diagnostic accuracy (96 vs. 90%), particularly for TIRADS class 4 thyroid nodules [37]. Another study compared the diagnostic performance of CEUS, acoustic radiation force impulse (ARFI) elastography, and the combined evaluation. CEUS yielded global diagnostic performance of 87.5%, ARFI of 88.6% and the combination of methods proved to be even better, with diagnostic rate of 90.9% [19].

Although most data are in favor of using CEUS in thyroid nodule evaluation, there are also isolated studies that found no benefit in adding CEUS to the US evaluation, concluding that CEUS data affirm subjective observations, yet they do not modify the initial pre-contrast analysis, the effectiveness of in differentiating thyroid nodules being constrained due to overlapping findings [38].

Currently, there is no universally accepted standard or criterion for interpreting the patterns of enhancement in CEUS for thyroid nodules, which limits its global applicability and widespread use. Additionally, CEUS has not been incorporated into any TIRADS guidelines. Thus, its role in routine thyroid nodule evaluation and classification remains uncertain and debated among clinicians.

5. Other applications in thyroid imaging: Before and after local therapy

For less intrusive treatment of proven benign thyroid nodules, recurrent thyroid cancer, and metastatic cervical lymph nodes, thermal ablation is commonly used in clinical thyroidology. Laser, radiofrequency ablation (RFA), microwave ablation, and, recently, high-frequency ultrasound (HIFU) are the most common treatments for solid and mixed-structure nodules with benign cytology findings. CEUS separates viable and nonviable tissue before and after treatment. This could help estimate the ablated area more accurately and reproducibly after ablation and in follow-up imaging [39, 40].

6. Challenges and limitations

The use of CEUS in evaluating thyroid nodules presents several challenges and limitations, which are important to consider in both clinical and research settings. The technical limitations refer to operator-dependent features such as the skill and experience of the operator, but also variations in the technique, such as the amount of contrast agent used or the settings of the ultrasound machine, can lead to inconsistent results. Additionally, the size of the nodules may affect the accuracy of the micro vascularity in very small nodules (smaller than 1 cm) or very large nodules (larger than 2–3 cm). Thus, the ideal evaluation is made in a nodule with sizes between 1 and 2.5 cm. Nevertheless, in some cases, even microcarcinomas present the typical features described previously [34, 41]. **Figure 7** displays a case of a micro-PTC with very low enhancement in CEUS but with the absence of suspicious features in B-mode ultrasound.

Some nodule features, such as intranodular calcifications may influence the CEUS appearance. When macrocalcifications are present inside a nodule, they generate posterior shadowing, limiting the interpretation of CEUS evaluation [28].

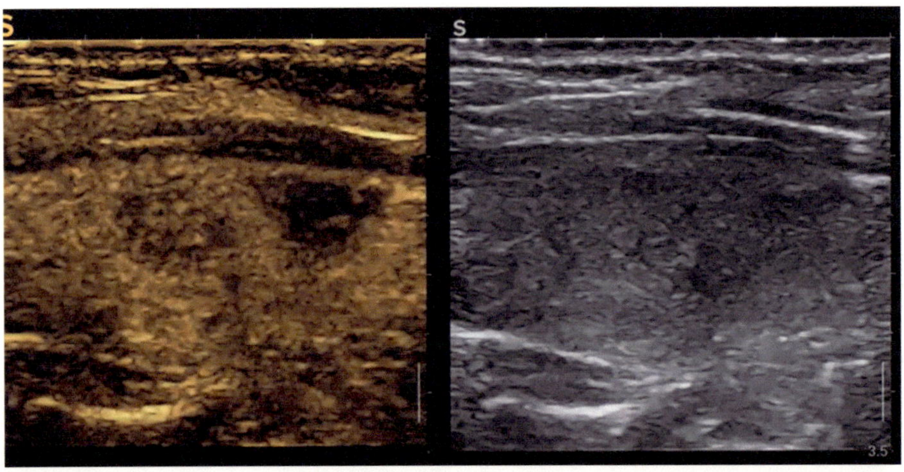

Figure 7.
A micro papillary thyroid carcinoma: left figure—CEUS: with very low enhancement (nodule in the right side of the image), right figure—B mode.

There is also a qualitative bias that has been described. While CEUS improves the visualization of vascularity in thyroid nodules, in the qualitative assessment its ability to distinguish benign from malignant nodules depends on the operator's interpretation of images, which may be subjective and can vary between observers, potentially leading to diagnostic uncertainty. It also involves additional costs for contrast agents and may require more sophisticated ultrasound equipment and trained personnel. This can limit its accessibility in resource-limited settings or in institutions where such resources are not readily available. Although there is a minimal risk of allergic reactions or side effects, especially in patients with certain medical conditions or allergies, the use of contrast agents used in CEUS is generally considered safe. In terms of evaluation time, the CEUS procedure can be more time-consuming compared to conventional ultrasound, as it requires a venous cannula, the preparation of the contrast agent, the actual scanning time, and additional time for image interpretation. In some regions, there may be regulatory hurdles related to the use of ultrasound contrast agents, and reimbursement for CEUS is not as straightforward as for conventional ultrasound, given that it is not a guideline procedure, which may be also limit its widespread use [30, 34, 42]. Importantly, given the lack of universally accepted protocols and criteria for the use and interpretation of CEUS in thyroid nodules [24]. This lack of standardization can lead to variability in how CEUS is used and interpreted across different centers.

7. Conclusion

In conclusion, CEUS represents a potentially valuable tool in differentiating malignant from benign thyroid nodules. Its enhanced ability to visualize nodule vascularity, namely microvessels, offers a unique advantage over traditional ultrasound imaging. However, the efficacy of CEUS relies on its technical limitations, the standardization of protocols, and further validation through comparative studies. While the technique shows promise, its practical application in clinical settings will depend on addressing these challenges, ensuring operator expertise, and confirming its diagnostic accuracy through comprehensive research. Ultimately, CEUS could become an integral component of thyroid nodule assessment, completing existing diagnostic modalities and contributing to more precise non-invasive diagnosis.

Author details

Andreea Bena, Luciana Moisa Luca* and Dana Liana Stoian
"Victor Babes" University of Medicine and Pharmacy, Timisoara, Romania

*Address all correspondence to: lucaluciana@umft.ro

References

[1] Pellegriti G, Frasca F, Regalbuto C, Squatrito S, Vigneri R. Worldwide increasing incidence of thyroid cancer: update on epidemiology and risk factors. Journal of Cancer Epidemiology. 2013;**2013**:965212. DOI: 10.1155/2013/965212

[2] Pellegriti G, Frasca F, Regalbuto C, Squatrito S, Vigneri R. Worldwide increasing incidence of thyroid cancer: Update on epidemiology and risk factors. Journal of Cancer Epidemiology. 2013. DOI: 10.1155/2013/965212

[3] Seib CD, Sosa JA. Evolving understanding of the epidemiology of thyroid cancer. Endocrinology and Metabolism Clinics of North America. 2019;**48**:23-35. DOI: 10.1016/j.ecl.2018.10.002

[4] Yi KH. The Revised 2016 Korean Thyroid Association Guidelines for Thyroid Nodules and Cancers: Differences from the 2015 American Thyroid Association Guidelines. Endocrinol Metab (Seoul). Sep 2016;**31**(3):373-378. DOI: 10.3803/EnM.2016.31.3.373

[5] Haugen BR, Alexander EK, Bible KC, Doherty GM, Mandel SJ, Nikiforov YE, et al. 2015 American Thyroid Association management guidelines for adult patients with thyroid nodules and differentiated thyroid cancer: The American Thyroid Association guidelines task force on thyroid nodules and differentiated thyroid cancer. Thyroid. 2016;**26**:1-133. DOI: 10.1089/thy.2015.0020

[6] Russ G, Bonnema SJ, Erdogan MF, Durante C, Ngu R, Leenhardt L. European Thyroid Association guidelines for ultrasound malignancy risk stratification of thyroid nodules in adults: The EU-TIRADS. European Thyroid Journal. 2017;**6**:225-237. DOI: 10.1159/000478927

[7] Koc AM, Adıbelli ZH, Erkul Z, Sahin Y, Dilek I. Comparison of diagnostic accuracy of ACR-TIRADS, American Thyroid Association (ATA), and EU-TIRADS guidelines in detecting thyroid malignancy. European Journal of Radiology. Dec 2020;**133**:109390. DOI: 10.1016/j.ejrad.2020.109390

[8] Gharib H, Papini E, Garber JR, Duick DS, Harrell RM, Hegedüs L, et al. American association of Clinical Endocrinologists, American college of endocrinology, and Associazione Medici Endocrinologi medical guidelines for clinical practice for the diagnosis and management of thyroid nodules - 2016 update. Endocrine Practice. 2016;**22**:1-60. DOI: 10.4158/EP161208.GL

[9] Grani G, Calvanese A, Carbotta G, D'Alessandri M, Nesca A, Bianchini M, et al. Intrinsic factors affecting adequacy of thyroid nodule fine-needle aspiration cytology. Clinical Endocrinology. 2013;**78**:141-144. DOI: 10.1111/J.1365-2265.2012.04507.X

[10] Shi M, Nong D, Xin M, Lin L. Accuracy of Ultrasound Diagnosis of Benign and Malignant Thyroid Nodules: A Systematic Review and Meta-Analysis. International Journal of Clinical Practice. 13 Sep 2022;**2022**:5056082. DOI: 10.1155/2022/5056082

[11] Cantisani V, Wilson SR. CEUS: Where are we in 2015? European Journal of Radiology. 2015;**84**:1621-1622. DOI: 10.1016/j.ejrad.2015.05.028

[12] Sorrenti S, Dolcetti V, Fresilli D, Del Gaudio G, Pacini P, Huang P, et al. The Role of CEUS in the Evaluation of

Thyroid Cancer: From Diagnosis to Local Staging. Journal of Clinical Medicine. 30 Sep 2021;**10**(19):4559. DOI: 10.3390/jcm10194559

[13] Zhang B, Jiang YX, Bin LJ, Yang M, Dai Q, Zhu QL, et al. Utility of contrast-enhanced ultrasound for evaluation of thyroid nodules. Thyroid. 2010;**20**:51-57. DOI: 10.1089/THY.2009.0045

[14] Piscaglia F, Bolondi L, Aiani L, Luigi Angeli M, Arienti V, Barozzi L, et al. The safety of Sonovue® in abdominal applications: Retrospective analysis of 23188 investigations. Ultrasound in Medicine & Biology. 2006;**32**:1369-1375. DOI: 10.1016/j.ultrasmedbio.2006.05.031

[15] Piscaglia F, Nolsøe C, Dietrich CF, Cosgrove DO, Gilja OH, Bachmann Nielsen M, et al. The EFSUMB guidelines and recommendations on the clinical practice of contrast enhanced ultrasound (CEUS): Update 2011 on non-hepatic applications. Ultraschall in der Medizin. 2012;**33**:33-59. DOI: 10.1055/S-0031-1281676

[16] Paefgen V, Doleschel D, Kiessling F. Evolution of contrast agents for ultrasound imaging and ultrasound-mediated drug delivery. Frontiers in Pharmacology. 15 Sep 2015;**6**:197. DOI: 10.3389/fphar.2015.00197

[17] Dietrich CF, Averkiou M, Nielsen MB, Barr RG, Burns PN, Calliada F, et al. How to perform contrast-enhanced ultrasound (CEUS). Ultrasound International Open. 2018;**4**:E2. DOI: 10.1055/S-0043-123931

[18] Eisenbrey JR, Daecher A, Kramer MR, Forsberg F. Effects of needle and catheter size on commercially available ultrasound contrast agents. Journal of Ultrasound in Medicine. 2015;**34**:1961-1968. DOI: 10.7863/ULTRA.14.11008

[19] He Y, Wang XY, Hu Q, Chen XX, Ling B, Wei HM. Value of contrast-enhanced ultrasound and acoustic radiation force impulse imaging for the differential diagnosis of benign and malignant thyroid nodules. Frontiers in Pharmacology. 2018;**9**:423345. DOI: 10.3389/FPHAR.2018.01363/BIBTEX

[20] Radzina M, Ratniece M, Putrins DS, Saule L, Cantisani V. Performance of Contrast-Enhanced Ultrasound in Thyroid Nodules: Review of Current State and Future Perspectives. Cancers (Basel). 30 Oct 2021;**13**(21):5469. DOI: 10.3390/cancers13215469

[21] Yuan Z, Quan J, Yunxiao Z, Jian C, Zhu H. Contrast-enhanced ultrasound in the diagnosis of solitary thyroid nodules. Journal of Cancer Research and Therapeutics. 2015;**11**:41-45. DOI: 10.4103/0973-1482.147382

[22] Zhang Y, Luo YK, Zhang MB, Li J, Li J, Tang J. Diagnostic accuracy of contrast-enhanced ultrasound enhancement patterns for thyroid nodules. Medical Science Monitor. 2016;**22**:4755. DOI: 10.12659/MSM.899834

[23] Petrasova H, Slaisova R, Rohan T, Stary K, Kyclova J, Pavlik T, et al. Contrast-Enhanced Ultrasonography for Differential Diagnosis of Benign and Malignant Thyroid Lesions: Single-Institutional Prospective Study of Qualitative and Quantitative CEUS Characteristics. Contrast Media Mol Imaging. 23 Apr 2022;**2022**:8229445. DOI: 10.1155/2022/8229445

[24] Sidhu PS, Cantisani V, Dietrich CF, Gilja OH, Saftoiu A, Bartels E, et al. The EFSUMB guidelines and recommendations for the clinical practice of contrast-enhanced ultrasound (CEUS) in non-hepatic applications:

Update 2017 (long version). Ultraschall in der Medizin. 2018;**39**:e2-e44. DOI: 10.1055/A-0586-1107/ID/JR513-18/BIB

[25] Jin L, Xu C, Xie X, Li F, Lv X, Du L. An algorithm of image heterogeneity with contrast-enhanced ultrasound in differential diagnosis of solid thyroid nodules. Ultrasound in Medicine & Biology. 2017;**43**:104-110. DOI: 10.1016/J.ULTRASMEDBIO.2016.05.011

[26] Giusti M, Orlandi D, Melle G, Massa B, Silvestri E, Minuto F, et al. Is there a real diagnostic impact of elastosonography and contrast-enhanced ultrasonography in the management of thyroid nodules? Journal of Zhejiang University. Science. B. 2013;**14**:195. DOI: 10.1631/JZUS.B1200106

[27] Zhang J, Zhang X, Meng Y, Chen Y. Contrast-enhanced ultrasound for the differential diagnosis of thyroid nodules: An updated meta-analysis with comprehensive heterogeneity analysis. PLoS One. 20 Apr 2020;**15**(4):e0231775. DOI: 10.1371/journal.pone.0231775

[28] Jiang J, Shang X, Wang H, Xu Y-B, Gao Y, Zhou Q. Diagnostic value of contrast-enhanced ultrasound in thyroid nodules with calcification. The Kaohsiung Journal of Medical Sciences. 2015;**31**:138-144. DOI: 10.1016/j.kjms.2014.12.001

[29] Moon HJ, Kwak JY, Kim MJ, Son EJ, Kim EK. Can vascularity at power Doppler US help predict thyroid malignancy? Radiology. 2010;**255**:260-269. DOI: 10.1148/RADIOL.09091284

[30] Kim BK, Choi YS, Kwon HJ, Lee JS, Heo JJ, Han YJ, et al. Relationship between patterns of calcification in thyroid nodules and histopathologic findings. Endocrine Journal. 2013;**60**:155-160. DOI: 10.1507/ENDOCRJ.EJ12-0294

[31] Liu MJ, Men YM, Zhang YL, Zhang YX, Liu H. Improvement of diagnostic efficiency in distinguishing the benign and malignant thyroid nodules via conventional ultrasound combined with ultrasound contrast and elastography. Oncology Letters. 2017;**14**:867-871. DOI: 10.3892/OL.2017.6245

[32] Wu Q, Wang Y, Li Y, Hu B, He Z-Y. Diagnostic value of contrast-enhanced ultrasound in solid thyroid nodules with and without enhancement. Endocrine. 2016;**53**:480-488. DOI: 10.1007/s12020-015-0850-0

[33] Wu Y, Zhou C, Shi B, Zeng Z, Wu X, Liu J. Systematic review and meta-analysis: Diagnostic value of different ultrasound for benign and malignant thyroid nodules. Gland Surgery. 2022;**11**:1067-1077. DOI: 10.21037/GS-22-254/COIF

[34] Trimboli P, Castellana M, Virili C, Havre RF, Bini F, Marinozzi F, et al. Performance of contrast-enhanced ultrasound (CEUS) in assessing thyroid nodules: A systematic review and meta-analysis using histological standard of reference. Radiologia Medica. 2020;**125**:406-415. DOI: 10.1007/S11547-019-01129-2/TABLES/3

[35] Ma X, Zhang B, Ling W, Liu R, Jia H, Zhu F, et al. Contrast-enhanced sonography for the identification of benign and malignant thyroid nodules: Systematic review and meta-analysis. Journal of Clinical Ultrasound. 2016;**44**:199-209. DOI: 10.1002/JCU.22311

[36] Yu D, Han Y, Chen T. Contrast-enhanced ultrasound for differentiation of benign and malignant thyroid lesions:

Meta-analysis. Otolaryngology–Head and Neck Surgery. 2014;**151**:909-915. DOI: 10.1177/0194599814555838

[37] Zhang Y, Zhou P, Tian S-M, Zhao Y-F, Li J-L, Li L. Usefulness of combined use of contrast-enhanced ultrasound and TIRADS classification for the differentiation of benign from malignant lesions of thyroid nodules. European Radiology. 2017;**27**:1527-1536. DOI: 10.1007/s00330-016-4508-y

[38] Bartolotta TV, Midiri M, Runza G, Galia M, Taibbi A, Damiani L, et al. Incidentally discovered thyroid nodules: Incidence, and greyscale and colour Doppler pattern in an adult population screened by real-time compound spatial sonography. La Radiologia Medica. 2006;**111**:989-998. DOI: 10.1007/s11547-006-0097-1

[39] Papini E, Monpeyssen H, Frasoldati A, Hegedüs L. 2020 European thyroid association clinical practice guideline for the use of image-guided ablation in benign thyroid nodules. European Thyroid Journal. 2020;**9**:172-185. DOI: 10.1159/000508484

[40] Bernardi S, Giudici F, Cesareo R, Antonelli G, Cavallaro M, Deandrea M, et al. Five-year results of radiofrequency and laser ablation of benign thyroid nodules: A multicenter study from the Italian minimally invasive treatments of the thyroid group. Thyroid. 2020;**30**:1759-1770. DOI: 10.1089/THY.2020.0202

[41] Wang J, Wei W, Guo R. Ultrasonic elastography and conventional ultrasound in the diagnosis of thyroid micro-nodules. Pakistan Journal of Medical Sciences. 2019;**35**:1526-1531. DOI: 10.12669/pjms.35.6.777

[42] Bartolotta TV, Midiri M, Galia M, Runza G, Attard M, Savoia G, et al. Qualitative and quantitative evaluation of solitary thyroid nodules with contrast-enhanced ultrasound: Initial results. European Radiology. 2006;**16**:2234-2241. DOI: 10.1007/S00330-006-0229-Y/METRICS

Section 2

Musculoskeletal

Chapter 5

Musculoskeletal Ultrasound in Inflammatory Myopathies

Carolina Solomon

Abstract

Idiopathic inflammatory myopathies (IIM) represent a special group of pathological conditions that represent a challenge for clinical practice and also for the patients' quality of life. Skeletal muscles represent a very suitable for ultrasound (US) examination, being superficial and very easily approachable through this examination. Musculoskeletal US, having the advantages of an accessible, non-radiating and easy-to-use imaging method, provides useful information about structure, echogenicity, vascularity or elasticity, useful for the diagnosis and the follow-up in the evolution of patients with IIM. This chapter briefly reviews the US characteristics of IIM, pointing out some particular aspects. The listed aspects are exemplified by images of some clinical cases from personal experience.

Keywords: ultrasound, myopathies, musculoskeletal, elastography, myositis

1. Introduction

Idiopathic inflammatory myopathies (IIM) (commonly called myositis) represent a heterogeneous group of acquired muscle diseases characterized by chronic muscle weakness, elevated muscle enzymes, inflammatory cellular infiltrates in skeletal muscles on biopsy, and other extra-muscular manifestations, mainly skin involvement and interstitial lung disease [1–3].

In recent years, clinical, serological, radiological, and pathological techniques have developed a lot, leading to a precise and complex diagnosis. Added to these are the development of myositis-specific antibodies (MSA), as well as new techniques, such as proteomics or transcriptomics.

Over time, there have been several classifications of IIM, starting from the classification made by Bohan and Peter. Currently, based on what was described above, detailed classifications of these pathological entities include dermatomyositis (DM), immune-mediated necrotizing myopathy (IMNM), anti-synthetase syndrome (ASyS) and inclusion body myositis (IBM), and overlap myositis. In the last years, with the emergence of the pandemic SARSCoV-2 (COVID-19) was described a new myopathy associated with this infection, which along with immune checkpoint inhibitors-related myositis represents emergency myopathies [2, 4].

Integration of polymyositis in the IIM group is currently controversial because most cases can be reclassified, based on the results of the clinical, serological and pathological exams, in other subtypes of inflammatory myopathies, especially IMNM and ASS. Also, in the case of polymyositis with mitochondrial pathology, which presents characteristics similar to IBM, it was reclassified as early IBM in the category of inclusion body myositis [4].

Idiopathic inflammatory myopathies with adult-onset are associated with an increased risk of cancer, especially in the previous 3 years and the 3 years after the onset of the disease. Inflammatory myopathies associated with cancers usually occur in ovarian, gastrointestinal tract, lung, breast, lymphoma, and nasopharyngeal cancers. Neoplasia is the main cause of death in patients with IIM, in part, most likely due to the late diagnosis and in advanced stages [2].

IIM are characterized by predominantly mononuclear inflammatory infiltrates with perivascular and perifascial location, changes in intramuscular vascularization (endothelial hyperplasia, intravascular thrombi with obliteration of the vascular lumen and reduction in capillary density), necrosis and microinfarcts of muscle fibers, which cause perifascicular muscle atrophy. In advanced forms of the disease, muscle structures are reduced in size, muscle fibers are replaced by fibrous or adipose tissue [5, 6].

The main symptom for which patients with IIM present to the doctor, less so those with IBM, is symmetrical muscle weakness, localized in the proximal skeletal muscles. In the case of DM, patients show skin changes, for example, erythema (heliotrope rash), periorbital edema or Gottron papules on the dorsal side of the hands and fingers. Rashes can also appear during development of the ASS [3].

Considering the complexity of IIM, the early diagnosis and subtype classification of these pathological conditions is very important for the establishment of appropriate therapy and optimal management of these patients, with improved long-term outcomes.

The classical diagnosis of IIM is based on the clinical examination, the determination of the serum level of muscle enzymes, electromyography and muscle biopsy.

Imaging examinations play a very important role in the diagnosis, evaluation of the degree of disease activity, of the response to the therapy, as well as monitoring the evolution of the disease. The most used imaging methods for muscle assessment in IIM are: magnetic resonance imaging (MRI), ultrasound (US), and positron emission tomography (PET) [3, 7, 8].

2. Ultrasound in IIM

Ultrasonography is a non-invasive, non-irradiating, easy to use, widely available method, having very good resolution on soft tissue structures, such as skeletal muscles [3].

Muscle US is used both for the assessment and diagnosis of diseases that affect muscles, as well as for the follow-up of these disorders [7, 8].

2.1 Normal muscle

On cross-sections, the normal muscle structure shows a hypoechoic fascicle separated by hyperechoic points, represented by connective tissue (perimysium, epimysium, fasciae)—coarse dotted appearance—"starry night sky." On longitudinal view, the muscle fibers are visualized parallel to the insertion, having appearance of a "comb structure" (**Figure 1**) [8].

US examinations can evaluate echogenicity, dimensions, vascularization (using Doppler techniques) and elasticity (using elastographic techniques).

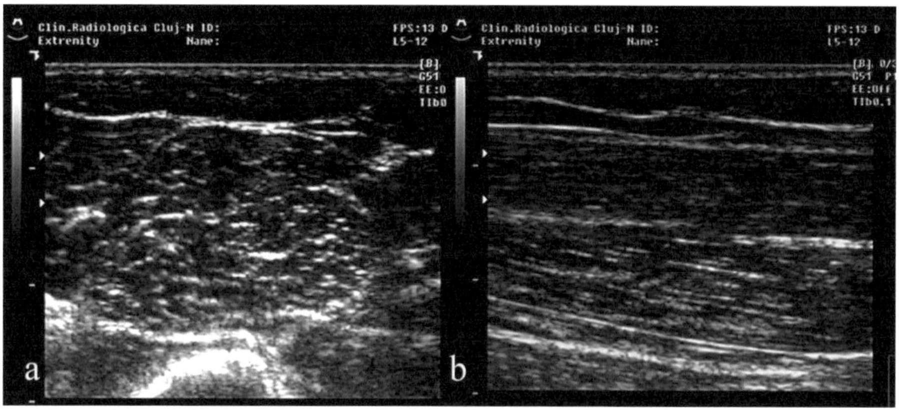

Figure 1.
Normal appearance of the muscular structure in transversal (a) and longitudinal (b) plane.

Muscle echogenicity can be assessed qualitatively and quantitatively. The visual qualitative analysis can be staged using the Heckmatt scale (**Table 1**), which is based on the degree of muscle echogenicity and visualization of deep bone structures [8–10].

There is also the possibility of quantitative evaluation of muscle echogenicity through software that allows the calculation of histograms, but these are not widely used in daily clinical practice.

2.2 Gray scale US

Classic US (also named gray scale US or bidimensional US—2D US) is frequently used for the exploration of muscle in various pathologies, implicitly in IIM. In these entities, US can detect edema-like changes, fatty infiltration, fibrosis or atrophy.

At the beginning of the disease, the muscle appearance on gray scale US may be normal (**Figure 2**).

Edema-like lesions represent a sign of acute muscle inflammation, and are important for establishing the biopsy site and the diagnosis. These lesions are characterized by changes in echogenicity and an increase in muscle size. The echogenicity of the area of muscle edema is assessed differently by various authors, from a slight decrease compared to normal muscle, to its increase, with a more hyperechoic

Grade	Echogenicity
Grade I	Normal, without attenuation and with the clear highlighting of the underlying bone
Grade II	A slightly increased, without architecture loss or attenuation, but with the distinct highlighting of the underlying bone
Grade III	Clearly increased muscle echogenicity, loss of muscle architecture, with reduced the visibility of deeper structures (the underlying bone)
Grade IV	Very increased muscle echogenicity (white muscle) with loss of muscle architecture and strong attenuation of ultrasound signal, with not highlighting of the underlying bone

Table 1.
Heckmatt scale for qualitative evaluation of muscle echogenicity.

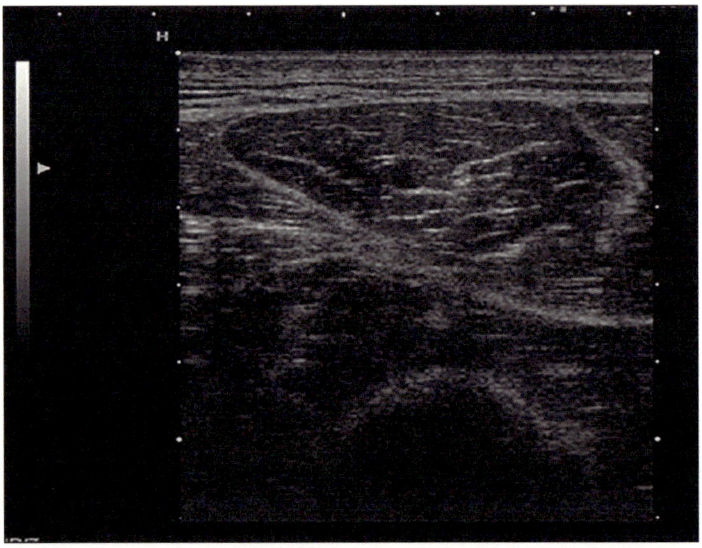

Figure 2.
2D US: Preserved muscle structure in the proximal third of the thigh, in a 60 years old female with DM.

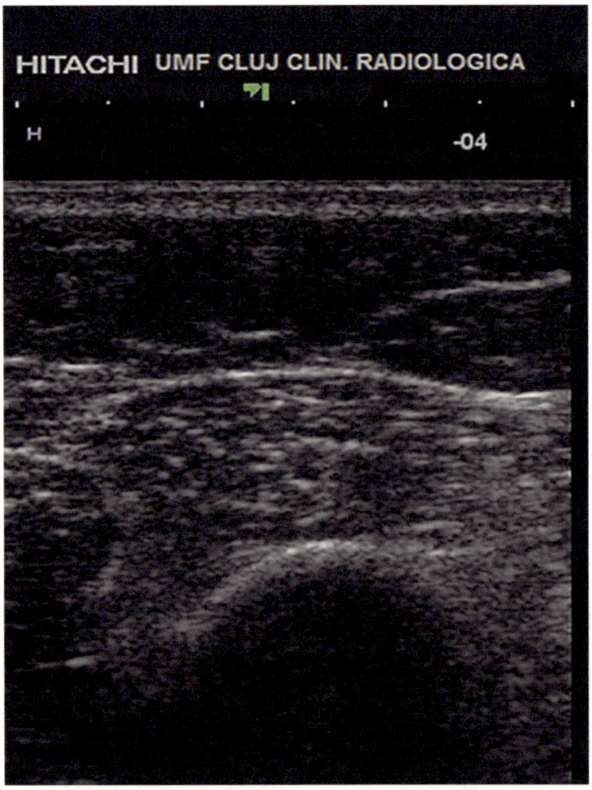

Figure 3.
2D US: Moderate increase in echogenicity, with preservation of the muscle structure at the level of the middle third of the right arm in a 54 years old female with DM.

appearance (**Figure 3**). According to some authors, US cannot identify edema-like lesions in the early stages or in mild myopathies, these being better highlighted by MRI, on T2 or STIR sequences [11].

Adipose or fibro-adipose infiltration of muscle tissue can determine, in the early stages, an appearance similar to edema-like lesions, the difference is made by the homogeneity of the image (homogeneous in edema-like and inhomogeneous in fatty infiltration).

In the acute phase of the disease, muscle edema can be observed in US as a global increase in echogenicity without attenuation of the underlying bone, named a "shine-through" appearance or "see-through echogenicity increase" [8]. This aspect is different from that determined by atrophy, found in the advanced stages of the disease or in muscular dystrophies [11].

Atrophy is present in the advanced stages of IIM, is characterized by a significant reduction in the size of the affected muscles, as well as by a significant increase in muscle echogenicity (**Figure 4**) [11].

A number of authors found changes in the muscle fascia in patients with IIM, especially in those with DM. The US appearance of fasciitis in grayscale is of thickening of fascia, and on PD examination is represented by increased vascular signal along the fascia [12].

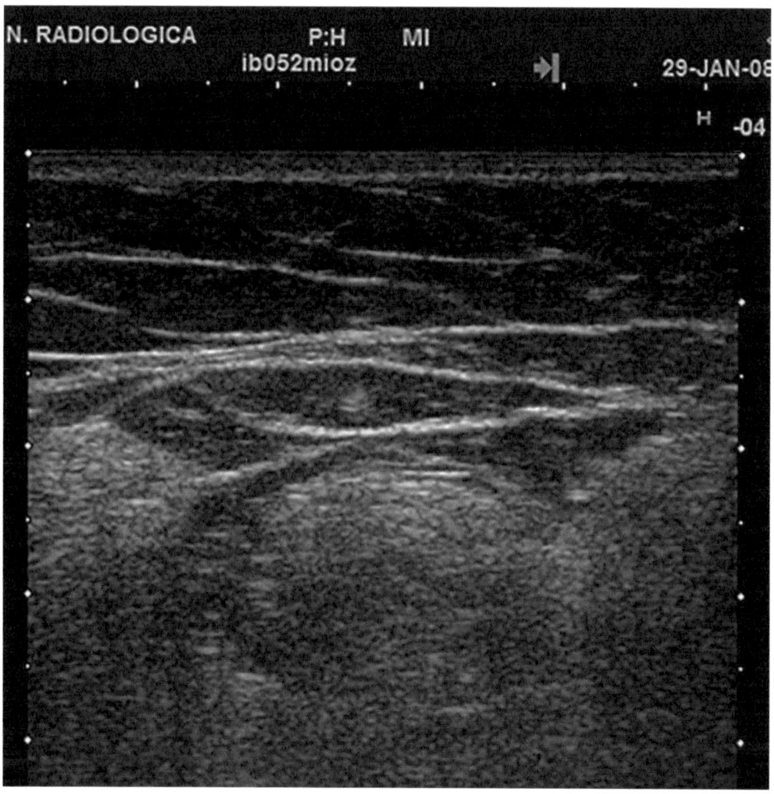

Figure 4.
2D US: Atrophy and significant increase in echogenicity at the level of the antero-superior right thigh in a 63 years old female with PM.

2.3 Doppler techniques

The use of Doppler techniques in the assessment of the vascularization of muscles affected in IIM is controversial and not routinely used, the most studied method is the power Doppler (PD). The accentuation of vascularization, expressed by the increase of the intramuscular PD signal, was associated with the presence of inflammation and correlated with the degree of disease activity [8].

In patients with chronic IIM, there is a poor correlation between PD signal and edema or inflammation and fatty infiltration. They suggest that PD value is weak in differentiating the vascularization between the normal and pathological muscle (**Figure** 5) [13].

In a recent study, Conticini et al. proposed a combined score between 2D US and PDUS for evaluation of patients with IIM, showing a positive statistical correlation between PDUS and edema and the degree of activity of the disease. Also, the authors found that PDUS represents a valuable method for the follow-up of these patients [14].

The availability of new Doppler techniques specific to microvessels (micro-V and superb microvascular imaging), having greater sensitivity than PDUS, will bring new and complex information in the muscle US evaluation of IIM [14].

2.4 Contrast-enhanced ultrasonography (CEUS)

PDUS cannot differentiate between arterial and venous circulation, nor can it measure capillary flow. The use of US contrast substances increases the performance of US in assessing tissue perfusion in a certain region but also for measuring blood flow.

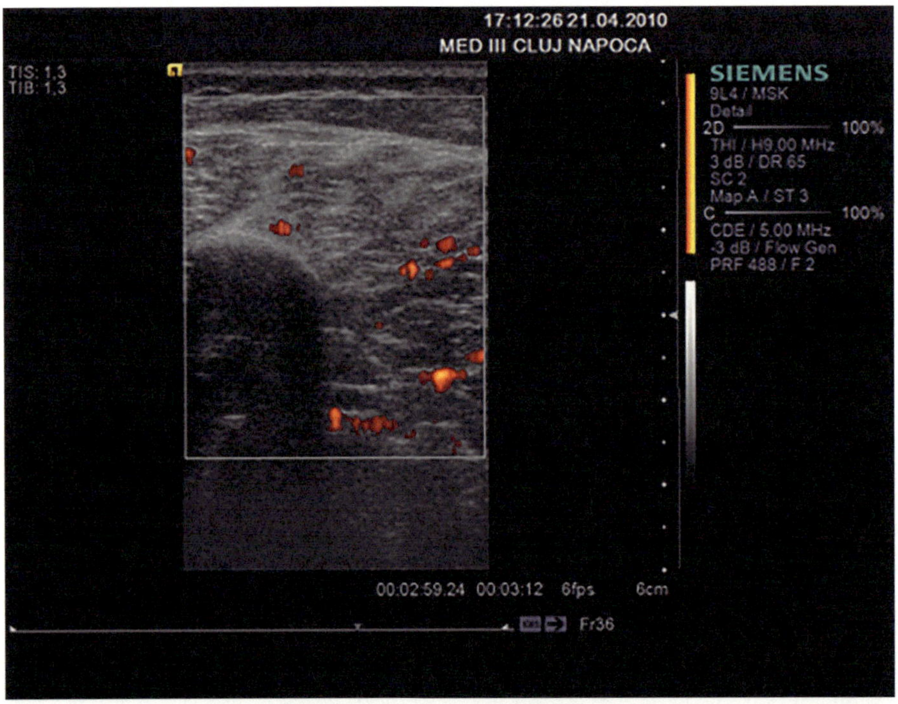

Figure 5.
PD US: Increased muscle vascularity in the proximal third of the left arm in a 50 years old female with PM.

Weber et al. studied, using CEUS, the changes determined by inflammation in muscle vascularization in patients with polymyositis and dermatomyositis. They found an increase in muscle perfusion in patients who presented edema during the MRI examination and who had histological confirmation of the disease, blood flow measured by CEUS being the best parameter for the diagnosis of PM and DM. The authors suggest that CEUS can be used as an additional method for the diagnosis of IIM [8, 15].

In another study, Weber et al. indicated that the blood flow decreased with the improvement of the other quantification parameters of the disease [8, 16].

2.5 Ultrasound elastography

Elastography is a new ultrasound technique, developed in recent years, which evaluates the elasticity/stiffness of tissues. Currently, there are two main types of elastography, according to the EFSUMB guidelines:

- strain elastography (SE)—quasi-static, qualitative technique and more operator dependent

- shear wave elastography (SWE)—dynamics and quantitative technique [3, 17].

Musculoskeletal structures represented some of the first *in vivo* applications of elastography, all available variants can be applied to evaluate the elasticity of the muscle tissue.

Regarding strain elastography, previous studies have shown an increase in muscle stiffness in patients with myositis compared to the group control group [8, 18–20].

SWE offers a quantitative assessment of muscle elasticity, starting from the differences in relative stiffness of soft tissues when an external force (the ultrasound beam) is applied to the boundary between the tissues. Alfuraih et al. showed that thigh muscle stiffness measured using SWE was lower in patients with active IIM compared to the healthy group. Also, they found that reduced muscle stiffness was accompanied by the presence of edema and atrophy on MRI, as well as weakness on clinical exam [20, 21].

New studies indicate that SWE can be used as an imaging biomarker that can support the diagnosis of IIM [3, 13, 22].

2.6 Ultrasound viscoelasticity

Viscosity represents a new parameter, recently introduced in the use of elastographic techniques, which is correlated to shear-wave dispersion. This technique is based in the viscoelastic properties of the tissues, starting from the premise that the presence of inflammation leads to changes in tissue viscosity. There are few published studies on muscle viscoelasticity until now, this technique not yet being available on all equipment.

2.7 US-guided muscular biopsy

The advantage of being a real-time exploration method as well as that of identifying pathological muscle changes, gives US the possibility of being used to guide muscle biopsies. These can be guided by 2D US, but also using elastography.

3. Special ultrasound aspects in IIM

The ultrasound changes encountered in IIM are variable, presenting themselves as a complex picture, which combines the changes of chronic disease with elements of acute exacerbation. Anatomical location and the predominance of a certain type of lesion with ultrasound expression can constitute the characteristic US patterns for certain diseases in the IIM group.

3.1 Polymyositis, dermatomyositis and inclusion body myopathy—2D US

Inflammatory myopathy in DM and PM is characterized by symmetrical localization to the proximal muscle groups, especially the deltoid and hip flexor muscles.

In DM and PM, changes appear as focal areas of increased echogenicity. Over time, these areas of hyperechogenicity expand, according to the evolution of the disease. In the acute phase of the disease, muscle edema is highlighted by slight increase of echogenicity with a shiny aspect. In the chronic phase, the increase in echogenicity becomes marked, being associated with the reduction of the size of the affected muscle groups (**Figure 6**) [3].

Muscle changes in DM can be associated with skin and subcutaneous soft tissue edema (dermis and hypodermis) (**Figure 7**), highlighted by their increased echogenicity. In some cases of DM, calcinosis can be found - calcifications in the hypodermis (**Figure 8**).

IBM is one of the most common myopathies of the elderly and is usually characterized with predilection on the quadriceps muscle and the deep flexor muscles of the fingers. In IBM, muscle can be affected asymmetrically, sometimes with a "moth-eaten" aspect.

3.2 Polymyositis, dermatomyositis, inclusion body myopathy—Elastography

Regarding the elastographic examination, SE revealed the increase in muscle stiffness, in correlation with the histological results. In PM, increased stiffness was

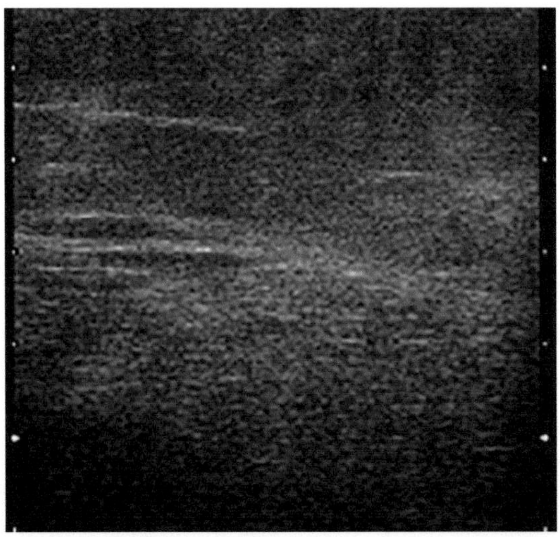

Figure 6.
2D US: Wiped muscle structure in the proximal third of the thigh in a 44 years old female with DM.

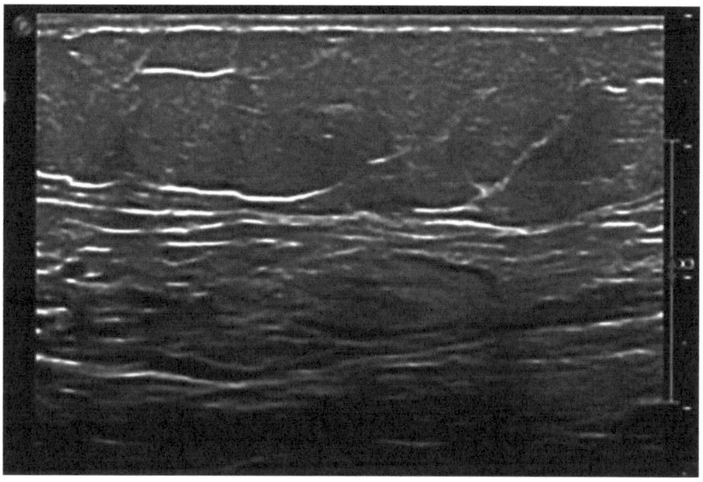

Figure 7.
2D US: Increased echogenicity of the subcutaneous tissue in the proximal third of the thigh, in a 55 years old female with DM.

associated with fibrosis and atrophy, while increased elasticity found in DM had as a histological substrate of the increased elasticity, fatty infiltration (**Figures 9–11**) [19, 20].

SWE, used more and more in recent years, showed lower stiffness in patients with more severe weakness. In some studies, the results obtained at SWE were correlated with muscle weakness and the appearance of edema and atrophy founded on MRI, but not with the CPK levels, disease duration or fatty infiltrations (**Figure 12**) [3, 21].

Although there are still not many studies regarding the evaluation of muscle viscoelasticity, this could have a role in the evaluation of patients with IIM (**Figure 13**).

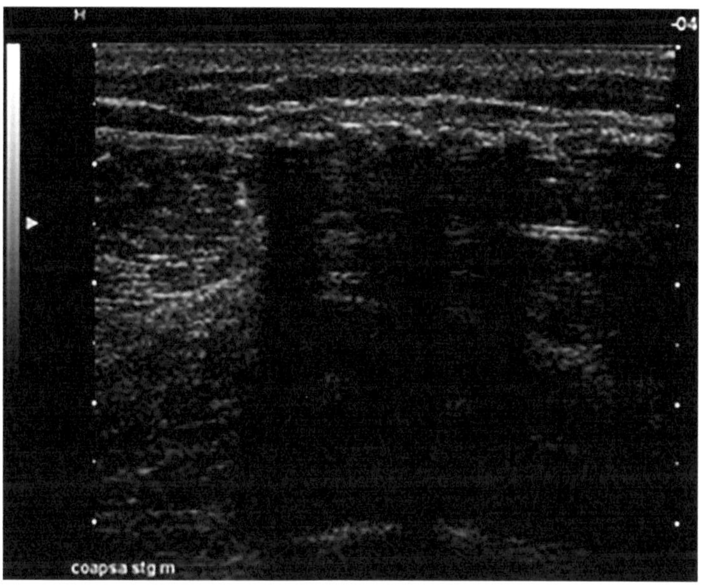

Figure 8.
2D US: Calcifications in the adipose tissue in the proximal third of the thigh, in a 41 years old male with DM.

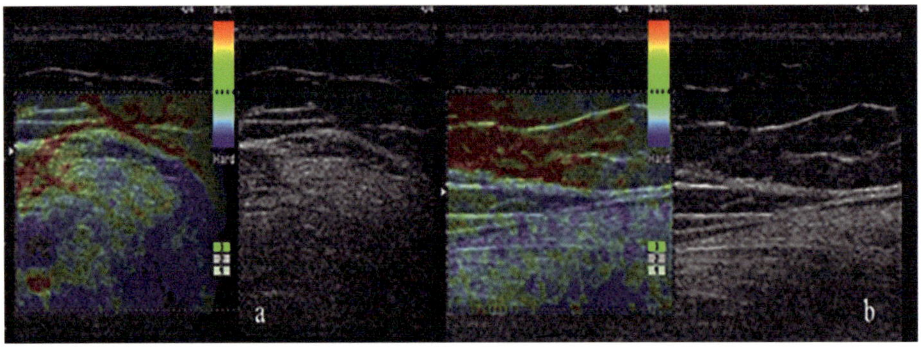

Figure 9.
SE: Increased stiffness in the proximal of the thigh in a 43 years old female with PM (a—transversal and b—longitudinal view).

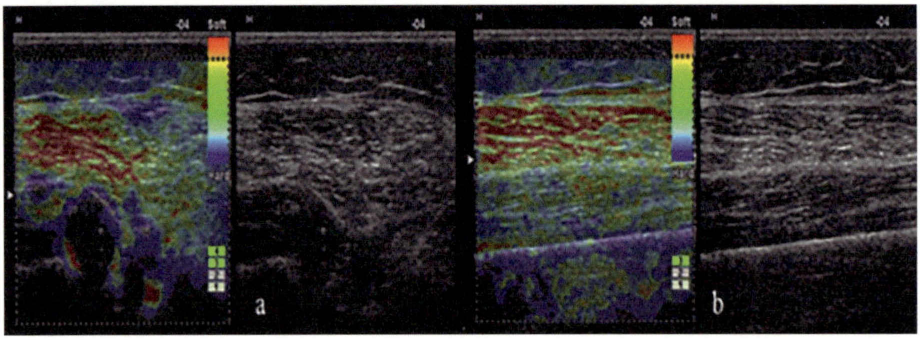

Figure 10.
Very increased elasticity in the proximal third of the thigh, in a 52 years old female with DM (a—transversal and b—longitudinal view).

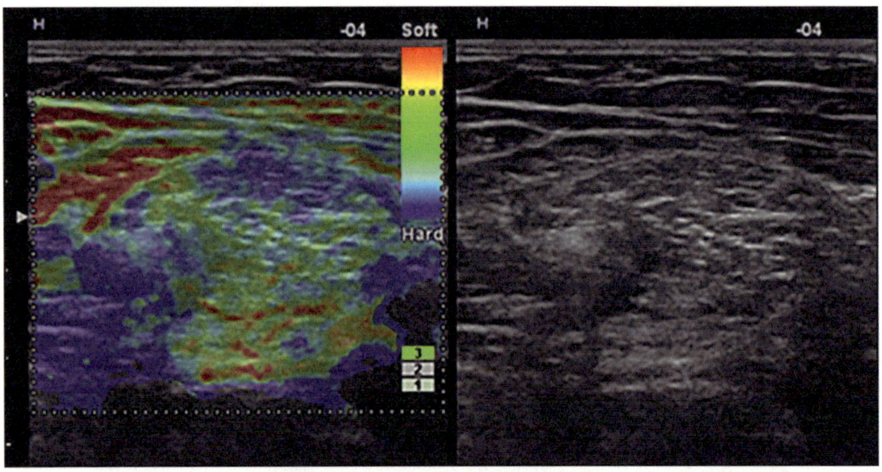

Figure 11.
SE: Inhomogeneous aspect, with area of increased stiffness and medium elasticity in a 77 years old male with IBM.

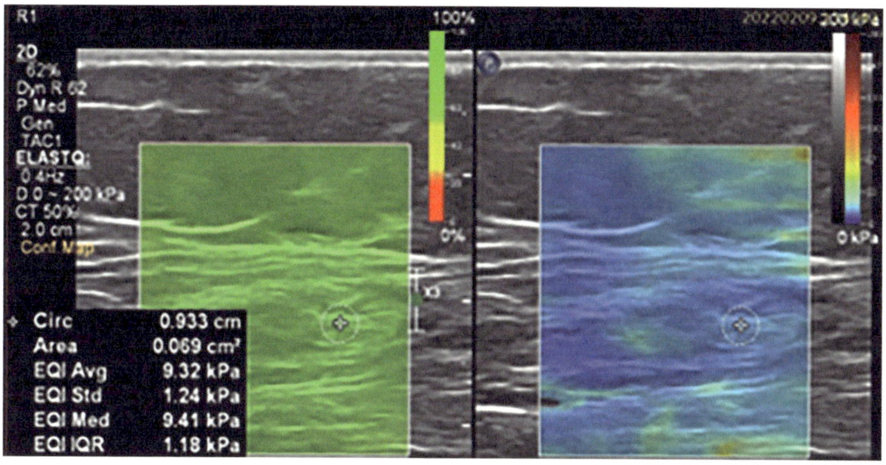

Figure 12.
SWE: Increased elasticity in the proximal third of the thigh, in a 58 years old female with DM.

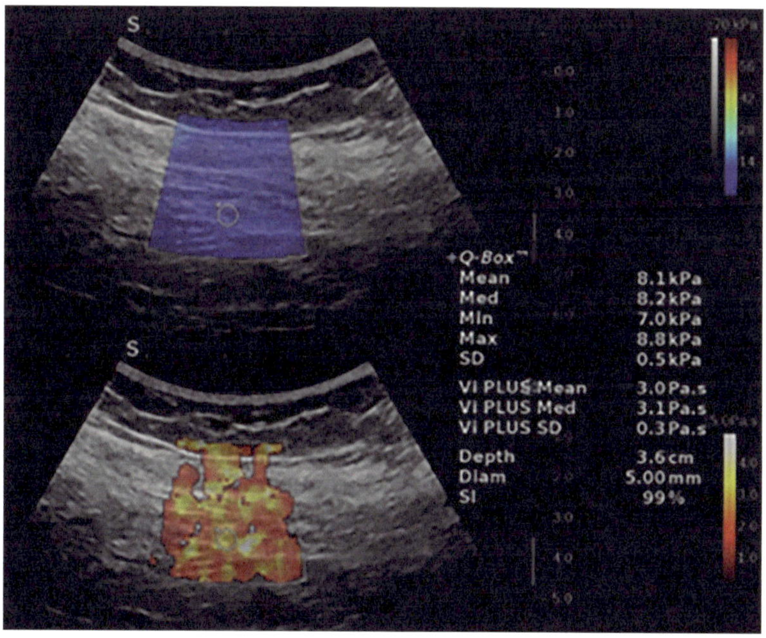

Figure 13.
Viscoelasticity: The same patient like in **Figure 11**.

4. Estimation of the evolution of the IIM

Monitoring patients with IIM represents a challenge in clinical practice. Several authors have shown that the ultrasound changes observed in patients with IIM are apparently correlated with the degree of activity of the disease evaluated clinically and biologically.

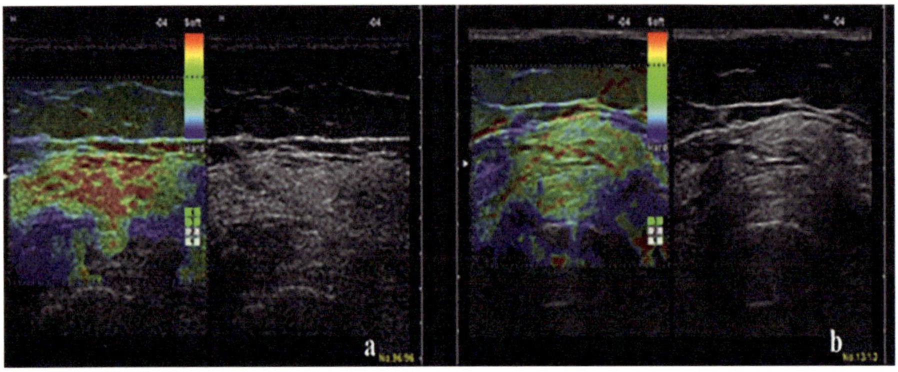

Figure 14.
SE: Changing the appearance of muscle elasticity in the medium 1/3 of the thigh, in a 50 years old patient with DM, first (a) and after a period of 4.5 months (b).

US represents an important tool also for the monitoring response to treatment. In the case of a favorable post-therapy evolution, the US and/or elastographic appearance resolves. In cases of mild damage, the muscles can return to normal (**Figure 14**).

5. Other imaging modalities

5.1 Magnetic resonance imaging

Currently, magnetic resonance imaging (MRI) represents the best imaging method for evaluation of skeletal muscle. Muscle edema and fat replacement, encountered in IIM, are best characterized using T1-weighted and T2-weighted fat suppression or STIR sequences. The presence, extensiveness and severity of chronic changes are assessed using T1-weighted spin-echo sequences, which occur hyperintense due to muscle fatty replacement. The inflammatory changes appear as hyperintensities on T2-weighted sequences.

In addition to qualitative changes, MRI could provide quantitative evaluation, using special sequences, such as Dixon sequences and the generation of water T2 parametric maps, not only for diagnosis, but especially for the follow-up of patients with IIM.

Diffusion-weighted imaging, functional imaging measures and spectroscopy, new MRI techniques, can offer additional information for the diagnosis and management of IIM.

Even if the MRI examination presents many advantages, is expensive, with a long examination time and is inaccessible to all patients.

5.2 Positron emission tomography (PET)

Positron emission tomography (PET) represents an imaging method that provides functional information about a tissue and can identify whether abnormal tissue, more or less active than normal tissues. PET offer useful information of the muscle function at cellular level. Fluorodeoxyglucose (FDG-PET) is used for diagnosis in IIM, identification of inflammation in IIM, by identifying pathological accumulation as a marker of inflammation. Currently, for inclusion body myositis are used as neurodegenerative markers.

6. Conclusions

In conclusion, there are multiple imaging modalities for the evaluation of IIM. US plays an important role in the detection and localization of muscle disease, quickly detecting fatty replacement and fibrosis. US offers also the possibility of guiding muscle biopsies.

The new US techniques increase the possibility of early diagnosis and can represent an objective tool for the evaluation and monitoring of patients with IIM.

Author details

Carolina Solomon[1,2]

1 "Iuliu Hațieganu" University of Medicine and Pharmacy, Cluj-Napoca, Romania

2 Emergency Clinical County Hospital Cluj-Napoca, Romania

*Address all correspondence to: carolinasolomon12@gmail.com

References

[1] Albayda J, Demonceau G, Carlier PG. Muscle imaging in myositis: MRI, US, and PET. Best Practice & Research. Clinical Rheumatology. 2022;**36**(2):101765. DOI: 10.1016/j.berh.2022.101765

[2] Oldroyd AGS, Callen JP, Chinoy H, et al. International Myositis Assessment and Clinical Studies Group Cancer Screening Expert Group; Aggarwal R. International guideline for idiopathic inflammatory myopathy-associated cancer screening: An international myositis assessment and clinical studies group (IMACS) initiative. Nature Reviews Rheumatology. Dec 2023;**19**(12):805-817. DOI: 10.1038/s41584-023-01045-w. Epub 2023 Nov 9. Erratum in: Nature Reviews Rheumatology. May 2024;**20**(5):315. DOI: 10.1038/s41584-024-01111-x. PMID: 37945774; PMCID: PMC10834225

[3] Zubair AS, Salam S, Dimachkie MM, Machado PM, Roy B. Imaging biomarkers in the idiopathic inflammatory myopathies. Frontiers in Neurology. 2023;**14**:1146015. DOI: 10.3389/fneur.2023.1146015

[4] Tanboon J, Needham M, Mozaffar T, Stenzel W, Nishino I. Editorial: Inflammatory muscle diseases: An update. Frontiers in Neurology. 2023;**14**:1259275. DOI: 10.3389/fneur.2023.1259275

[5] Dalakas M, Hichlfeld R. Polymyositis and dermatomyositis. Lancet. 2003;**362**:971-982

[6] Reimers CD, Finkanstaedt M. Muscle imaging in inflammatory myopathies. Current Opinion in Rheumatology. 1997;**9**:475-485

[7] Fodor D, Rodriguez-Garcia S, Cantisani V, et al. The EFSUMB guidelines and recommendations for musculoskeletal ultrasound-part I. Ultraschall in der Medizin. 2022;**43**(01):34-57

[8] Albayda J, van Alfen N. Diagnostic value of muscle ultrasound for myopathies and myositis. Current Rheumatology Reports. 2020;**22**:82. DOI: 10.1007/s11926-020-00947-y

[9] Leeuwenberg KE, Albyda J. Muscle ultrasound in inflammatory myopathies: A critical review. Journal of Rheumatic Diseases and Treatment. 2019;**5**:069. DOI: 10.23937/2469-5726/1510069

[10] Heckmatt JZ, Leeman S, Dubowitz V. Ultrasound imaging in the diagnosis of muscle disease. The Journal of Pediatrics. 1982;**101**:656-680. DOI: 10.1016/s0022-3476(82)80286-2

[11] Zaidman CM, van Alfen N. Ultrasound in the assessment of myopathic disorders. Journal of Clinical Neurophysiology. 2016;**33**:103-111. DOI: 10.1097/WNP.0000000000000245

[12] Yoshida K, Nishioka M, Muatsushima S, et al. Power Doppler ultrasonography for detection of increased vascularity in the fascia: A potential early diagnostic tool in fasciitis of dermatomyositis. Arthritis and Rheumatism. 2016;**68**:2986-2991. DOI: 10.1002/art.39798

[13] Paramalingam S, Needham M, Harris S, et al. Muscle B mode ultrasound and shear-wave elastography in idiopathic inflammatory myopathies (SWIM): Criterion validation against MRI and muscle biopsy findings in an incident patient cohort. BMC Rheumatology. 2022;**6**(1):47. DOI: 10.1186/s41927-022-00276-w

[14] Conticini E, Falsetti P, Grazzini S. Accuracy of power Doppler ultrasonography in the diagnosis and monitoring of idiopathic inflammatory myopathies. Rheumatology. 2023;**62**:766-774. DOI: 10.1093/rheumatology/keac351

[15] Weber MA, Jappe U, Essig M, et al. Contrast-enhanced ultrasound in dermatomyositis- and polymyositis. Journal of Neurology. 2006;**253**:1625-1632. DOI: 10.1007/s00415-006-0318-5

[16] Weber M-A, Krix M, Jappe U, Huttner HB, Hartmann M, Meyding-Lamadé U, et al. Pathologic skeletal muscle perfusion in patients with myositis: Detection with quantitative contrast enhanced US—Initial results. Radiology. 2006;**238**:640-649. DOI: 10.1148/radiol.2382041822

[17] Bamber J, Cosgrove D, Dietrich CF, et al. EFSUMB guidelines and recommendations on the clinical use of ultrasound elastography. Part 1: Basic principles and technology. Ultraschall in der Medizin. 2013;**34**(2):169-184. DOI: 10.1055/s-0033-1335205

[18] Botar-Jid C, Damian L, Dudea SM, Vasilescu D, Rednic S, Badea R. The contribution of ultrasonography and sonoelastography in assessment of myositis. Medical Ultrasonography. 2010;**12**:120-126

[19] Song Y, Lee S, Yoo DH, Jang K-S, Bae J. Strain sonoelastography of inflammatory myopathies: Comparison with clinical examination, magnetic resonance imaging and pathologic findings. The British Journal of Radiology. 2016;**89**:20160283. DOI: 10.1259/bjr.20160283

[20] Săftoiu A, Gilja OH, Sidhu PS, et al. The EFSUMB guidelines and recommendations for the clinical practice of elastography in non-hepatic applications: Update 2018. Ultraschall in der Medizin. 2019;**40**:425-453. DOI: 10.1055/a-0838-9937

[21] Alfuraih AM, O'Connor P, Tan AL, Hensor EMA, Ladas A, Emery P, et al. Muscle shear wave elastography in idiopathic inflammatory myopathies: A case-control study with MRI correlation. Skeletal Radiology. 2019;**48**:1209-1219. DOI: 10.1007/s00256-019-03175-3

[22] Li M, Guo R, Tang X, Huang S, Qiu L. Quantitative assessment of muscle properties in polymyositis and dermatomyositis using high-frequency ultrasound and shear wave elastography. Quantitative Imaging in Medicine and Surgery. 2023;**13**:428-440. DOI: 10.21037/qims-22-423

Chapter 6

Perspective Chapter: Musculoskeletal Ultrasound in Inflammatory Joint Diseases

Razvan Adrian Ionescu and Florentin Ananu Vreju

Abstract

Musculoskeletal ultrasound is a very important and useful tool in daily activity as a rheumatologist. It is also called "the stethoscope of rheumatologists." It enables the clinician to "see" into and around the joint, as ultrasound can penetrate any tissue except for bone. Even though ultrasound cannot penetrate bone, they are completely reflected by bony surfaces, which allows for the appreciation of bone integrity and the visualization of erosions. Another important aspect of using ultrasound for the evaluation of inflammatory joint diseases is the fact that it can depict inflammation within the musculoskeletal system (by depicting new vessel formation, using the Doppler effect), thus being able to contribute to the early and, even, very early diagnosis of inflammatory joint diseases and, conversely, to the early initiation of treatment that enables the prevention of irreversible disability.

Keywords: inflammation, joint, ultrasound, Doppler effect, B mode

1. Introduction

Ultrasonography (US) is a very important tool to be used in medicine. In rheumatology, its use is embedded in routine daily clinical practice and is called "the stethoscope of the rheumatologist."

There are some situations in which the "standard" approach to joint disease (i.e., anamnesis, clinical examination, lab tests, and radiographic examination) does not allow making the distinction between inflammatory and degenerative joint diseases, let alone the exact diagnosis of the diseases itself [1]. In such instances, there is a need for additional investigations to make the diagnosis. That is when the US was very helpful.

There are many advantages to using the US in rheumatology, especially inflammatory joint diseases. It is easy to use, it may be used on the bedside, it can be repeated, and it is sensitive to change. Musculoskeletal ultrasound (MSK-US) is the only rheumatological imaging modality that offers a dynamic examination while being a real-time examination, acquiring information as it happens. It is safe, fast, and non-invasive, while allowing for diagnostic procedures (e.g., arthrocentesis and biopsy) and treatment procedures (e.g., injection of different substances into the targeted area). But probably the most important advantage of MSK-US over any other imaging modality is its ability to diagnose the presence of inflammation, via using the Doppler

Multiple advantages of using MSK-US	
Reproducible	Very good acceptance
Good cost/effectiveness ratio	Easy doable
Improves sensitivity of clinical exam	Early detection of pathology
Real-time images	Very good acceptance
No radiation	Improved effectiveness of interventions

Table 1.
Advantages of MSK-US (modified from [2]).

module, as soon as the pathogenic process begins. Last, but not least, MSK-US allows simultaneous examination of multiple anatomical structures and increases the sensitivity of the clinical examination (**Table 1**) [2].

MSK-US is validated as a diagnostic tool for rheumatoid arthritis, crystal-induced arthritis, and psoriatic arthritis. It has also been validated for use as a follow-up tool in rheumatoid arthritis and psoriatic arthritis. Very important, because of its sensitivity to change, MSK-US is useful in evaluating response to treatment as well, in rheumatoid arthritis [3, 4]. When evaluating the metacarpophalangeal (MCP) joint for erosions, the intraobserver kappa statistic quotient is 0.75, while the interobserver kappa statistic quotient (which interprets agreement among different observers) is 0.76 [5]. Those quotients imply a good reliability of the observations and are comparable to those of radiologists scoring lesions on mammograms [5]. These reliabilities are dependent on multiple factors, one being the joint that is examined. Therefore, the kappa statistical quotient is 0.76 for the shoulder but 0.28 for the ankle/toes [6]. Another factor is the lesion that is evaluated: the overall agreement for tendon lesions and joint effusions is 91%. It is 83.5% for bursitis, 84% for tenosynovitis, and 87% for erosions [7]. In detecting knee synovitis, MSK-US is more sensitive than clinical examination [8].

There are some downsides to the use of MSK-US, too. The most important one is that it is operator-dependent. As shown above, sometimes, the inter-operator reliability is not that good. As such, there is a need for long, thorough, specialized, and continuous, time-consuming training to achieve expert levels, as it is a very dynamic field. Apart from the specialized operator, expert use of MSK-US involves the use of high-end machines, which are still quite expensive in some parts of the world. Due to the physical properties of ultrasound, they cannot penetrate bone. Consequently, MSK-US cannot be used to describe intra-osseous lesions, only cortical ones. Moreover, some anatomical regions are very difficult to explore on ultrasound [2].

The importance of MSK-US use in the context of inflammatory joint diseases is emphasized by its inclusion in EULAR's (European Alliance of Associations for Rheumatology) recommendations for the use of imaging in some of the inflammatory diseases management [9, 10].

2. Performing ultrasound examination

2.1 General principles

The most important thing about inflammatory joint diseases is to make the correct diagnosis and treatment as early as possible to avoid irreversible structural damage to the joints. US can produce high-resolution images, distinguishing between different tissues and being able to assess bursae, tendons, ligaments, articular capsules, synovial proliferation, cartilage, and bone surface. Additionally, and of paramount importance, is the ability to assess inflammatory angiogenesis that characterizes inflammatory joint diseases.

EULAR's standardized procedures for ultrasound imaging in rheumatology [11] provide the general frame for a standardized MSK-US examination. Additionally, OMERACT (Outcome Measures in Rheumatology, former Outcome Measures in Rheumatoid Arthritis Clinical Trials) provides definitions for pathologic US findings [12].

When performing MSK-US, it is recommended we use linear transducers with a frequency ranging between 6 and 14 MHz for deep and intermediate structures and above 15 MHz for superficial ones [10]. There are two main modes to be used when performing MSK-US: B-mode, also termed gray scale (GS) mode, can provide anatomical information of the targeted region, and the Doppler mode (color Doppler or power Doppler) that allows for assessment of inflammatory angiogenesis [13]. When using Doppler mode, as little compression as possible is mandatory to avoid compression of very small vessels newly formed. Because blood flow in these vessels is very slow, the pulse repetition frequency should be less than 1 kHz.

Scanning joints should be performed with the probe oriented parallel or perpendicular to the surface of the bone (bony acoustic landmark) so that the cortical bone appears hyperechoic, bright, and sharp [11]. To avoid anisotropy, the probe should be tilted, angulated, and continually adjusted to maintain the ultrasound beam as perpendicular to the structure (usually a tendon) as possible, especially when the structure changes direction (as happens at the insertion site of tendons).

The probe can be used for compressing the region of interest, distinguishing between a liquid (compressible, that is displaceable) and a solid structure (non-compressible, that is non-displaceable) [11].

When performing MSK-US, a fair amount of gel should be used, especially when scanning superficial structures (e.g., extensor tendons of the hand). The orientation of the transducer is of paramount importance. If the structure to examine has a long axis in the craniocaudal orientation, then its most proximal part is placed on the left side of the screen. When in short axis view, the targeted region should be oriented on the screen as if the sonographist is looking at the patient [11].

MSK-US is a dynamic technique in that it can assess the region of interest in movement (passive or active) but also in that the probe should be translated, rotated, angulated, and tilted to allow the best assessment of the targeted region [11].

2.2 Structure examination and normal appearance

2.2.1 Tendons

The US examination of tendons shall be performed using linear probes with a frequency higher than 10 MHz. Because tendons are prone to anisotropy, care should be taken to maintain a perpendicular position of the probe onto the region of interest. This is particularly true for the attachment of the tendon to the bone (enthesis), where some tendons slightly change their orientation and any change of course of the tendon. Like any other structure examined in MSK-US, tendons should be examined in both longitudinal and transverse planes. In the transverse plane, one should be

Structure	US appearance
Tendon	Hyperechoic (to the subcutaneous surrounding tissue) fibrillar structure; L-parallel hyperechoic lines T-hyper/hypoechoic dots ("salt and pepper") No Doppler signal

Table 2.
US appearance of tendons. L, longitudinal view; T, transverse view (modified from [14, 15]).

aware of the small transonic image on the sides of the tendon, which is an artifact (tangential shadow) due to the curved shape of tendons in the transverse view. For tendons with synovial sheath, little probe pressure should be applied to avoid displacement (and missing) of small amounts of fluid in the sheath.

The normal appearance of a transverse scan of a tendon is that of a round/oval-shaped structure, resembling "salt and pepper" (hyper and hypoechoic) due to the fibrillar normal structure of a tendon. In longitudinal scans, they appear like fibrillar linear hyperechoic structures with a parallel disposition (**Table 2**).

Tendons must be examined on a gray scale (B-mode) and in Doppler mode to check for abnormal vascularization. Normal tendons do not have visible vessels. The examiner should pay attention to the Doppler settings for superficial or intermediate/profound tendons.

2.2.2 Enthesis

Enthesis is the complex region where a tendon, ligament, joint capsule, fascia, or muscle attaches to the bone [2]. Enthesis of interest in MSK-US are the fibrocartilaginous ones as they represent the target organ in spondylarthritis where the pathogenic process originates. Fibrocartilaginous entheses are a histologically complex structure of attachment to bone, so complex that the term "entheseal body" was coined at the beginning of the century [16, 17]. By the ultrasonographic definition, enthesis is the region where tendon, ligament, and joint capsule insert over the bone with regular edges and the same appearance and width as the rest of the tendon/ligament/capsule, having a fibrillar linear homogenous echogenicity [18]. The probe used for assessing enthesis is one with high frequency (>10 MHz). The normal US aspect of an enthesis in longitudinal view was aforementioned. In the transverse view, it is similar to the tendon/ligament/capsule it inserts. Nevertheless, when assessing an enthesis using US, one must assess all the components of the "entheseal body": the tendon, the bone underneath, the bursa (that frequently exists to lower friction between the tendon and the bone), and periarticular tissue [19]. For example, in the case of tendons, the US examination of the enthesis must consider the curvature enthesis usually taken when inserted into the bone. This can translate into malalignment of the transducer with the fibers of the enthesis, thus producing anisotropy. Therefore, whenever examining an enthesis, the probe must be slightly and continuously adjusted in its position over the enthesis. Doppler mode is mandatory, especially if spondyloarthritis is suspected (pay attention to the settings of the Doppler mode). Normal enthesis does not have visible vessels. The enthesis of interest in the evaluation of spondyloarthropathies is the insertion of the tricipital tendon on the olecranon, the insertion of the common extensor of the fingers tendon of the lateral humeral epicondyle, the insertion of the quadricipital tendon on the patella, the superior and inferior insertions of the patellar tendon on the patella and the tibial tuberosity, respectively, the insertion of the Achilles tendon on the calcaneus, and the insertion of the plantar fascia on the inferior aspect of the calcaneus.

2.2.3 Cartilage

As normal cartilage is mainly made of water and has no intrinsic vasculature, the US beam will pass through it without almost any reflection; its normal appearance is, consequently, an intense hypoechoic structure. There are two types of cartilage that are of interest in MSK-US: hyaline cartilage and fibrocartilage. As hyaline cartilage lies over bones, which are totally impenetrable to US (thus constituting bony acoustic landmarks), it can be easily recognized because the profound interface between two structures with highly different acoustic impedance (bone and cartilage) produces an intense echo. Because of the very same physical reasons, the superficial border of the cartilage is more difficult to recognize since the difference in acoustic impedance between the cartilage and the surrounding intraarticular space is less [20]. Depicting the fibrocartilage is even more complicated (e.g., triangular fibrocartilage complex (TFFC) of the wrist). When assessing the cartilage, the choice of the probe's frequency depends on the depth of the region of interest: the deeper the region, the lower the frequency. The most frequently assessed hyaline cartilages in rheumatic inflammatory diseases are the femoral condyles cartilage and the cartilage of the head of the metacarpal bones. For both, the best position to assess them is in maximum flexion of the knee and of the metacarpophalangeal joints, respectively, because in this position they are best exposed from within other bony structures. As usual, they are examined in longitudinal and transverse view. The US examination must describe its transparency, homogeneity, thickness, the continuity of the interfaces (cartilage/adjacent soft tissue and cartilage/bone), and the subjacent bone profile. The most frequently assessed fibrocartilage is the triangular fibrocartilage complex of the wrist and the menisci of the knees. For the TFFC examination, the hand should be pronated and slightly deviated to the radial side, thus exposing the complex. It is examined only in the longitudinal view because the transverse approach does not bring much supplementary information [21]. As the TFFC is deep, the acoustic window is represented by the tendon of the sixth compartment of the extensor tendons of the hand, the extensor carpi ulnaris tendon, viewed in the longitudinal axis as well. The TFFC is viewed as a triangular, homogenous, hypoechoic (compared to the tendon above) structure lying between the distal head of the ulna and the triquetrum. Because the menisci are between the femur and the tibia, they are not completely depictable in any position. To view the external portion, the knee must be in a neutral position (extension) or slightly flexed (around 30 degrees), with the patient lying in dorsal decubitus [20]. They normally appear triangular shaped (basis—superficial, peak—deep), hypoechoic, homogenous structures. Normally, Doppler mode examination reveals no vessels in the cartilage.

2.2.4 Bone

Due to its abundance in calcium, bones cannot be assessed by US. Nevertheless, MSK-US is very accurate in assessing bone surface [22]. The frequency of the probe depends on the depth at which the bone is localized. The normal appearance of the cortical bone is as a hyperechoic continuous line that generates posterior acoustic shadowing and, sometimes, reverberation artifacts. Bones are examined on a gray scale for the continuity and sharpness of their surface. Special attention must be given to the normal irregularities produced by the foramen nutritive, grooves for tendons or nerves, and sesamoid bones. Usually, most of these structures can be easily recognized, and the foramen nutritive is smooth and oblique to the diaphysis. Doppler mode is helpful in differentiating between nutritive vessels and inflammatory neoangiogenic vessels [23].

2.2.5 Joint capsule, synovial membrane, and joints

The joint capsule, which attaches to the bone at the end of the cartilage and is usually strengthened by ligaments, appears on MSK-US examination as a hypo/hyper-echoic curved line above the joint visible in longitudinal view in B-mode examination. Its insertions (enthesis) are better seen than the mid portion.

Under normal conditions, the synovial membrane is extremely thin, so it cannot be visualized by US. It is visible only when it becomes thicker, as in chronic inflammatory joint disease. It is then when Doppler mode is most needed.

Examining a joint with US means examining the profile of the two bones that compose the articulation, the cartilage in between, the capsule, and the synovial membrane. In 2017, EULAR standardized procedures for ultrasound imaging [11]. As per these, the best way to perform wrist joint examination, bearing in mind that we are assessing two joints (radio-carpal and inter-carpal), is placing the transducer longitudinally, on the dorsal aspect, at the level of the radio-lunate and luno-capitate joints (corresponding to the third finger). For the metacarpophalangeal joint, the transducer is placed longitudinally over the midline of the joint and for the elbow joint the transducer is placed longitudinally on the anterior aspect over the coronoid fossa. All these techniques will allow for all or most of the above-mentioned structures to be visualized. The capsule of the glenohumeral joint is merely visible over the posterior recess of the joint. At the level of the ankle, the transducer should be placed over the anterior tibiotalar joint recess, while at the knee, the capsule is visible at the lateral and medial aspect of the tibiofemoral joint [11]. For the hip joint, the transducers should have low frequency and should be large enough to visualize the joint as much as possible. One should be aware that low-frequency transducers are not very reliable for Doppler mode use [24].

2.3 Pathological US findings

To understand and practice MSK-US in inflammatory joint diseases, it is mandatory to know the pathological findings that must be searched for.

Since MSK-US is operator-dependent, it should be as standardized as possible. In this respect, OMERACT has developed standardized definitions to be used when assessing and reporting an MSK-US examination to ensure maximum uniformity of reports [11]. Additionally, in 2005, the OMERACT Ultrasound Working Group (WG) initiated research on definitions and scoring of elementary lesions and US-detected pathologies [12] that have been updated along with the combined EULAR-OMERACT scoring system [25]. The result is a series of definitions and scoring systems for some of the inflammatory joint diseases and other rheumatic inflammatory or degenerative diseases that serve as a basis for diagnosing inflammatory joint diseases using MSK-US in clinical daily practice (**Tables 3** and **4**) [25].

There are inflammatory joint diseases in which some of the elementary US lesions are useful for diagnosis and/or treatment and are not inflammatory in nature but structural. Since they are used in daily clinical practice, their OMERACT definitions follow (**Table 5**).

Type of pathology	Description of US findings
Synovitis	Presence of hypoechoic synovial hypertrophy (SH) (regardless of presence of effusion or Doppler signal)
Tenosynovitis	Abnormal anechoic and/or hypoechoic (relative to the tendon) tendon sheath widening, related to tenosynovial abnormal fluid/hypertrophy. Doppler mode should be used only if there is peritendinous synovial sheath widening on B-mode; Doppler signal can be considered if in two perpendicular planes, within the peritendinous synovial sheath, excluding normal feeding vessel
Enthesitis	Hypoechoic and/or thickened insertion of the enthesis close to the bone (<2 mm from bony cortex) with Doppler signal (if active) and possible structural lesions
Erosion	Intra- and/or extra-articular discontinuity of bone cortex visible in two perpendicular planes (step-down discontinuity in [19])

Table 3.
OMERACT definitions for US-detected pathologies (modified after [25]).

US pathology	Elementary lesion
Synovitis	SH is defined as the presence of abnormal hypoechoic synovial tissue within the capsule that is not displaceable and poorly compressible and that may exhibit Doppler signals
Enthesitis	Hypoechoic increased thickness of enthesis (i.e., tendon insertion <2 mm from bony cortex) that exhibits Doppler signal
Tenosynovitis	Tenosynovial hypertrophy is the presence, in two perpendicular planes, within the synovial sheath, of abnormal hypoechoic (relative to tendon) tissue, not displaceable and poorly compressible, that may exhibit Doppler signal

Table 4.
OMERACT definitions of inflammatory elementary lesions composing the inflammatory US pathologies (modified from [25]).

Pathology	Structural elementary lesion
Enthesitis	Erosions, calcifications, enthesophytes at the level of the enthesis
Gout double contour	Abnormal hyperechoic band over the superficial margin of the hyaline cartilage, independent of the angle of insonation, regular/irregular, continuous/intermittent, that can be distinguished from the cartilage interface sign
Gout aggregate	Heterogenous hyperechoic foci maintain their high degree of reflectivity when the gain is minimized or the insonation angle is changed, which occasionally can generate posterior acoustic shadow
Gout tophus	Circumscribed, inhomogeneous, hyperechoic and/or hypoechoic aggregation, with/without posterior shadowing, which may be surrounded by a small anechoic rim
CPPD fibrocartilage	Hyperechoic deposits of variable shape, within the cartilage, fixed or moving along with the fibrocartilage during dynamic assessment
CPPD hyaline cartilage	Hyperechoic deposits of variable size and shape, without posterior shadowing, within the cartilage, fixed or moving along with the hyaline cartilage during dynamic assessment
CPPD tendon	Hyperechoic linear structures, generally without posterior shadowing, within the tendon, fixed or moving along with the tendon during dynamic assessment
CPPD synovial fluid	Hyperechoic deposits of variable size, without posterior shadowing, within the synovial fluid, mobile with joint movement and probe compression

Table 5.
Definitions of structural elementary lesions composing the inflammatory US pathologies (modified from [25]).

Based on those definitions, as previously mentioned, there is a EULAR-OMERACT combined scoring system [25], considering together gray scale appearance and Doppler signal, for synovitis (**Tables 6** and 7), tenosynovitis (**Table 8**), and enthesitis (**Tables 9** and **10**), separately.

Gray scale (SH) appearance	Grade 0 (normal)	No SH (irrespective of effusion)
	Grade 1 (minimal)	Minimal hypoechoic SH, up to the joint line
	Grade 2 (moderate)	Moderate hypoechoic SH protruding beyond the joint line with concave surface
	Grade 3 (severe)	Severe hypoechoic SH protruding beyond the joint line with convex surface
Doppler (PD) appearance	Grade 0 (normal)	No signals
	Grade 1 (minimal)	<3 single signals OR 1 confluent +2 single OR 2 confluent
	Grade 2 (moderate)	>grade1 BUT <50% of SH area covered by signals
	Grade 3 (severe)	>50% of SH area covered by signals

Table 6.
OMERACT scoring system for synovitis. SH, synovial hypertrophy; PD, power Doppler (modified from [25]).

Grade 0: normal	No SH + no PD
Grade 1: minimal synovitis	Grade 1 SH and/or ≤ grade 1PD
Grade 2: moderate synovitis	Grade 2 SH and/or ≤ grade 2 PD or Grade 1 SH + grade 2 PD
Grade 3: severe synovitis	Grade 3 SH and/or ≤ grade 3 PD or Grade 1 or 2 SH + grade 3 PD

Table 7.
EULAR-OMERACT combined scoring system for synovitis. EULAR, European Alliance of Associations for Rheumatology; OMERACT, Outcome Measures in Rheumatology; SH, synovial hypertrophy; PD, power Doppler (modified from [25]).

Grade	**B-mode (GS)**	**Doppler mode**
Grade 0	No tenosynovial widening	No Doppler signal
Grade 1	Minimal amount of an–/hypoechoic material within the tenosynovial sheath, in two perpendicular planes, localized or displaceable	Signals in one area of the widened sheath, in two perpendicular planes, excluding normal feeding vessel
Grade 2	Moderate amount of an–/hypoechoic material within the tenosynovial sheath	Signals in >1 area of the widened sheath, in two perpendicular planes, excluding normal feeding vessel
Grade 3	Severe amount of an–/hypoechoic material within the tenosynovial sheath	Signals filling most of the widened sheath in two perpendicular planes, excluding normal feeding vessel

Table 8.
OMERACT combined scoring system for tenosynovitis. GS, gray scale (modified from [25]).

Doppler	0–3
Hypoechogenicity	0/1
Thickened enthesis	0/1
Bone erosion	0/1
Enthesophyte or calcification	0/1

Table 9.
OMERACT combined scoring system for enthesitis with semiquantitative Doppler grading—part 1 (modified from [25]).

Grade 0	0 Doppler signal
Grade 1	< 2 punctiform Doppler signals with no confluent Doppler signal
Grade 2	2–4 punctiform Doppler signal OR 1 confluent Doppler signal
Grade 3	>4 punctiform Doppler signal OR > 1 confluent Doppler signal

Table 10.
OMERACT combined scoring system for enthesitis with semiquantitative Doppler grading—part 2 (modified from [25]).

All this data is mandatory for performing high-quality MSK-US. On one hand, they guide on "speaking the same language," and on the other hand, they allow appreciation of the efficacy of management of the disease, as they allow comparisons in the same patient between different points in time.

3. Ultrasound examination in rheumatic inflammatory joint diseases

3.1 Rheumatoid arthritis (RA)

The use of MSK-US in rheumatoid arthritis is frequent because it can provide valuable information on diagnosis, differential, disease severity, and monitoring disease course on treatment [26].

As a diagnostic tool, MSK-US can be used in undifferentiated arthritis to help a positive or a differential diagnosis [27]. This is especially important in seronegative patients whose disease could thus remain undiagnosed for a long time.

The features that US can depict in RA are synovial hypertrophy, cortical bone erosions, tenosynovitis and effusion. Padovano et al. showed that effusion without synovial hypertrophy should not be considered inflammatory in nature [28]. The presence of a Doppler signal within the thickened synovium is indicative of active inflammatory disease [29]; it, as well as features of tenosynovitis, predicts the risk of imaging progression of RA [30]. MSK-US is a more sensitive imaging modality for detecting erosions than X-ray examination [31]. MSK-US is very useful in depicting erosion on the fifth MTP joint and the second and fifth MCP joints. Even though the clinical relevance of a discovered erosion is variable (depending on its dimension and location), erosion at the fifth MTP increases the probability of RA diagnosis in arthritic patients [26].

MSK-US can also be used to evaluate disease progression in RA. It has been proven that a high baseline power Doppler US signal at the MCP level is predictive of the development of radiographic erosions over the next year [32].

It is well known that some patients, despite being in clinical remission, continue to progress radiologically [26]. Studies have shown that MSK-US is a very good imaging modality in assessing residual activity in RA patients: patients in clinical remission with residual power Doppler active synovitis are at high risk of progressive joint disease [33]. Moreover, these patients are at increased risk of relapse as compared to those power Doppler negative [34].

MSK-US scanning can be quite a time-consuming approach; that is why the number of joints to scan is always a question. This number depends on the clinical presentation, but there are studies pertaining to the choice and number of joints to be scanned in RA. Naredo et al. suggest the assessment of 12 joints (bilateral wrists, metacarpophalangeal, and proximal interphalangeal II and III of hands and knees) using power Doppler US, as it provides an overall assessment of joints' inflammation [35].

US has been proven to be useful in monitoring disease activity and response to treatment. It correlates strongly with disease activity score 28 joints (DAS28) and inflammatory serum markers (C-reactive protein and erythrocyte sedimentation rate) [36], and it is also sensible to therapy-induced change, thus being able to influence treatment decisions [37].

Combining clinical examination and MSK-US improves the diagnosis of RA patients, especially when radiology assessment is not conclusive. This allows for an early diagnosis, which is the key to avoiding permanent structural joint damage. It is useful in monitoring disease and appreciating the risk of disease flare (in patients in clinical remission) as well as in guiding treatment decisions.

3.2 Spondylarthritis (SpA)

US use in SpA is merely confined to peripheral SpA since in axial SpA, the US examination of the sacroiliac joints is limited to the posterior part of the joints, thus making magnetic resonance imaging the preferred modality to assess these joints [26]. In fact, US imaging has a greater sensitivity than other imaging modalities and clinical examination to detect peripheral involvement in SpA [33].

Using MSK-US in SpA is peripheral SpA is endorsed by EULAR in its recommendations for the use of imaging modalities in the diagnosis and management of SpA [9]. Published in 2015, these recommendations state that, in peripheral SpA, US can and should be used in diagnosing, monitoring disease activity, and evaluating structural damage.

The features associated with peripheral SpA that are assessable using MSK-US are arthritis, enthesitis, tenosynovitis, and dactylitis.

The US appearance of SpA arthritis is no different than RA's (**Table 3**). Using Doppler mode can confirm the intense inflammatory vascularization of the hypertrophied synovium, confirming active disease. This is also true for the US aspect of SpA tenosynovitis, with the additional comment that, in SpA, tenosynovitis is more frequent than in RA.

Enthesitis is considered the hallmark of SpA, since the pathogenic process of the disease appears to start at the level of the enthesis [38]. The definition, the US aspect, and the combined scoring system of enthesis have been described previously (see **Tables 3**, **9**, and **10**). Assessing entheseal inflammation has been long shown to have a very good diagnostic value in peripheral SpA [39]. It is noteworthy that, to define it as inflammatory, the lesion should be confined to less than 2 mm from the bone cortex [40], and that structural bone lesions (enthesophytes and erosions) are seen in later stages, while the earlier lesions are those related to the tendon [41]. It should be emphasized that some structures are considered as "functional enthesis," even though they do not respect the "anatomical" definition in that we cannot find a fibrocartilaginous structure (e.g., the tendon areas around the pulleys) [10]. It is also noteworthy that peritendon inflammation of the extensor digitorum tendon (PTI pattern) and central slip tendon enthesitis at the level of the proximal interphalangeal joint are features specific for psoriatic arthritis (as a form of peripheral SpA) [38]. There are multiple US scores that can be used in assessing enthesitis as per the selection of sites to be assessed: MASEI (Madrid Sonography Enthesitis Index) [42], OMERACT US [40], and GUESS (Glasgow Ultrasound Enthesitis Score) [43].

Dactylitis is a very complex US inflammatory lesion, as it involves many structures; it consists of soft tissue edema, enthesitis of the superficial flexor of the finger tendon, peritendinous inflammation (PTI pattern of the extensor tendon), tenosynovitis of the flexor tendon and arthritis, all located in the same finger or toe, making it a pandigital involvement [44]. There is also a scoring system for dactylitis [45].

3.3 Crystal-induced arthritis

The use of MSK-US in crystal-related joint diseases is supported by its high sensitivity and specificity [46]. Both types of crystal deposits generate reflectivity, thus forming the US image.

Monosodium urate crystal deposits on the surface of the articular cartilage [47]. Because of that, they generate a hyperechoic band on that surface parallel to the contour of the head of the bone and move along with the bone, confirming it belongs to the cartilage. This is the "double contour" sign. The band is visible, irrespective of the angle of insonation (see also **Table 5**). Also, it is visible along the contours of the cartilage. The double contour sign is visible in most long-standing gouty patients; it is also reversible with treatment. Another US appearance of monosodium urate is the so-called "snowstorm appearance," which is the presence of numerous hyperechoic spots within an area of echogenicity. This is usually depicted when monosodium urate crystals are present within a synovial effusion. Another possible US finding that may be depicted in chronic gout is gout tophus, which appears as a heterogeneous mass containing hyperechoic foci. Sometimes, they must be differentiated from rheumatoid nodules. Tophi may be found inside tendons, joints, and bursae [46, 48].

In diagnosing calcium pyrophosphate deposits, MSK-US is an accurate tool with a high likelihood ratio and better sensitivity than X-rays [49, 50]. Calcium pyrophosphate crystals deposit inside the hyaline cartilage of the joints (intraarticular), in contrast to monosodium urate crystals (which, as previously noted, are located on the surface of the cartilage). Their appearance is classical at the wrist level, where they can be depicted inside the triangular cartilage and at the knee level (inside the cartilage and the menisci). They can also be viewed inside the hip and the acromioclavicular joints [49, 50].

As with all other MSK-US examinations, the evaluation of deposits must be done both in B-mode and in Doppler mode to assess the presence of inflammation associated with the deposit itself. Also, the evaluation must be performed in 2 perpendicular planes, especially when it is referring to the consequences of the presence of crystal deposits, that is, erosion; as well as with other MSK pathologies potentially producing erosions, lesions produce by crystal deposits must be confirmed in both perpendicular planes.

4. Discussion

Having such a versatile imaging tool in rheumatology as MSK-US represents a very good advantage for clinician rheumatologists. Knowing how to use it is mandatory nowadays. As it is validated for diagnosis in its early stages of inflammatory joint diseases, as well as for follow-up and evaluation of treatment efficacy, MSK-US has to be and is incorporated into daily routine practice.

On the other hand, one must not over-emphasize the role of MSK-US in inflammatory joint diseases since there are some downsides to it. Probably the most important problem with this imaging technique is the need for good training, especially long training. Moreover, no matter the quality of the training, any US image is clearly operator-dependent. This is illustrated by the differences in agreement that arise when several experimented experts examine the same joint in the same patient. It is noteworthy, though, that these "disagreements" also depend on other factors, such as the joint examined.

One of the important advantages of MSK-US is the possibility of exploring joints dynamically. The possibility of examining joint movement while it happens allows for viewing details that can provide diagnostic clues. Moreover, MSK-US is the only at-hand imaging method that permits interventional maneuvers, whether diagnostic or therapeutic.

Of course, MSK-US cannot examine every joint in the body, even in the context of inflammatory joint diseases. That is because of the anatomical situation of some joints, as is the case of the sacroiliac joint, whose inflammatory state in the context of spondyloarthritis is US accessible with great difficulty, even though they are superficially located under the skin. This brings us to the fact that MSK-US, like any other investigation, should be carefully chosen, in the appropriate context, of an inflammatory joint disease. The previous example, pertaining to the sacroiliac joints, is conclusive: in case of suspicion of involvement of those joints, as part of a axial spondyloarthritis, one should prefer magnetic resonance imaging over any other imaging technique, including MSK-US, for diagnostic purposes. On the other hand, if there is a suspicion of enthesitis also in the context of spondyloarthritis, one should choose US over any other imaging method for confirming the peripheral involvement.

5. Conclusions

Ultrasound is a very useful tool for the practicing rheumatologist. It is at hand, rapid, non-invasive, cost-effective, repeatable and allows for dynamic evaluation. It can be used for diagnosis, monitoring and treatment decision making. Its use has opened a new window to the diagnosis and also to a more profound understanding of pathogenetic mechanisms of inflammatory joint diseases, thus allowing for an early diagnosis, followed by an early treatment and, hence, avoidance of irreversible joint damage and disability. It has become an extension of the clinical examination ("rheumatologist's extended finger" [51]) enabling the treating physician with a more profound view of processes to be influenced by the various and effective treatments of inflammatory joint diseases. Thus, performing musculoskeletal ultrasound is mandatory for any clinician working in the field of rheumatology.

Conflict of interest

The authors declare no conflict of interest.

Author details

Razvan Adrian Ionescu[1*] and Florentin Ananu Vreju[2]

1 "Carol Davila" University of Medicine and Pharmacy, Colentina Clinical Hospital, Bucharest, Romania

2 Craiova University of Medicine and Pharmacy, Craiova County Emergency Hospital, Craiova, Romania

*Address all correspondence to: tane67@gmail.com

References

[1] Kaeley GS, Bakewell C, Deodhar A. The importance of ultrasound in identifying and differentiating patients with early inflammatory arthritis: A narrative review. Arthritis Research & Therapy. 2020;**22**(1):1-10. DOI: 10.1186/s13075-019-2050-4

[2] Mata Arnaiz MC, de Miguel ME. Utilidad de la ecografia en la evaluacion de las entesis perifericas en las espondiloarthritis. Reumatologia Clinica. 2014;**10**:113-119

[3] Haavardsholm EA, AgaAB OIC, et al. Ultrasound in management of rheumatoid arthritis: ARCTIC randomized controlled strategy trial. BMJ. 2016;**354**:i4205

[4] Dale J, Stirling A, Zhang R, et al. Targeting ultrasound remission in early rheumatoid arthritis: The results of the TaSER study, a randomized clinical trial. Annals of the Rheumatic Diseases. 2016;**75**:1043

[5] Antonio AL, Crespi CM. Predictors of interobserver agreement in breast imaging using the brest imaging reporting and data system. Breast Cancer Research and Treatment. 2010;**120**:539

[6] Scheel AK, Schmidt WA, Hermann KG, et al. Interobserver reliability of rheumatologists performing musculoskeletal ultrasonography: Results from a EULAR "train the trainers" course. Annals of the Rheumatic Diseases. 2005;**64**:1043

[7] Naredo E, Moller I, Moragues C, et al. Interobserver reliability in musculoskeletal ultrasonography: Results from a "Teach the Teachers" rheumatologist course. Annals of the Rheumatic Diseases. 2006;**65**:14

[8] Karim Z, Wakefield RJ, Qiunn M, et al. Validation and reproductibility of ultrasonography in the detection of synovitis in the knee: A comparison with arthroscopy and clinical examination. Arthritis and Rheumatism. 2004;**50**:387

[9] Mandl P, Navarro-Compan V, Terslev L, et al. EULAR recommendations for the use of imaging in the diagnosis and management of spondylarthritis in clinical practice. Annals of the Rheumatic Diseases. 2015;**74**(7):1327-1339

[10] Colebatch AN, Edwards CJ, Østergaard M, et al. EULAR recommendations for the use of imaging of the joints in the clinical management of rheumatoid arthritis. Annals of the Rheumatic Diseases. 2013;**72**(6):804-814. DOI: 10/1136/annrheumdis-2012-203158

[11] Moller I, Janta I, Backhaus M, et al. The 2017 EULAR standardized procedures for ultrasound imaging in rheumatology. Annals of the Rheumatic Diseases. 2017;**0**:1-6

[12] Wakefield RJ, Balint PV, Szkudlarek M, et al. Musculoskeletal ultrasound including definitions for ultrasonographic pathology. The Journal of Rheumatology. 2005;**32**(12):2485-2487

[13] Vreju F, Ciurea M, Rosu A, et al. Power Doppler sonography, a non-invasive method of assessment of the synovial inflammation in patients with early rheumatoid arthritis. Romanian Journal of Morphology and Embryology. 2011;**52**(2):637-643

[14] Naredo E, d'Agostino MA, Wakwfield RJ, et al. OMERACT ultrasound task force. Reliability of a consensus based ultrasound score for

tenosynovitis in rheumatoid arthritis. Annals of the Rheumatic Diseases. 2013;**72**:1328-1334

[15] Micu M. Tendoanele. In: Fodor D, editor. Ecografie Musculoscheletala vol 1: Semiologia normala si patologica a structurilor musculoscheletale. Bucuresti: Librex Publishing; 2017. pp. 37-48

[16] Benjamin M, McGonagle D. The anatomical basis for disease localization in seronegative spondyloarthropathy at enthesis and related sites. Journal of Anatomy. 2001;**199**:503-526

[17] Benjamin M, Moriggl B, Brenner E, et al. The enthesis organ concept. Why enthesopathies may not present as a focal insertional disorder. Arthritis and Rheumatism. 2004;**50**:3306-3313

[18] Terslev L, Naredo E, Iagnocco A, et al. Defining enthesitis in spondyloarthritis by ultrasound: Results of a Delphi process and of a reliability reading exercise. Athritis Care Research. 2014;**66**:741-748

[19] Vlad V. Enteza. In: Fodor D, editor. Ecografie Musculoscheletala vol 1: Semiologia normala si patologica a structurilor musculoscheletale. Bucuresti: Librex Publishing; 2017. pp. 57-64

[20] Felea I, Tamas M-M. Cartilajul. In: Fodor D, editor. Ecografie Musculoscheletala vol 1: Semiologia normala si patologica a structurilor musculoscheletale. Bucuresti: Librex Publishing; 2017. pp. 71-80

[21] Taljanovic MS, Goldberg MR, Sheppard E, et al. US of intrinsic and extrinsic wrist ligaments and triangular fibrocartilage complex—Normal anatomy and imaging technique. Radiographics. 2011;**e44**:1-26

[22] Zamorani MP, Valle M. Bone and joint. In: Bianchi S, Martinoli C, editors. Ultrasound of the Musculoskeletal System. Springer Science & Business Media. Germany: Springer-Verlag Berlin Heidelberg; 2007. pp. 137-185

[23] Vreju FA. Osul, periostul. In: Fodor D, editor. Ecografie Musculoscheletala vol 1: Semiologia normala si patologica a structurilor musculoscheletale. Bucuresti: Librex Publishing; 2017. pp. 103-110

[24] Vlad V, Berghea F. Articulatiile sinoviale. In: Fodor D, editor. Ecografie Musculoscheletala vol 1: Semiologia normala si patologica a structurilor musculoscheletale. Bucuresti: Librex Publishing; 2017. pp. 91-101

[25] Bruyn GA, Iagnocco A, Naredo E, et al. OMERACT definitions for ultrasonographic pathologies and elementary lesions of rheumatic disorders 15 years on. The Journal of Rheumatology. 2019;**46**(10):1388-1393. DOI: 10.3899/jrheum.181095

[26] D'Agostino MA, Padovano I, Iagnocco A. Imaging. In: Bijlsma JWJ, Hahula E, editors. EULAR Textbook on Rheumatic Diseases. 3rd ed. London: BML Publishing Group Ltd; 2018. pp. 122-157

[27] Gutierrez M, Bertolazzi C, Castillo E, et al. Ultrasound as a useful tool on the diagnosis of rheumatoid arthritis in patients with undifferentiated arthritis. Journal of Clinical Rheumatology. 2019;**25**(5):203-208. DOI: 10.1097/RHU.0000000000001034

[28] Padovano I, Constantino F, Breban M, et al. Prevalence of ultrasound synovial inflammation in heathy subjects. Annals of the Rheumatic Diseases. 2016;**75**(10):181901823. DOI: 10.1136/annrheum dis-2015-208103

[29] Iagnocco A, Ceccarelli F, Perricone C, et al. The role of ultrasound in rheumatology. Seminars in Ultrasound, CT, and MR. 2011;**32**(2):66-73. DOI: 10.1053/j.sult.2010.11.004

[30] Lillegraven S, Bøyesen P, Hammer HB, et al. Tenosynovitis of the extensor carpi ulnaris tendon predicts erosive progression in early rheumatoid arthritis. Annals of the Rheumatic Diseases. 2011;**70**(11):2049-2050. DOI: 11.1136/ard.2011.151316

[31] Grassi W, Filippucci E. Ultrasonography and the rheumatologist. Current Opinion in Rheumatology. 2007;**19**(1):55-60. DOI: 10.1097/BOR.0b013e3280119648

[32] Taylor PC, Steure A, Gruber J, et al. Comparison of ultrasonographic assessment of synovitis and joint vascularity with radiographic evaluation in a randomized, placebo-controlled study of infliximab therapy in early rheumatoid arthritis. Arthritis and Rheumatism. 2004;**50**(4):1107-1116. DOI: 10.1002/art.20123

[33] Brown AK, Quinn MA, Karim Z, et al. Presence of significant synovitis in rheumatoid arthritis patients with disease-modifying antirheumatic drug-induced clinical remission: Evidence from an imaging study may explain structural progression. Arthritis and Rheumatism. 2006;**54**(12):3761-3773. DOI: 10.1002/art.22190

[34] Foltz V, Gandjbakhch F, Etchepare F, et al. Power Doppler ultrasound, but not low-field magnetic resonance imaging predicts relapse and radiographic disease progression in rheumatoid arthritis patients with low levels of disease activity. Arthritis and Rheumatism. 2012;**64**(1):67-76

[35] Naredo E, D'Agostino MA, Wakefield RJ, et al. Reliability of a consensus-based ultrasound score for tenosynovitis in rheumatoid arthritis. Annals of the Rheumatic Diseases. 2013;**71**(8):1328-1334. DOI: 10.1136/annrheumdis-2012-202092

[36] Damjaniv N, Radunovic G, Prodanovic S, et al. Construct validity and reliability of ultrasound disease activity score in assessing joint inflammation in RA: Comparison with DAS28. Rheumatology. 2012;**51**(1):120-128. DOI: 10.1093/rheumatology/ker255

[37] Sifeuntes-Cantu C, Contrearas-Yanez I, Saldarriaga L, et al. The added value of musculoskeletal ultrasound to clinical evaluation in the treatment decision of rheumatoid arthritis outpatients: Physician experience matters. BMC Muculoskeletal Disorder. 2017;**18**(1):1-10. DOI: 10.1186/s12891-017-1747-2

[38] Zabotti A, Salvin S, Quartuccio L, et al. Differentiation between early rheumatoid and early psoriatic arthritis by the ultrasonographic study of the synovio-entheseal complex of the small joints of the hands. Clinical and Experimental Rheumatology. 2016;**34**(3):459-465

[39] D'Agostina MA, Said-Nahal R, Hacquard-Bouder C, et al. Assessment of peripheral enthesitis in the spondylarthropathies by ultrasonography combined with power Doppler: A cross sectional study. Arthritis and Rheumatism. 2003;**48**(2):523-533. DOI: 10.1002/art.10812

[40] Balint PV, Terslev L, Aegerter P, et al. OMERACT ultrasound task force members. Reliability of a consensus-based ultrasound definition and scoring for enthesitis in spondyloarthritis and psoriatic arthritis. Annals of the Rheumatic Diseases.

2018;**77**(2):1730-1735. DOI: 10.1136/annrheumdis-2018-213609

[41] Gutierrez M, Filippucci E, De Angelis R, et al. A sonographic spectrum of psoriatic arthritis: "The five targets". Clinical Rheumatology. 2010;**29**(2):133-142. DOI: 10.1007/s10067-009-1292-y

[42] Macia-Villa C, Falcao S, Medina J, et al. A descriptive and reliability analysis of elemental lesions and power Doppler subtypes. Scandinavian Journal of Rheumatology. 2019;**48**(6):454-459

[43] Balint PV, Kane D, Wilson H, et al. Ultrasonography of entheseal insertions in the lower limb in spondylarthropathy. Annals of the Rheumatic Diseases. 2002;**61**(10):905-910. DOI: 10.1136/ard.61.10.905

[44] Kaeley GS. Enthesitis in psoriatic arthritis (part 2): Imaging. Rheumatology. 2020;**59**(1):i5-i20

[45] Zabotti A, Sakellariou G, Tinazzi I, et al. Novel and reliable DACTylitis global Sonographic (DACTOS) score in psoriatic arthritis. Annals of the Rheumatic Diseases. 2020;**79**:1037-1043

[46] Christiansen RN, Ostergaard M, Terslev L. Ulttasonography in gout: Utility in diagnosing and monitoring. Clinical and Experimental Rheumatology. 2018;**36**:S61-S67

[47] Grassi W, Meenagh G, Pascual E, et al. "Crystal-clear" sonographic assessment of gout and calcium deposition disease. Seminars in Arthritis and Rheumatism. 2006;**36**(3):197-202. DOI: 10.1016/j.semarthrit.2006.08.001

[48] Neogi T, Jansen TLTA, Dalbeth N, et al. 2015 gout classification criteria: An America College of Rheumatology/European League Against Rheumatism collaborative initiative. Annals of the Rheumatic Diseases. 2015;**74**(10):1789-1798

[49] Zhang W, Doherty M, Bardin T, et al. European league against rheumatism recommendations for calcium pyrophosphate deposition. Part I: Terminology and diagnosis. Annals of the Rheumatic Diseases. 2011;**70**(4):563-570. DOI: 10.1136/ard.2010.139105

[50] Filipou G, Scanu A, Adinolfi A, et al. Criterion validity of ultrasound in the identification of calcium pyrophosphate crystal deposits at the knee: An OMERACT ultrasound study. Annals of the Rheumatic Diseases. 2020;**80**(2):261-267. DOI: 10.1136/annrheumdis-2020-217998

[51] Manger B, Kalden J. Joint and connective tissue ultrasonography—A bedside rheumatological procedure? Arthritis and Rheumatism. 1995;**38**:736-742

Section 3

Breast

Chapter 7

Perspective Chapter: Breast Imaging in Clinical Practice – Point of Care Ultrasound in Breast Symptomatic Patients

Anca I. Ciurea

Abstract

Breast ultrasound is the main imaging method used for the assessment of patients with positive screening mammography or, in symptomatic patients, to evaluate the clinical changes or anomalies depicted on the mammogram. It is usually performed by radiologists; however, because it is a fast and cheap imaging method, theoretically with no contraindications, it can also be performed by those who first examine the symptomatic patients, allowing a fast diagnosis and treatment (point of care ultrasound). Ultrasound is an ideal imaging method for a fast assessment of breast pathology. In most of the cases, women with symptoms will present for clinical evaluation to the general practitioners, gynecologists, or surgeons. In certain situations (e.g., trauma, inflammation, palpable masses), it can be used to initiate a specific treatment or to further recommend a correct investigation. In the present chapter, the ultrasound appearance of the most frequent breast pathologies is presented, and the imaging features that allow the differentiation of benign from malignant lesions are discussed.

Keywords: point of care ultrasound, breast ultrasound, breast nodules, mastitis, breast abscess, breast trauma, galactocele, breast cancer, pregnancy, lactation, male breast

1. Introduction

Breast ultrasound is the main imaging method used for the assessment of patients with positive screening mammography, to further evaluate any anomaly detected, including calcifications. As a screening method it is used only in conjunction with mammography, in patients with dense breasts, in which the sensitivity of mammography is lower due to the masking effect of the overlying dense breast tissue.

Ultrasound is also recommended as a first-step examination for the evaluation of palpable masses in young patients (under 35 years) or in those for whom mammography cannot be performed due to intense pain or marked breast edema (patients with breast inflammation or after trauma). Other indications for breast ultrasound are the evaluation of the axilla and the diagnosis of tumoral lymph nodes (with the highest specificity of all breast imaging methods), evaluation of breast implants, nipple discharge, chest wall recurrence, and guidance for interventional procedures (percutaneous biopsy, insertion of tissue marking clip or wire localization). It is also preferred for the examination of newborns or young male patients presenting with symptoms of gynecomastia, due to its lack of irradiation.

It is a fast and cheap imaging method, theoretically with no contraindications, and because it is non-iradiating, it can be repeated whenever necessary.

In screening and evaluation settings, ultrasound is performed by radiologists, but in most of the cases, women with symptoms will present for clinical evaluation to the general practitioners, gynecologists, or surgeons.

Because the use of the method is more and more clinically oriented for various pathologies involving different organs and symptoms and clinicians become familiar with the technique and its applications, in breast pathology, it can be used to initiate a specific treatment or to further recommend a correct investigation. In certain situations (e.g., trauma, inflammation, palpable masses), it can be performed by those who examine first the symptomatic patients, ultrasound being an ideal imaging method for a fast assessment of breast pathology.

Clinicians performing breast ultrasounds should be aware of the limitations of the method. Ultrasound is inefficient in the big breast because it is performed with high-frequency transducers (7–15 MHz), therefore will not properly evaluate the deep portions of the breast (close to the chest wall). It is also inefficient in the adipose breast, in which small, isoechoic lesions can be overlooked and missed.

However, targeted ultrasound for the clinical anomaly has higher sensitivity compared with screening ultrasound. Therefore, in symptomatic patients, it can be used with high confidence.

2. Breast lumps

According to the American College of Radiology, Breast Imaging Reporting and Data System (ACR-BIRADS) lexicon, when a breast lump is evaluated with ultrasound, just like with any other method, shape and margins are the most important features in the differential diagnosis. A regular shape and circumscribed margins suggest benign nature while an irregular shape and non-circumscribed contour suggest malignancy.

Lesions with regular shape are oval or round (**Figure 1a** and **b**), and any lesion with a shape that cannot be assessed as oval or round should be described as having an irregular shape (**Figure 1c** and **d**). Lesions with two or three discrete lobulations can also be considered to have a regular shape [1].

Well-defined margins, sometimes with a thin, echogenic wall, are encountered in circumscribed, benign lesions. Any other margins, spiculated, ill-defined, microlobulated, or angulated suggest a malignant nature (**Figure 2**) [1].

When analyzing the shape and margins of a mass, one should keep in mind that the more aggressive a cancer is, the more likely it is to mimic a benign lesion due to the lack of desmoplastic reaction [2–4]. The age of the patient, the recent appearance of the palpable lump (in postmenopausal women), and the associated clinical and ultrasound elements may aid in the differential diagnosis.

In addition to shape and margins, at ultrasound, method specific features are described.

Orientation represents the direction of the longest diameter of the lesion compared to the skin: parallel to the skin suggests that the lesion is benign, tending to develop between the anatomical structures, while a perpendicular direction (lesions "taller than wide") is characteristic for malignant lesions, which invade the normal structures of the breast (**Figure 3**). However, orientation alone has a lower positive

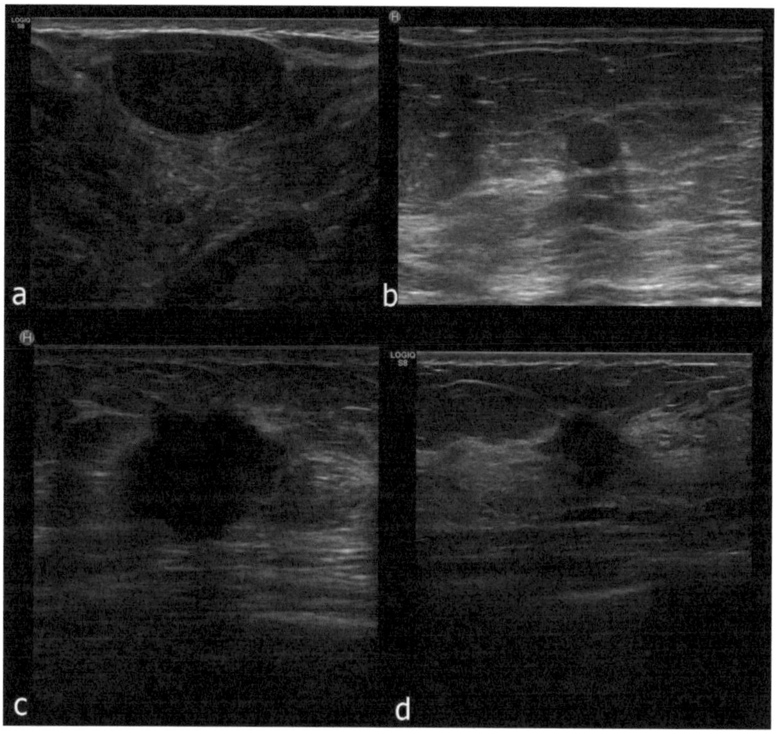

Figure 1.
Lesions with regular shape, oval (a) or round (b), and lesions with irregular shape (c and d).

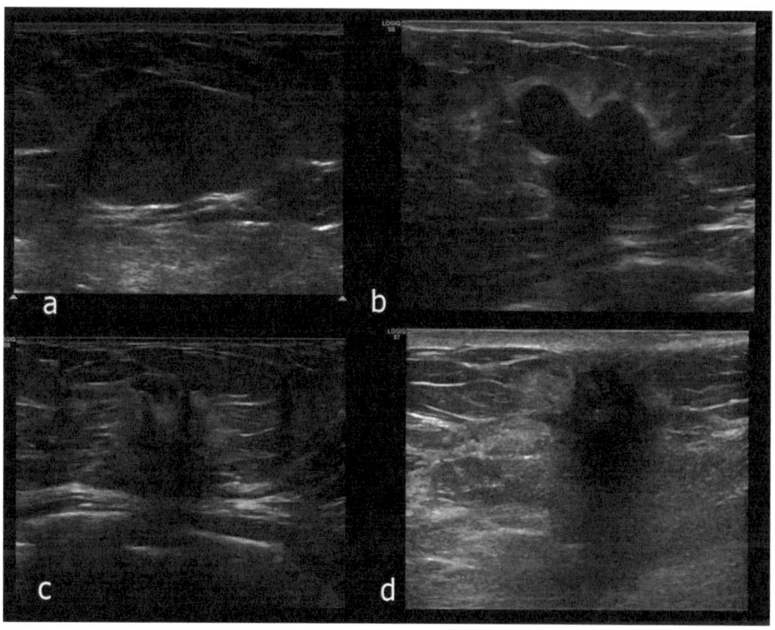

Figure 2.
Oval, circumscribed mass with a visible echogenic wall (a) and non-circumscribed masses: lobulated (b), spiculated (c), angulated and ill-defined (d).

predictive value compared with morphological features and should be used only in combination with the morphological characteristics when classifying a mass as benign or suspicious [1].

The glandular tissue is always hyperechoic, and the echogenicity of the lesions, which is another ultrasound characteristic of the masses, is described comparatively with that of the pre-glandular adipose tissue. The lesions can be anechoic (breast simple cysts, oil cysts, seromas), hypoechoic, isoechoic (**Figure 4**), hyperechoic, complex cystic masses, and heterogeneous [1].

Marked hypoechogenicity (**Figure 4b**) is suggestive of malignancy, but unfortunately, only one-third of breast cancers are intense hypoechoic, most of them being only moderately hypoechoic or isoechoic [1, 4]. Isoechoic lesions can be easily missed in fatty breasts (**Figure 5**), especially when small, if ultrasound is performed for screening in asymptomatic women [1]. Hyperechoic lesions are usually benign (angiomyolipoma), but colloid carcinoma (a special type of invasive ductal carcinoma) can also be hyperechoic compared with the fatty lobules (**Figure 6**). The final decision should be based in this situation on other morphological features (shape and margins).

Complex cystic masses are always suspicious and require biopsy unless the patient has a recent trauma or surgery when the mass may represent a hematoma or seroma. They can represent benign as well as malignant lesions (intracystic papilloma, encapsulated papillary carcinoma or carcinoma with extensive necrosis) (**Figure 7**) [1].

Masses with heterogeneous structures are lesions with hypo-, iso-, and hyperechoic areas. They can also be benign or malignant (**Figure 8**). Hamartomas (benign fibroepithelial lesion), composed of normal but disorganized components of breast tissue, are encapsulated and well-defined [5–7]. Any other lesion with a heterogeneous echostructure, if non-circumscribed, is suspicious and should be biopsied because they can represent carcinomas with liquefaction or coagulation necrosis [1].

The posterior features of a mass can also suggest the nature of the lesion. Attenuation, highly suggestive of malignancy, is encountered only in about 30% of breast cancers. Because it is due to the fibrosis accompanying the lesions it can appear

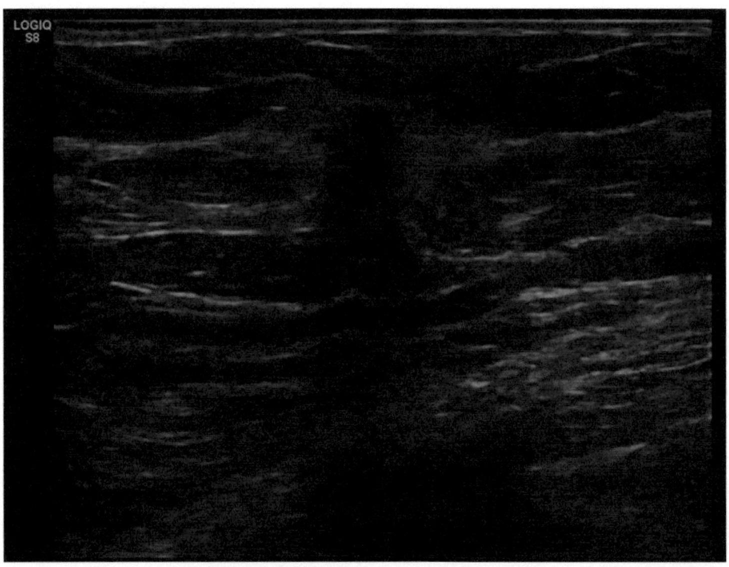

Figure 3.
The perpendicular orientation of a suspicious mass proved to be an invasive ductal carcinoma.

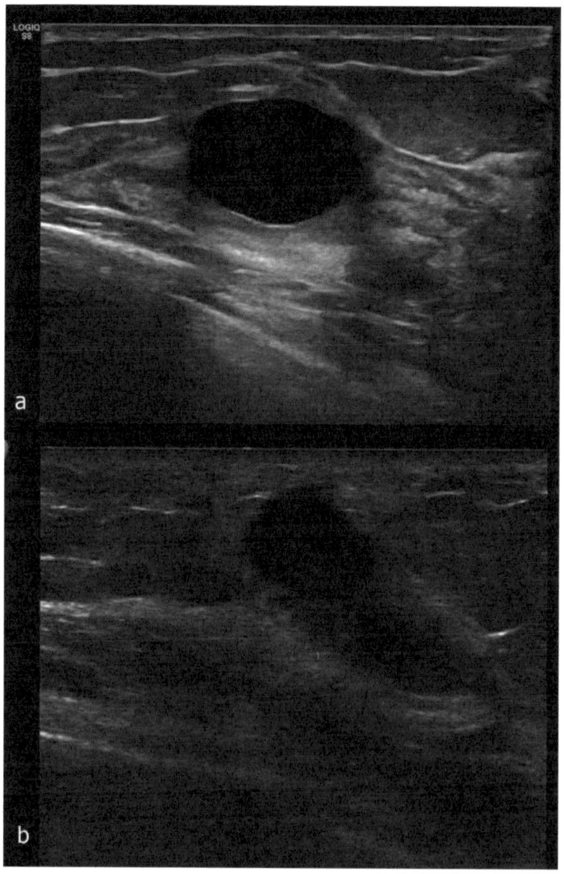

Figure 4.
Simple cyst presenting as an anechoic mass (a). Medullary invasive breast carcinoma, intense hypoechoic comparatively with the surrounding adipose tissue (b).

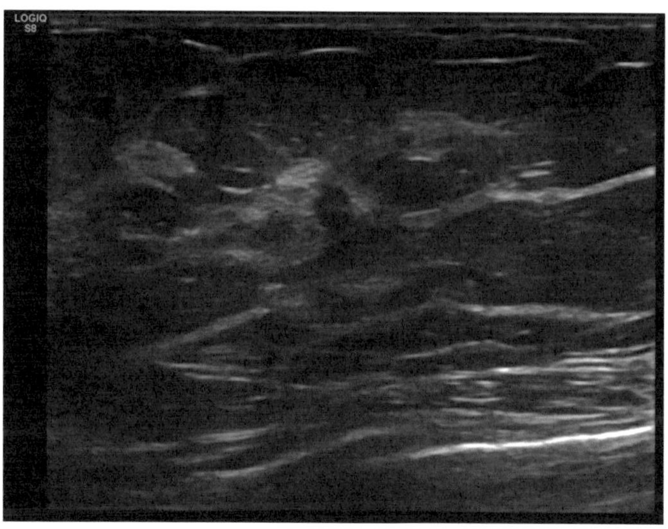

Figure 5.
A small, isoechoic lesion proved to be an invasive ductal carcinoma after ultrasound-guided biopsy.

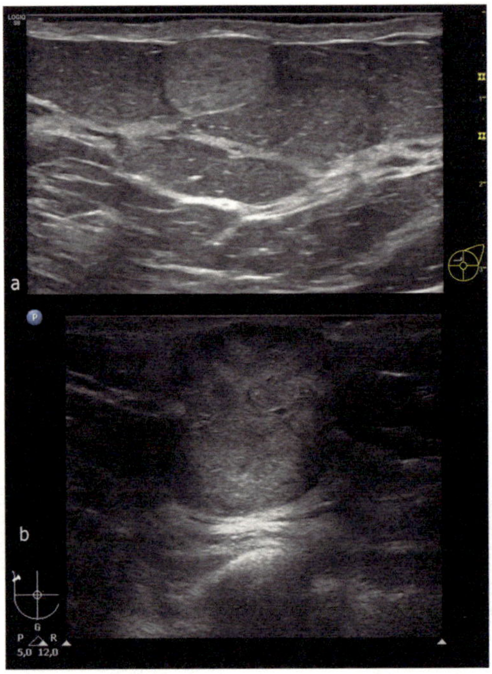

Figure 6.
Hyperechoic lesions: well-defined in an angiomiolipoma (a) and lobulated in a mucinous carcinoma (b).

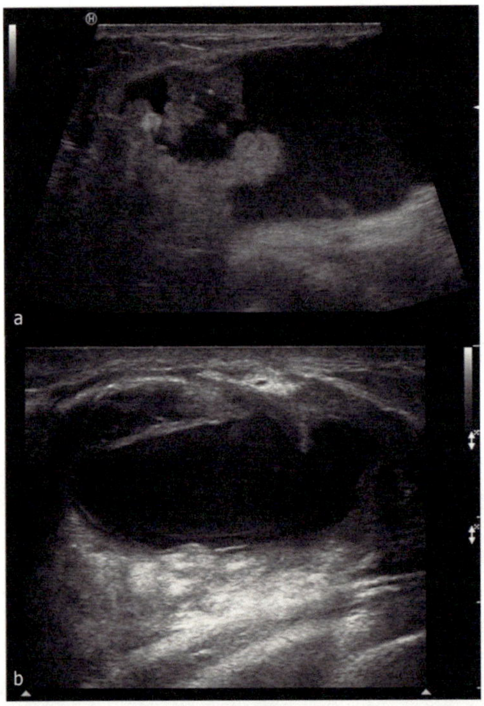

Figure 7.
Encapsulated papillary carcinoma (a) and galactocele (b), both appear as complex cystic masses with cystic and parenchymal components.

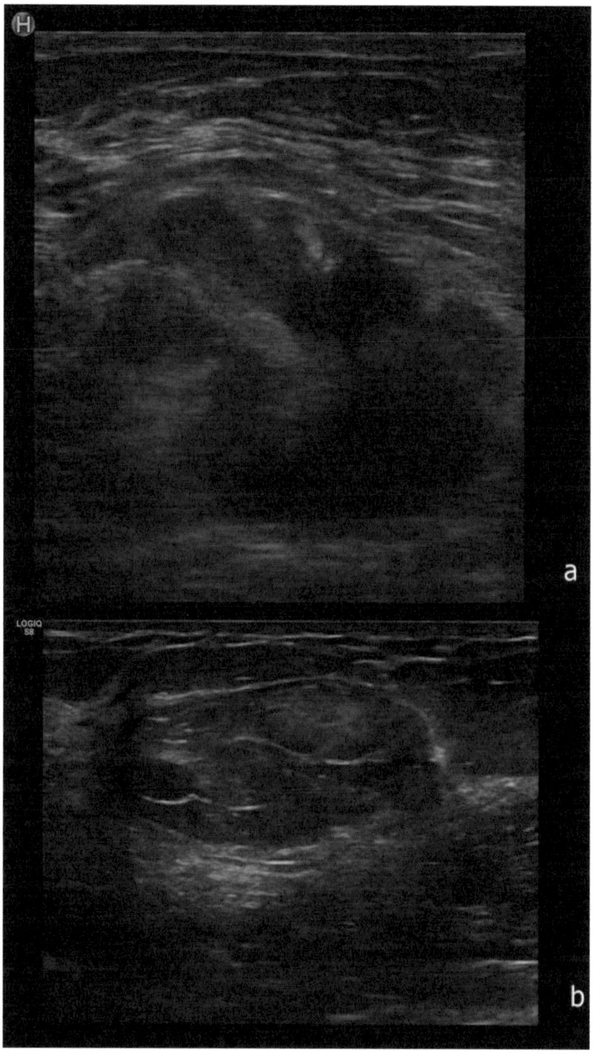

Figure 8.
Breast cancer with heterogeneous echostructure, irregular shape and non-circumscribed (ill-defined) margins (a) and hamartoma with heterogeneous echostructure but with regular shape and circumscribed margins (b).

in benign lesions as well (old fibroadenomas, focal fibrosis, fibrocystic changes). However, most fibroadenomas and breast cancers have no posterior features (do not alter the transmission of the ultrasound beam), and the acoustic enhancement, even if it is typically encountered in the benign, cystic lesions, can also appear in hypercellular fibroadenomas or cancers (**Figure 9**) [4, 8].

Any other features associated with the breast nodule (associated features) should be carefully analyzed (**Figure 10**). They include architectural distortion, surrounding edema, dilatation of the ducts in the vicinity of the lesion, skin edema, thickening or retraction, calcifications, vascularization, and elasticity [1].

The architectural distortion is seen as the attraction of Cooper ligaments toward the lesion.

Edema around a mass determines the appearance of the hyperechoic halo (**Figure 2b–d**). Unless it is seen in an inflammatory cyst or after trauma, masses with

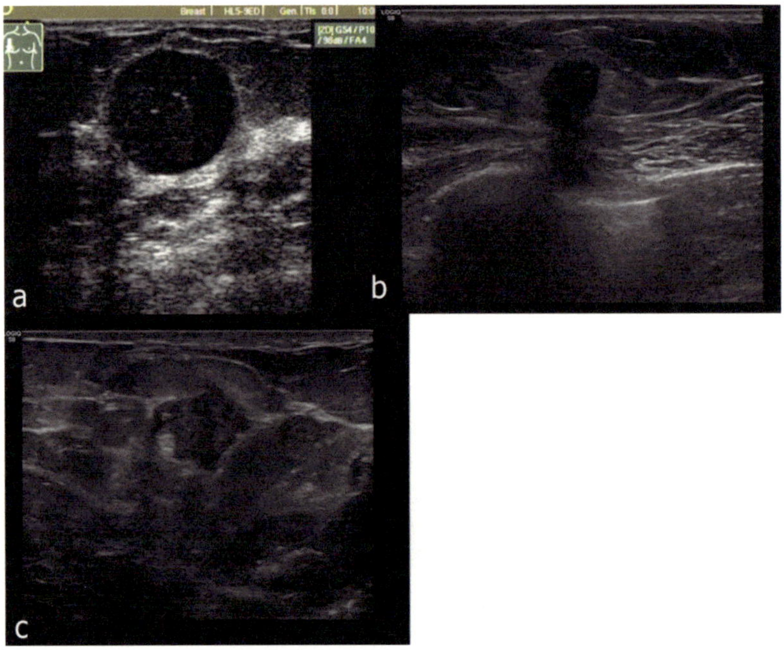

Figure 9.
Breast cancers exhibiting posterior enhancement (mucinous carcinoma) (a), posterior shadowing (b), and no posterior features (c).

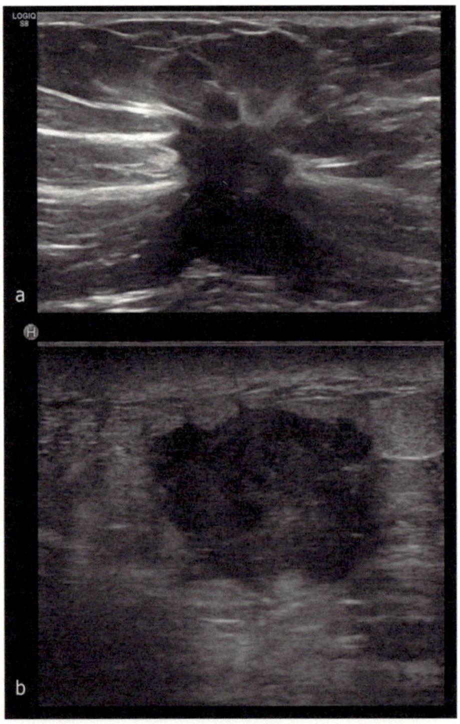

Figure 10.
Irregular and non-circumscribed masses, associated with architectural distortion (a) and skin thickening and edema (b), both proved to be invasive ductal carcinomas.

hyperechoic halo should be further investigated. In malignancy, it is due to the desmoplastic reaction or to the peritumoral inflammatory infiltrate and microinvasion.

Even if ultrasound has a low sensitivity in the detection of calcifications, sometimes they may be seen with performant devices or if they are superimposed with the hypoechoic background of the lesions. They can be seen associated with the masses or outside a mass (around it or in breast parenchyma) as small hyperechoic foci without attenuation (**Figure 11**). In breast cancer, calcifications are associated mainly with the necrotic intraductal component (*in situ* breast carcinoma, comedo type). Any suspicion of calcifications on ultrasound, associated or not with a mass, should be confirmed with mammography, no matter the age of the patient. Mammography allows the visualization and correct evaluation of their extension and, most of all, is the only method that allows the morphological characterization of calcifications and the correct assessment as benign or suspicious [1].

Vascularization and elasticity are considered associated features, and they have value only in association with the morphology of the masses [1]. When evaluating the vascularization, attention should be paid to the correct settings of the ultrasound machine and to the compression during the examination. Even if the examination is correctly performed, one should keep in mind that some benign lesions can have hypervascularization (hypercellular fibroadenomas), while some cancers may show no blood supply at all (cancers with extensive necrosis or very small in size). Also, there is no vascular pattern suggestive of the benign or malignant nature of a lesion. Yet, a circumferential blood supply, surrounding entirely or only partially a mass, suggests that the mass is benign in nature and pushes the blood vessel away, while a plunging blood vessel, having a perpendicular direction to the surface of the mass suggests the malignant nature (**Figures 12** and **13**) [1].

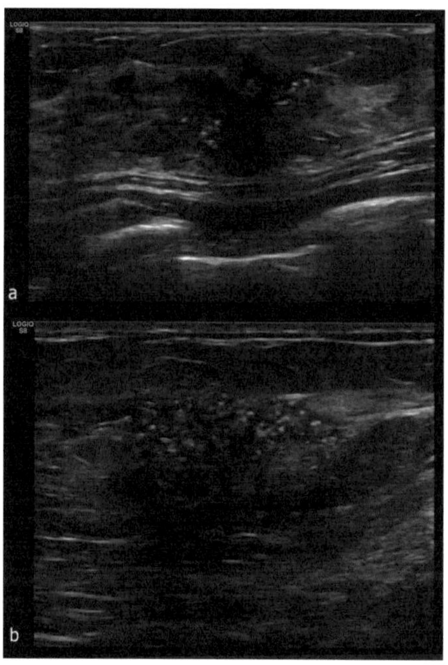

Figure 11.
Calcifications are seen as small, hyperechoic foci, with no posterior shadowing inside a mass (a) and outside a mass, in the breast parenchyma, with no associated lesion (b).

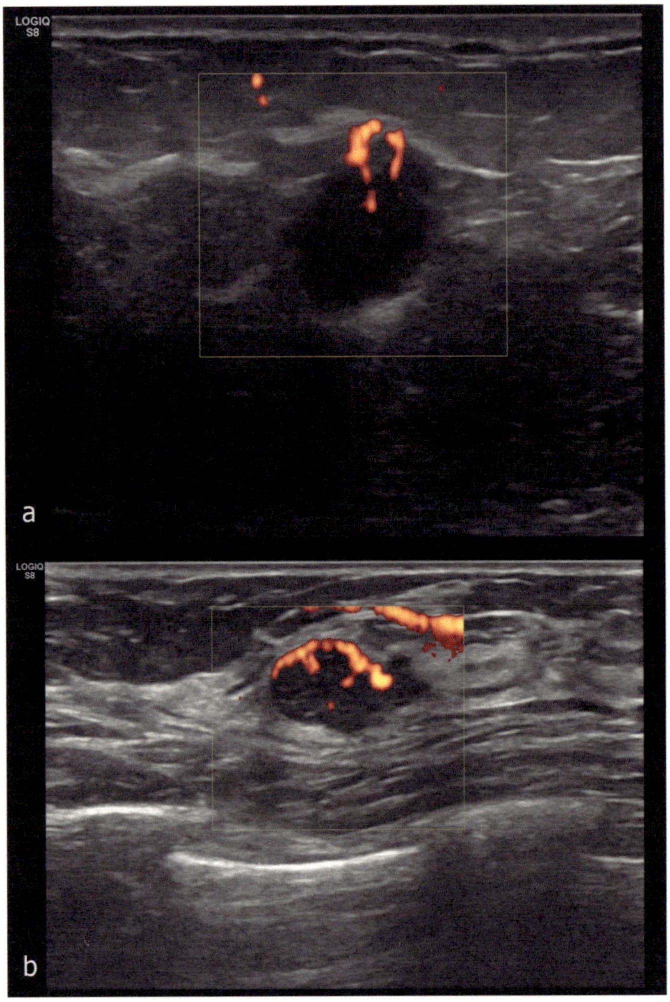

Figure 12.
Malignant lesion with vascularization, the blood vessels having a perpendicular direction to the surface of the lesion (a). Benign lesion (fibroadenoma) with circumferential vascularization (b).

Regarding elasticity, any technique can be used in the assessment of breast masses (strain elastography, ARFI, or shear wave elastography) [1, 9–11]. Lesions are described as soft (with same elasticity as the breast tissue or having the specific blue-green-red color artifact suggestive for the cystic nature), with intermediate elasticity (lesions having a stiff center and a soft peripheral rim) or stiff (with stiffness of the entire lesion or stiffness of the lesion as well as of the surrounding parenchyma, due to the desmoplastic reaction) (**Figure 14**). Stiff lesions are suspicious, and 16% of the lesions with intermediate elasticity may also be malignant [12]. There are also some benign lesions that may exhibit stiffness on elastography evaluation (fibroadenomas, oil cysts, papilloma, and radial scars). On the other hand, in a small proportion of cases, breast cancer may appear soft (**Figure 15**). Therefore, like Doppler evaluation, elasticity should not

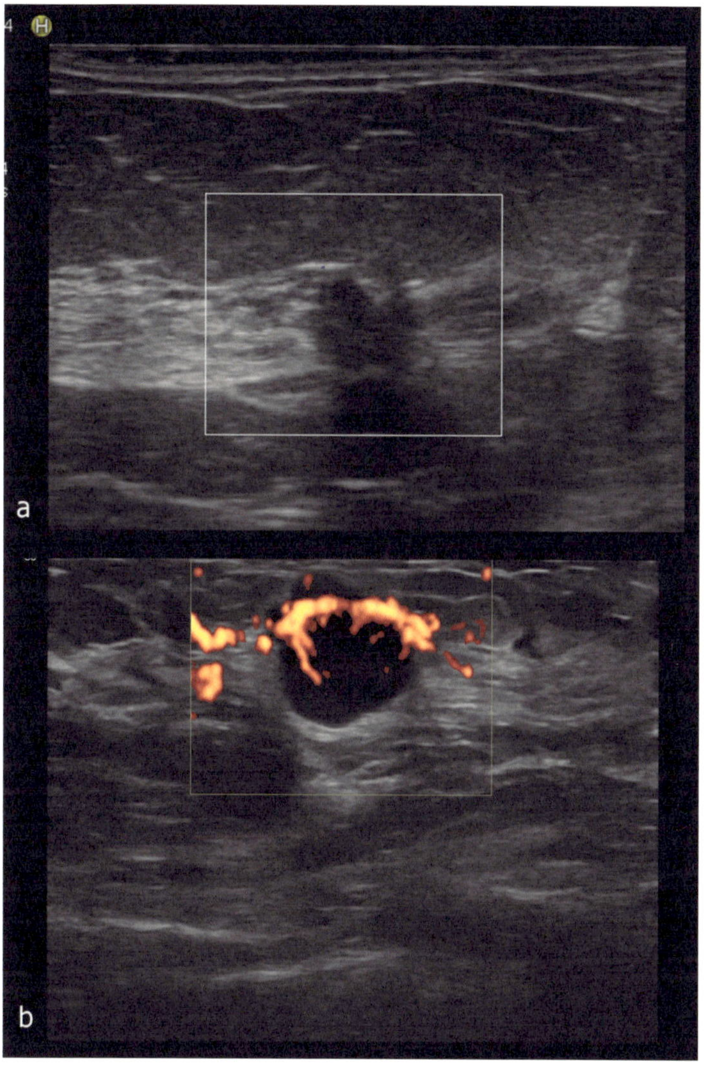

Figure 13.
A triple-negative breast cancer with no blood supply (a) and a Her2+ positive breast cancer with a peripheral blood vessel, suggestive of a benign nature (b).

be used as an independent predictor for the benign or malignant nature of lesions, only in combination with the other morphological criteria. The value of elastography lies in the fact that it increases the diagnosis confidence, especially in small lesions, and allows a regrading of BI-RADS 3 and 4A lesions, with the biopsy of the pseudo-benign breast cancers or short-term follow-up of otherwise biopsied lesions with ultrasound features of fibroadenomas [1, 13, 14].

Examination of the axilla is mandatory in all cases with suspicious masses and is an important part of the evaluation of all patients with breast cancer, considering that the presence or absence of lymph nodes metastasis influences the therapy of the patients. In patients with any breast lesions, evaluation of the axilla can offer

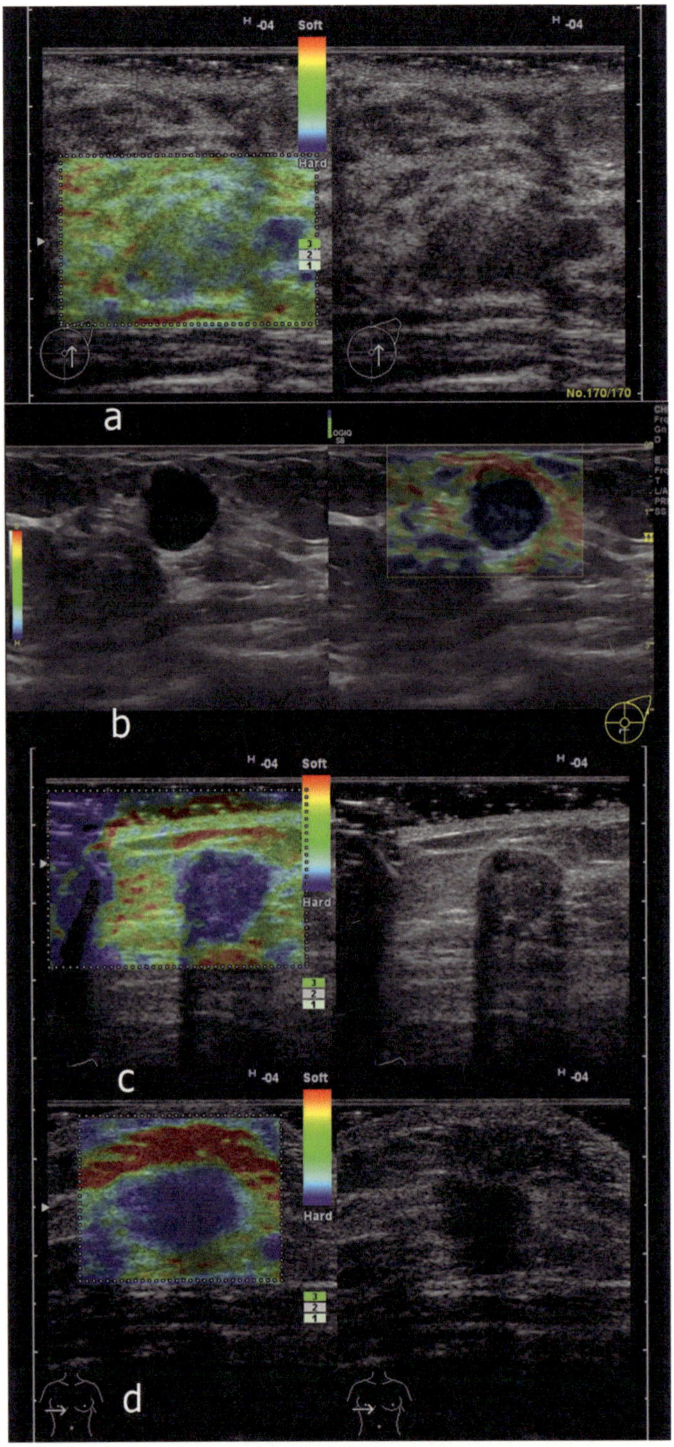

Figure 14.
(a) Benign fibroadenoma, soft at elastography (score 1). (b) Triple negative breast cancer, with intermediate elasticity (score 3). (c) Stiff mucinous carcinoma (score 4). (d) Stiff lobular carcinoma (score 5).

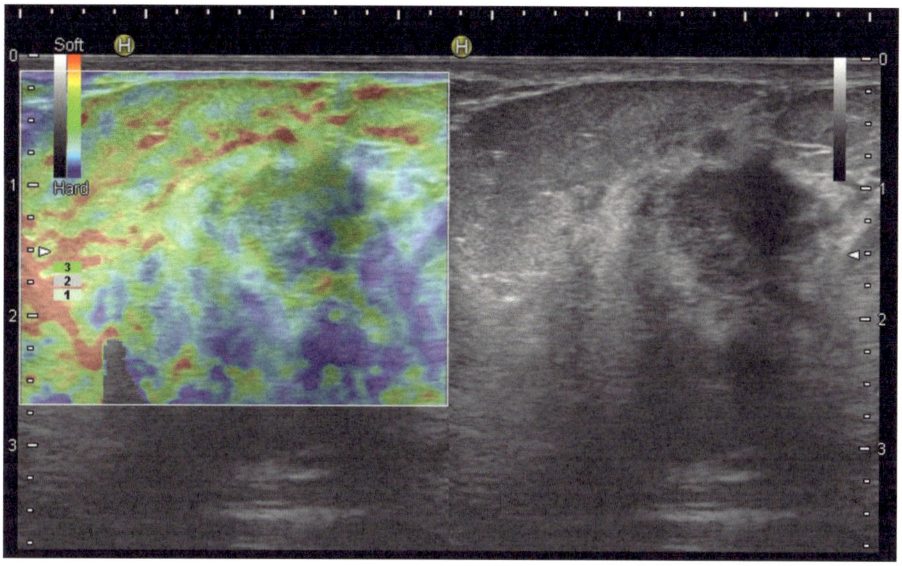

Figure 15.
Invasive ductal carcinoma, soft on elastography, with the same elasticity as the surrounding breast tissue (score 1).

supplementary information regarding the nature of the lesions and the appropriate attitude. Moreover, ultrasound is the method of choice for imaging the axilla, with higher sensitivity and specificity compared with mammography and magnetic resonance imaging [15, 16].

Lymph nodes appear as oval structures with a hyperechoic central hilum surrounded by a thin hypoechoic cortex, with a single vascular pole at color Doppler examination. Metastatic lymph nodes are round, with cortical thickening or focal bulging of more than 3 mm, with no central hyperechoic hilum, and with multiple vascular poles at Doppler interrogation (**Figure 16**) [15]. Inflammatory lymph nodes may, however, mimic malignancy, as can be seen in mastitis, cat scratch fever, rheumatoid arthritis, osteomyelitis, or scapulohumeral periarthritis. In the absence of any clinically benign conditions that can explain the appearance of the changes in the axillary lymph nodes, any suspicious lymph node should be biopsied, even if the lesion seen in the breast is most probably benign.

The lesions that can be diagnosed as benign in the breast are simple cysts (round or oval anechoic masses, with posterior enhancement and thin echogenic wall) (**Figure 4a**), lipomas (isoechoic oval masses corresponding to the palpable lump – undiagnosed if not palpable), angiomyolipoma (hyperechoic round or oval lesions, well-defined, with no blood supply) (**Figure 6a**) and, sometimes, hamartomas (**Figure 8b**). Complicated cysts (cystic lesions with low densities echoes inside, mobile or with a vertical fluid–fluid level or with mobile sediment and circumferential, regular wall thickening), parenchymal lesions with ultrasound appearance of a fibroadenoma, complex cystic masses after surgery or trauma may be assessed in BI-RADS 3 category (<2% risk of malignancy) with recommendation for short-term follow-up (4–6 months) (**Figure 17**) [1]. Any other lesions should be further investigated by a dedicated breast radiologist to rule out malignancy.

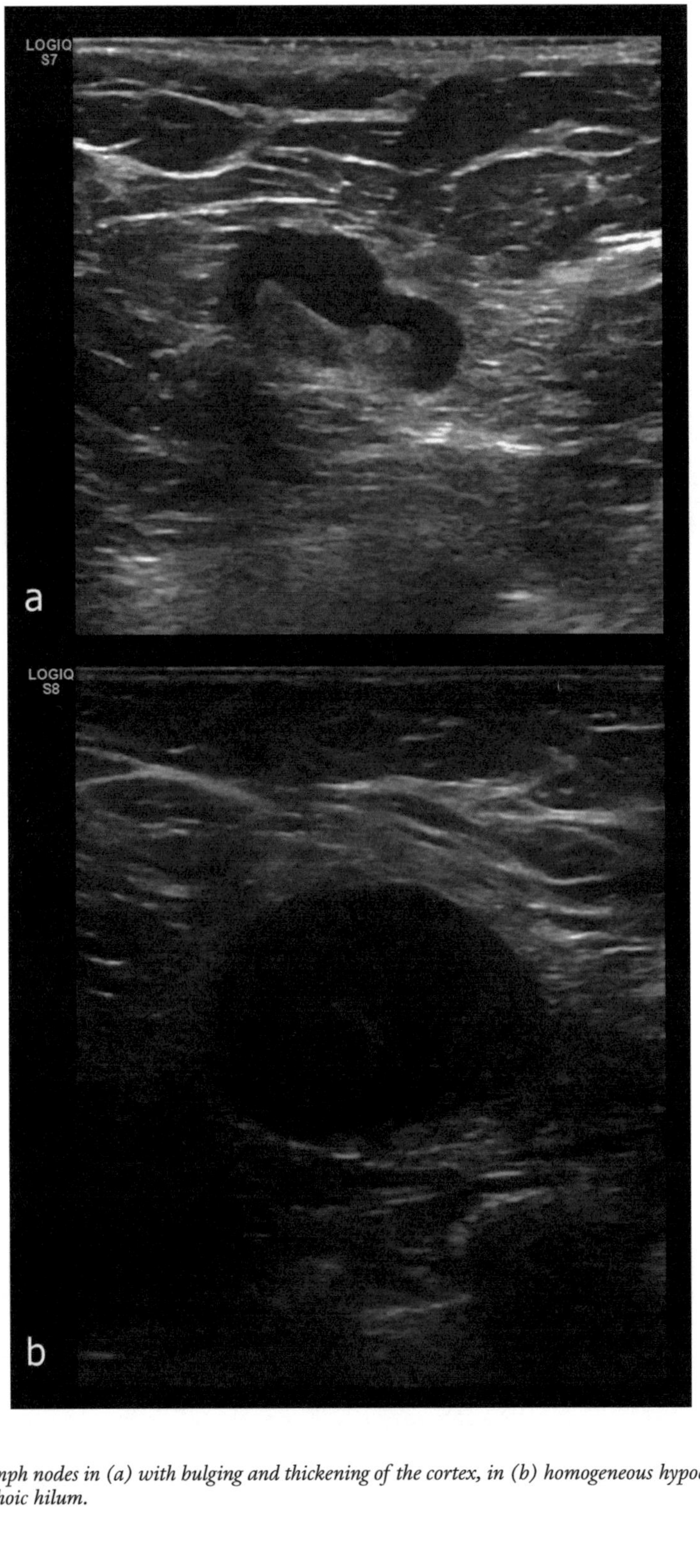

Figure 16.
Metastatic lymph nodes in (a) with bulging and thickening of the cortex, in (b) homogeneous hypoechoic, with no fatty, hyperechoic hilum.

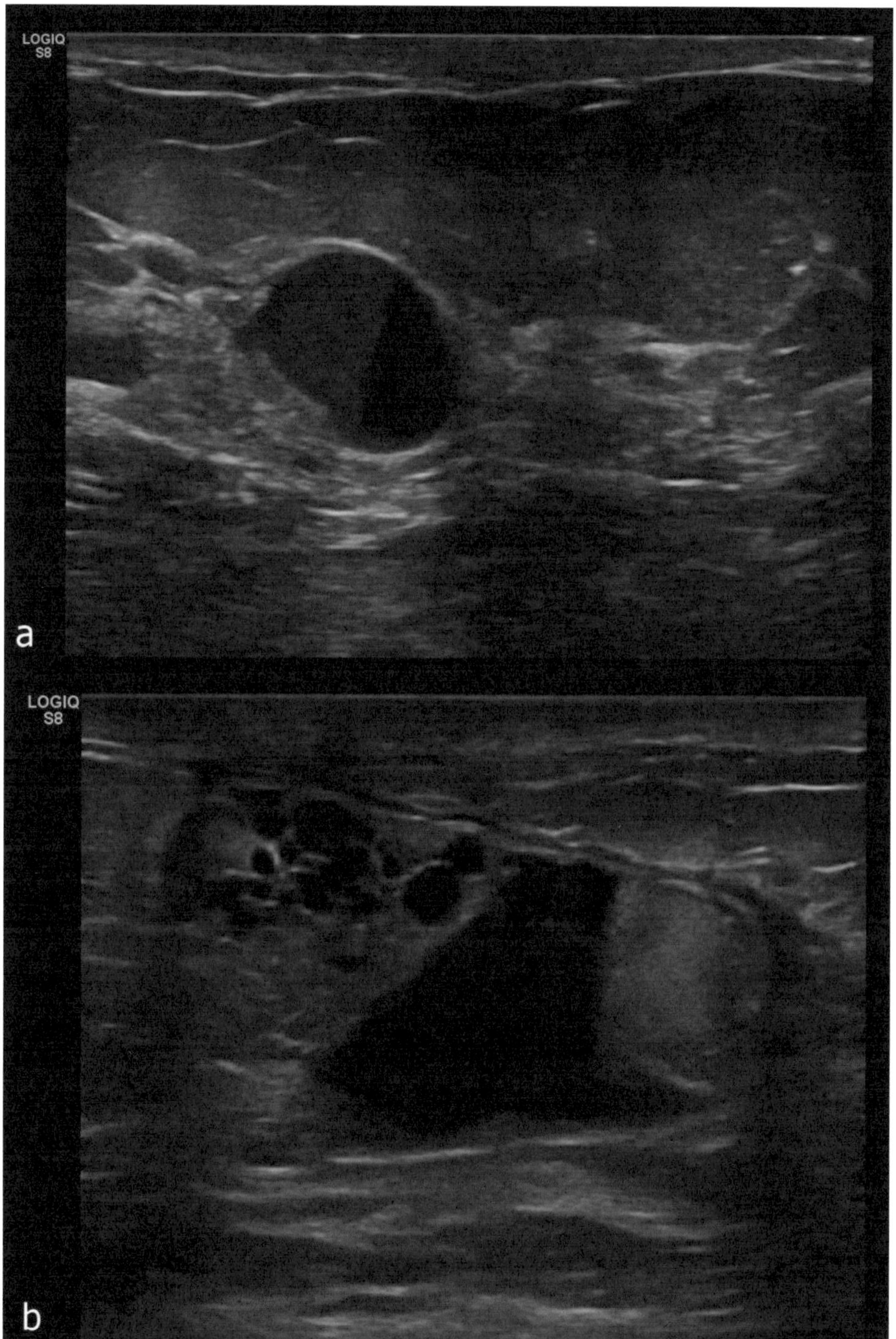

Figure 17.
Cyst with fluid–fluid level (a) and seroma after surgery (b).

3. Mastitis and breast abscess

Mastitis is an inflammatory condition of the breast, associated or not with infection. It appears more frequently during breastfeeding (lactational mastitis), when bacteria enter the breast through the cracks in the nipple, but it can also appear in non-lactating women and even in men (non-lactational mastitis).

In early phases, at ultrasound, signs of edema are seen: thickening of the skin and hyperechogenicity of all breast structures (adipose and glandular tissue). Also, reactive axillary lymph nodes may be present. In this stage, with proper treatment, the inflammation resolves with no complications. In cases with delayed treatment, the process may progress, with the formation of abscess [17]. Abscess appears as an irregular, non-circumscribed complex cystic mass, with intense blood supply around the lesion (**Figure 18**). Under ultrasound guidance, the collection in the abscess may be aspirated, and the cavity washed with saline until complete removal. Cases that cannot be solved by percutaneous aspiration should be referred to surgery [18].

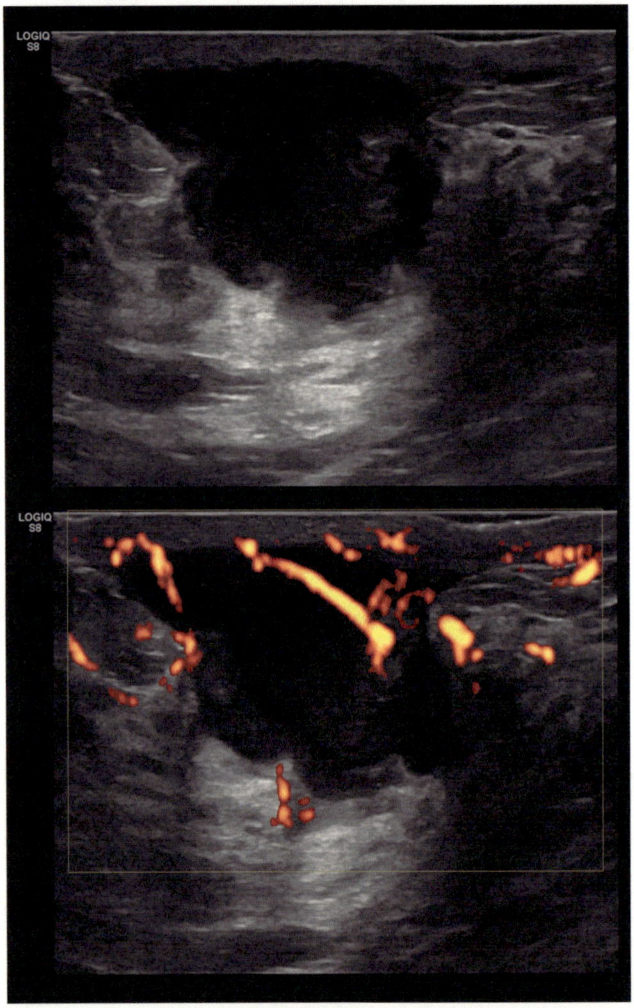

Figure 18.
Breast abscess: irregular, non-circumscribed complex cystic mass with intense blood supply.

Not all cases of mastitis are due to infection. Signs of mastitis may appear in inflammatory cysts, ductal ectasia, granulomatous mastitis and in carcinomatous mastitis [17, 19, 20]. Any inflammatory process that is not solved after treatment with antibiotics or non-steroidal anti-inflammatory drugs, especially if in postmenopausal women, should be further investigated to rule out malignancy.

4. Breast trauma

After breast trauma, regardless of the patient's age, due to the pain, it is difficult to evaluate the breast with mammography. In these situations, ultrasound is the first imaging option. It has the advantage of allowing the examination of a sensitive breast and, during the same examination, the aspiration of hematomas or seromas.

In the acute phase of breast trauma (in the first 4–5 days) signs of edema are seen (skin thickening and hyperechoic appearance of breast structures). Also, in this phase, small hypoechoic areas with superficial location may be present (**Figure 19**), areas that may represent areas of laceration or oil cysts [21].

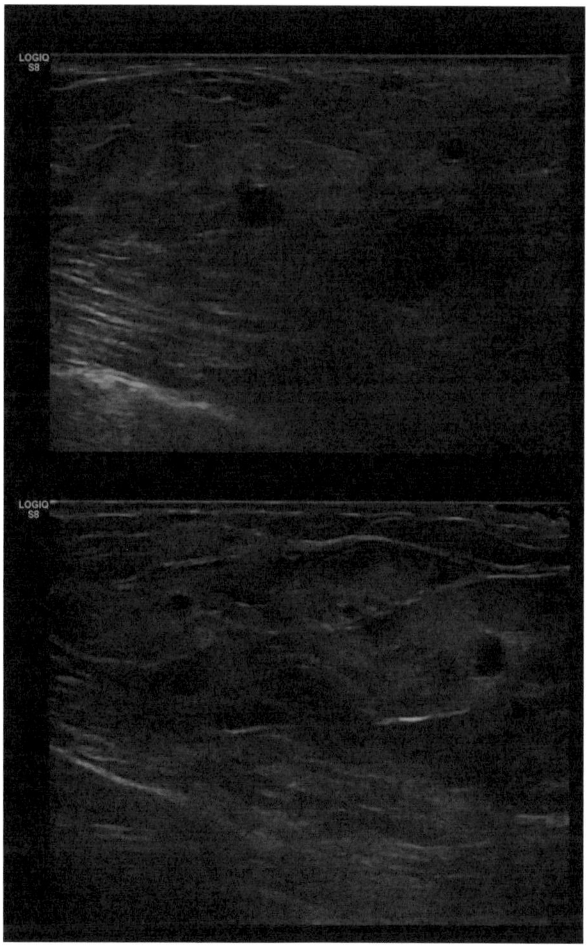

Figure 19.
Acute trauma, with edema and small anechoic lesions.

The intermediate phase (2 weeks after trauma) is characterized by the presence of fluid collections, which may be seromas or hematomas. Seromas are anechoic collections located superficially in the breast, with an orientation parallel to the skin, while hematomas appear as complex cystic masses (**Figure 20**). The diagnostic is usually straightforward in this phase due to the patient's history of trauma [22, 23].

In the late phase (1 year) oil cysts are usually seen as anechoic, round, and well-defined lesions, homogeneous or, less frequently, inhomogeneous (**Figure 21**). They may show posterior shadowing and can be stiff at elastography. However, the final diagnosis is based on mammography, which reveals lucent lesions, with or without rim calcifications [24].

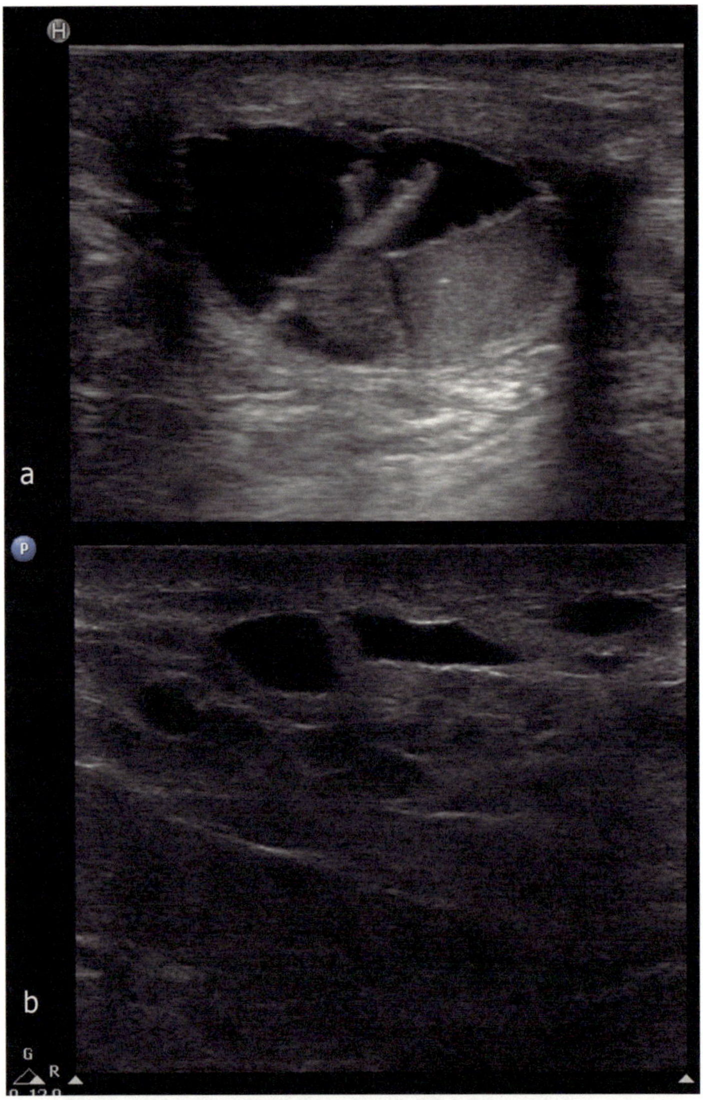

Figure 20.
Hematoma after breast trauma, presenting as a complex cystic mass (a) and fluid collections compatible with post-traumatic seromas (b).

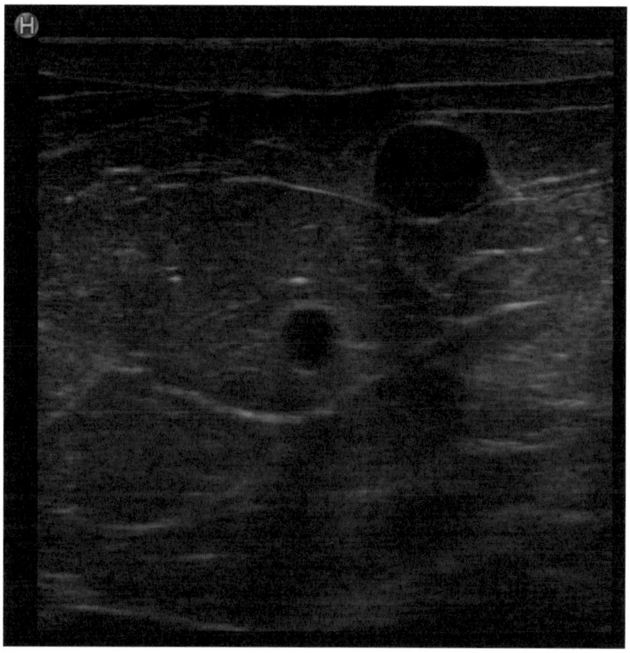

Figure 21.
Oil cysts are incidentally discovered 1 year after breast trauma and confirmed with mammography.

5. Pathological changes during pregnancy and lactation

In pregnancy and lactation, breast evaluation is difficult due to physiological changes. Mammography and MRI have limitations in these patients, and ultrasound is the first-step examination of these patients. The proliferation of epithelial and stromal components and the increased vascularization will determine a diffuse hypoechoic appearance of the breast tissue during pregnancy and a hyperechoic appearance, with dilated ducts and increased vascularization during lactation (**Figure 22**) [25].

In pregnancy and lactation, the existence of accessory glandular tissue may become clinically symptomatic as a palpable, tender mass, located most frequently in the axilla, easily diagnosed with ultrasound, which will reveal an area of breast parenchyma with visible ducts. On the accessory breast tissue, pathological lesions may develop anywhere else in the breast: cyst, fibroadenomas, galactocele, or cancer (**Figure 23**).

Mastitis and breast abscess in lactating breasts have the same appearance and features as described above.

Galactocele can be another cause of palpable lumps during breastfeeding. They represent milk-filled collections, and the appearance is different depending on the age of the collection. A recent galactocele appears as simple or complicated cysts or as an area with multiple dilatated ducts filled with hypoechoic fluid and mobile echoes inside. Old galactocele are inhomogeneous, with anechoic and hyperechoic areas inside, due to milk degradation (**Figure 24**) and may finally mimic oil cysts [25, 26].

Breast cancer in pregnancy and lactation is rare. In most cases, the ultrasound features are suggestive of malignancy (**Figure 25**), but because it is usually aggressive and fast growing, it can mimic benign conditions (**Figure 26**).

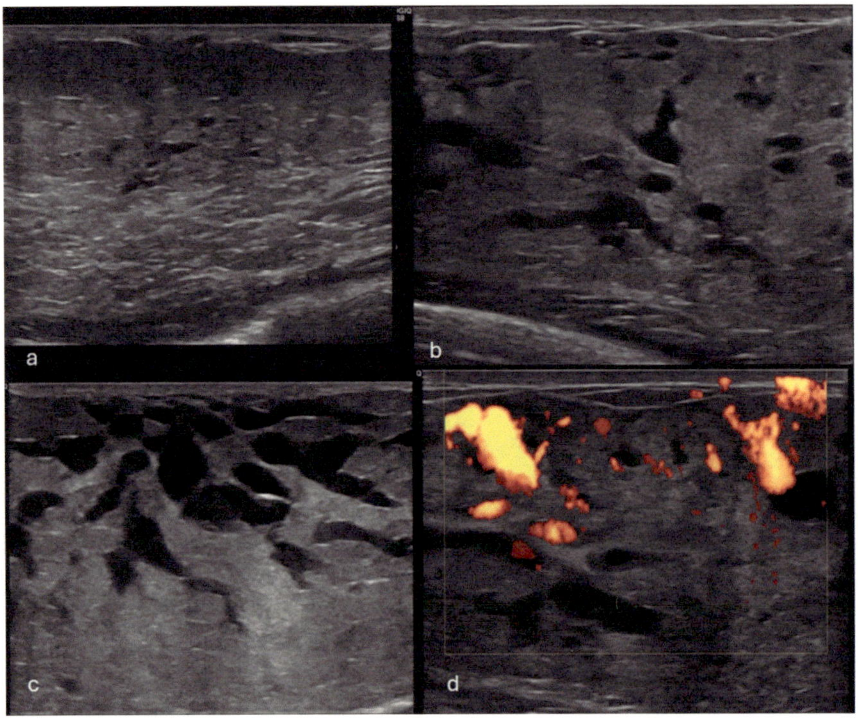

Figure 22.
Diffuse hypoechoic breast tissue in pregnancy (a). Ultrasound appearance of the breast during lactation: diffuse hyperechoic (b), with dilated, anechoic ducts (c) and hypervascularization (d).

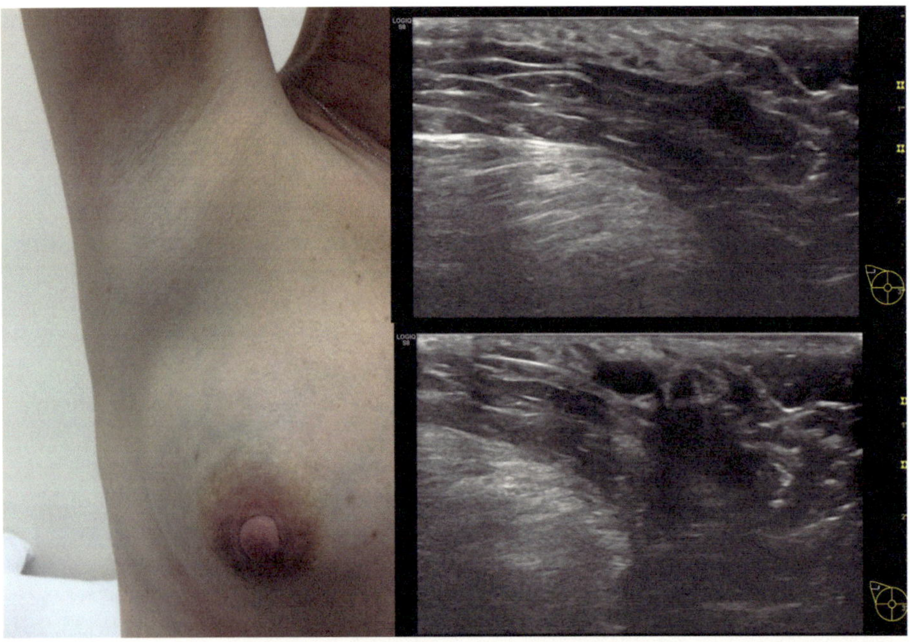

Figure 23.
Palpable, tender lump in the right axilla, with onset during the 2nd trimester of pregnancy (a). Ultrasound reveals accessory breast tissue in the axilla (b), with a small cyst (c).

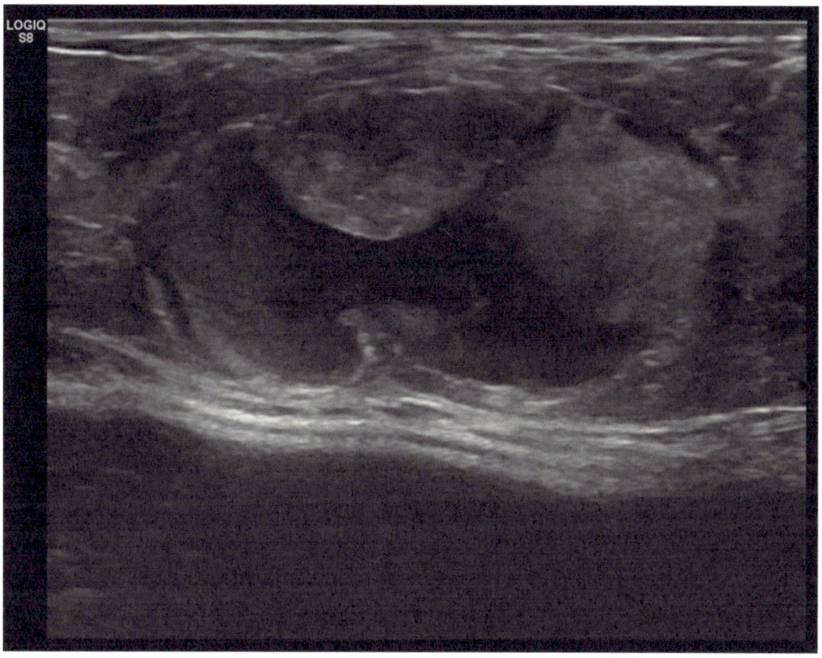

Figure 24.
Old galactocele in a patient with breast augmentation, having at ultrasound a heterogeneous echostructure.

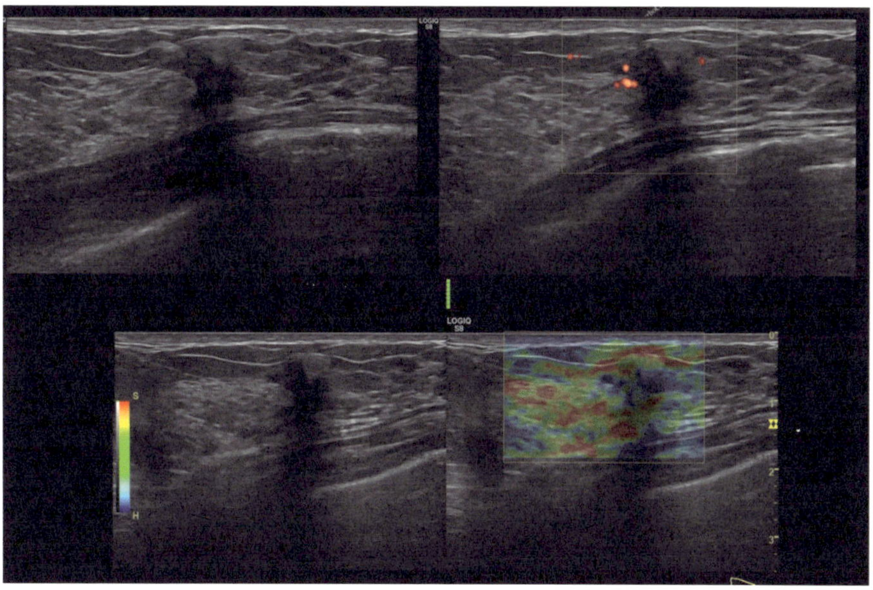

Figure 25.
Breast cancer during lactation, with typical morphological features on 2D ultrasound. Note the lack of blood vessels at power Doppler and the elastic appearance at elastography.

Careful evaluation should be performed for any palpable mass developing in this period, and further investigations are recommended for all cases in which the benign nature of a lump cannot be established with certainty. Mammography,

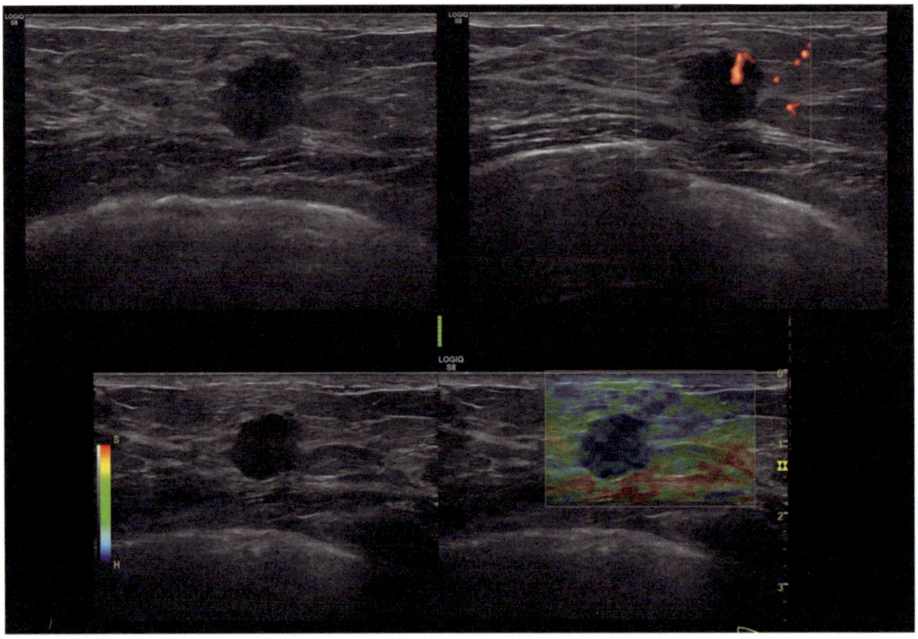

Figure 26.
A triple negative breast cancer in pregnancy, round, with a few discrete lobulations. The suspicion of malignancy was raised mainly by the blood vessel perpendicular to the surface and the stiff appearance at elastography.

even with low sensitivity, may reveal associated findings suggestive of malignancy (architectural distortion or calcifications), and the ultrafast sequences at MRI examination may also aid in the differential diagnosis. In all cases with uncertain lesions, biopsy should be performed even if there is a risk of developing fistulas after percutaneous biopsy [27]. Risks and benefits should be considered when deciding the management of these patients, especially that breast cancer during this period has a poor prognosis and a negative impact on both mother's and the baby's life.

6. Male breast lesions

In males, the most frequent pathologies are pseudo gynecomastia (breast enlargement due to adipose tissue), gynecomastia (proliferation of the ductal, lobular, and stromal components), and breast cancer. A tender and mobile lump in the retro areolar region represents gynecomastia, while breast cancer presents clinically as a stiff and non-tender mass. In the case of gynecomastia, ultrasound reveals the presence of glandular tissue, with the same appearance as in the female breast (**Figure 27**).

Breast cancer in males is also easily diagnosed, having the same morphological features and ultrasound appearance as in women (**Figure 28**). However, other lesions can also be encountered (lipomas, breast abscesses, metastasis from cancers with other location, neurofibromas) (**Figure 29**). Fibro-epithelial lesions of the breast and invasive lobular carcinoma are very rare in men due to the absence of lobules in male breast [28].

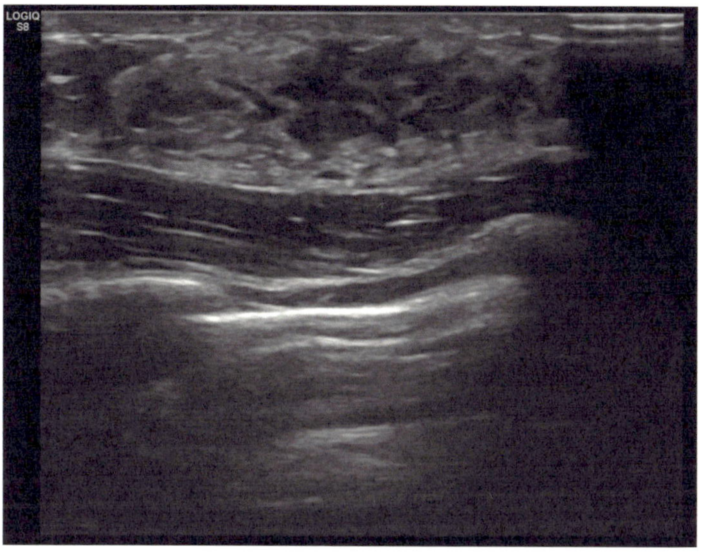

Figure 27.
Retro areolar breast tissue on ultrasound in a young patient with gynecomastia.

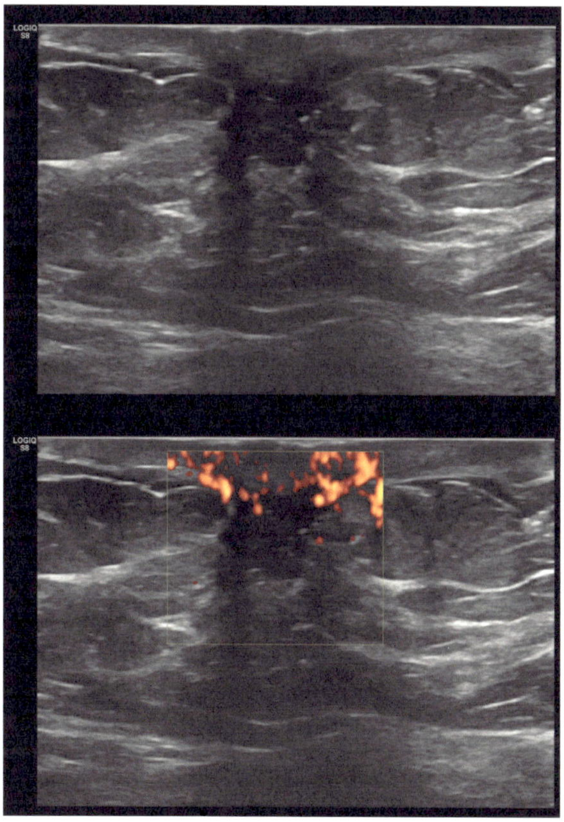

Figure 28.
Breast cancer in a male patient: centrally located irregular mass, non-circumscribed, with no posterior features, with intense blood supply.

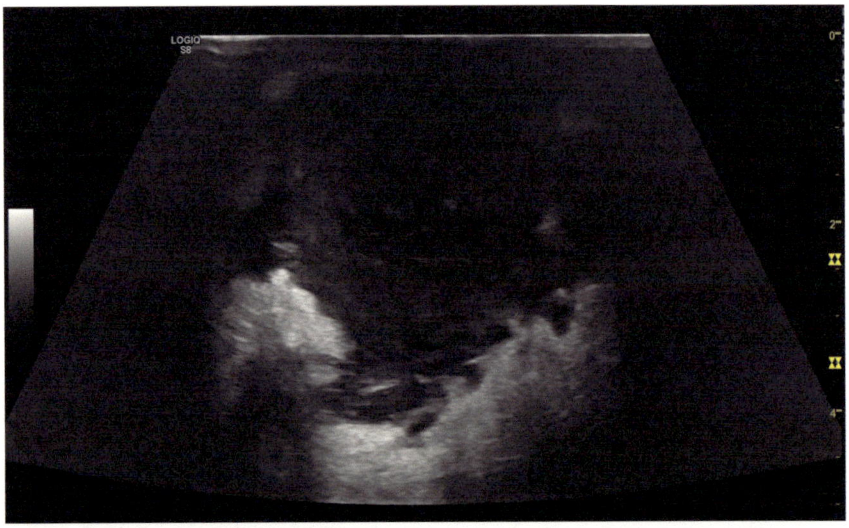

Figure 29.
Impure fluid collection in a male patient with clinical signs of mastitis (abscess).

7. Conclusion

Ultrasound is a useful imaging technique that allows a rapid assessment of clinical changes and a correct decision regarding the treatment, follow-up, or referral of patients for further investigations. Careful examination is required for a correct diagnosis and decision. Limitations of the method should always be kept in mind in order to minimize the false negative results. Any suspicious findings at ultrasound should prompt further imaging and investigations (mammography +/− percutaneous aspiration or biopsy).

Author details

Anca I. Ciurea
University of Medicine and Pharmacy "Iuliu Hațieganu", Cluj-Napoca, Romania

*Address all correspondence to: ancaciurea@elearn.umfcluj.ro

References

[1] Mendelson EB, Böhm-Vélez M, Berg WA, et al. ACR BI-RADS® ultrasound. In: ACR BI-RADS® Atlas, Breast Imaging Reporting and Data System. Reston, VA: American College of Radiology; 2013

[2] Hamilton LJ, Evans AJ, Wilson AR, Scott N, Cornford EJ, Pinder SE, et al. Breast imaging findings in women with BRCA1- and BRCA2-associated breast carcinoma. Clinical Radiology. 2004;**59**(10):895-902. DOI: 10.1016/j.crad.2004.03.013s

[3] Schrading S, Kuhl CK. Mammographic, US, and MR imaging phenotypes of familial breast cancer. Radiology. 2008;**246**(1):58-70. DOI: 10.1148/radiol.2461062173

[4] Karbasian N, Sohrabi S, Omofoye TS, Le-Petross H, Arun BK, Albarracin CT, et al. Imaging features of triple negative breast cancer and the effect of BRCA mutations. Current Problems in Diagnostic Radiology. 2021;**50**(3):303-307. DOI: 10.1067/j.cpradiol.2020.01.011

[5] Liu G, Wang ZL, Zhang MK, He Y, Liu Y. Breast hamartoma: Ultrasound, elastosonographic, and contrast-enhanced ultrasound features. Journal of Cancer Research and Therapeutics. 2019;**15**(4):864-870. DOI: 10.4103/jcrt.JCRT_711_18

[6] Presazzi A, Di Giulio G, Calliada F. Breast hamartoma: Ultrasound, elastosonographic, and mammographic features. Mini pictorial essay. Journal of Ultrasound. 2015;**18**(4):373-377. DOI: 10.1007/s40477-015-0175-0

[7] Tazeoğlu D, Dağ A, Arslan B, Berkeşoğlu M. Breast hamartoma: Clinical, radiological, and histopathological evaluation. European Journal of Breast Health. 2021;**17**(4):328-332. DOI: 10.4274/ejbh.galenos.2021.2021-3-6

[8] Boisserie-Lacroix M, Bullier B, Hurtevent-Labrot G, Ferron S, Lippa N, Mac GG. Correlation between imaging and prognostic factors: Molecular classification of breast cancers. Diagnostic and Interventional Imaging. 2014;**95**(2):227-233. DOI: 10.1016/j.diii.2013.12.013

[9] Barr RG. Breast Elastography: How to perform and integrate into a "best-practice" patient treatment algorithm. Journal of Ultrasound in Medicine. 2020;**39**(1):7-17. DOI: 10.1002/jum.15137

[10] Sigrist RMS, Liau J, Kaffas AE, Chammas MC, Willmann JK. Ultrasound Elastography: Review of techniques and clinical applications. Theranostics. 2017;7(5):1303-1329. DOI: 10.7150/thno.18650

[11] Barr RG, Nakashima K, Amy D, Cosgrove D, Farrokh A, Schafer F, et al. WFUMB guidelines and recommendations for clinical use of ultrasound elastography: Part 2: Breast. Ultrasound in Medicine & Biology. 2015;**41**(5):1148-1160. DOI: 10.1016/j.ultrasmedbio.2015.03.008

[12] Itoh A, Ueno E, Tohno E, Kamma H, Takahashi H, Shiina T, et al. Breast disease: Clinical application of US elastography for diagnosis. Radiology. 2006;**239**(2):341-350. DOI: 10.1148/radiol.2391041676

[13] Sinha D, Kundaragi NG, Sharma S, Kale SK. Can strain elastography be used in reclassification of indeterminate breast lesions in BIRADS lexicon?: A

prospective study. Indian Journal Of Radiology And Imaging. 2020;**30**(4):493-499. DOI: 10.4103/ijri.IJRI_425_19

[14] Cantisani V, David E, Barr RG, Radzina M, de Soccio V, Elia D, et al. US-Elastography for breast lesion characterization: Prospective comparison of US BIRADS, strain Elastography and shear wave Elastography. Ultraschall in der Medizin. 2021;**42**(5):533-540. DOI: 10.1055/a-1134-4937

[15] Marino MA, Avendano D, Zapata P, Riedl CC, Pinker K. Lymph node imaging in patients with primary breast cancer: Concurrent diagnostic tools. The Oncologist. 2020;**25**(2):e231-e242. DOI: 10.1634/theoncologist.2019-0427

[16] Chen MY, Gillanders WE. Staging of the axilla in breast cancer and the evolving role of axillary ultrasound. Breast Cancer (Dove Med Press). 2021;**17**(13):311-323. DOI: 10.2147/BCTT.S273039

[17] Muller KE. Acute Mastitis/Abscess. PathologyOutlines.com Website. Available from: https://www.pathologyoutlines.com/topic/breastacutemastitis.html [Accessed: March 10, 2024]

[18] Rashid T, Sae-Kho TM, Heuvelhorst KL, Glazebrook KN. Breast imaging of infectious disease. The British Journal of Radiology. 2023;**96**(1143):20220649. DOI: 10.1259/bjr.20220649

[19] Wu JM, Turashvili G. Cystic Neutrophilic Granulomatous Mastitis. PathologyOutlines.com Website. Available from: https://www.pathologyoutlines.com/topic/breastcysticgranulomatousmastitis.html [Accessed: March 10, 2024]

[20] Marotti J. Idiopathic Granulomatous Mastitis. PathologyOutlines.com Website. Available from: https://www.pathologyoutlines.com/topic/breastgranulomatousmastitis.html [Accessed: March 10, 2024]

[21] Bhatt AA, Woodard GA, Lee CU, Hesley GK. Urgent and emergent breast lesions - a primer for the general radiologist, on-call resident and sonographer. Australasian Journal of Ultrasound in Medicine. 2022;**25**(2):54-65. DOI: 10.1002/ajum.12296

[22] Molière S. Multimodality imaging of breast hematomas and their mimickers. The British Journal of Radiology. 2022;**95**(1133):20210514. DOI: 10.1259/bjr.20210514

[23] Mahoney MC, Ingram AD. Breast emergencies: Types, imaging features, and management. AJR. American Journal of Roentgenology. 2014;**202**(4):W390-W399. DOI: 10.2214/AJR.13.11758

[24] Taboada JL, Stephens TW, Krishnamurthy S, Brandt KR, Whitman GJ. The many faces of fat necrosis in the breast. AJR. American Journal of Roentgenology. 2009;**192**(3):815-825. DOI: 10.2214/AJR.08.1250

[25] Haliloglu N, Ustuner E, Ozkavukcu E. Breast ultrasound during lactation: Benign and malignant lesions. Breast Care. 2019;**14**(1):30-34. DOI: 10.1159/000491781

[26] Lee SE, Bae YK. Breast lesions during pregnancy and lactation: A pictorial essay. Ultrasonography. 2020;**39**(3):298-310. DOI: 10.14366/usg.19070

[27] Johnson HM, Mitchell KB. Low incidence of milk fistula with continued breastfeeding following radiologic and surgical interventions on the lactating breast. Breast Disease.

2021;**40**(3):183-189. DOI: 10.3233/BD-201000

[28] Kanakis GA, Nordkap L, Bang AK, Calogero AE, Bártfai G, Corona G, et al. EAA clinical practice guidelines-gynecomastia evaluation and management. Andrology. 2019;7(6):778-793. DOI: 10.1111/andr.12636

Section 4

Torax

Chapter 8

Endobronchial Ultrasound: Pioneering Advances in Mediastinal Lymphadenopathy Diagnosis

Arda Kiani, Fatemehsadat Rahimi, Pegah Soltani, Siamak Afaghi, Mehdi Kazempour Dizaji and Atefeh Abedini

Abstract

Endobronchial ultrasound (EBUS) represents a significant advancement in the diagnosis and management of mediastinal lymphadenopathy, offering a less invasive yet highly effective alternative to traditional methods. This chapter delves into the comprehensive role of EBUS, highlighting its diagnostic accuracy and clinical implications. It focuses on EBUS's capability to analyze sonographic features of lymph nodes, including size, shape, echogenicity, and the presence of necrosis. These characteristics, when correlated with histopathological findings, are instrumental in differentiating between malignant and benign nodes, thereby enhancing diagnostic precision. The chapter also discusses the intricacies of endobronchial ultrasound-guided transbronchial needle aspiration (EBUS-TBNA), emphasizing its diagnostic parameters such as sensitivity, specificity, positive predictive value (PPV), and negative predictive value (NPV). The convergence and discrepancies between EBUS and conventional diagnostic methods like spiral chest computed tomography (CT) scans are critically analyzed, underscoring EBUS's role as both a screening and confirmatory tool in varied clinical scenarios, including tuberculosis prevalence and lung cancer staging. Ultimately, this chapter provides a forward-looking perspective on EBUS, advocating for ongoing technological advancements and research to enhance its specificity and application in modern pulmonology and thoracic oncology.

Keywords: endobronchial ultrasound, EBUS, CT scan, sonographic future, lymphadenopathy, mediastinal lymphadenopathy, transbronchial needle aspiration

1. Introduction

Mediastinal lymphadenopathy (ML) is frequently observed in pulmonary medicine. Common causes include tuberculosis, sarcoidosis, metastatic carcinomas, and lymphoma [1]. However, the symptoms associated with these conditions are often non-specific and prevalent across various disorders that result in lymphadenopathy [2]. Consequently, it is essential to conduct pathological and microbiological assessments to determine the precise etiology of ML [2]. Additionally, lymph node enlargement may arise as a response to non-malignant or infectious comorbid conditions, a process referred to as reactive lymphadenopathy [3]. This condition often accompanies obstructive or interstitial lung diseases, chronic heart failure (CHF), or pulmonary arterial hypertension (PAH) [3]. ML is present in approximately half of the patients with bronchitis/emphysema and in about two-thirds of those diagnosed with usual interstitial pneumonia (UIP) and CHF [4]. **Table 1** illustrates the prevalence of mediastinal lymphadenopathy (ML) etiologies using the cumulative frequency data from 11 studies, including 2455 patients [1, 5–8]. Accordingly, the mycobacterial infections, malignancies (including carcinomas and lymphoma), and sarcoidosis were respectively the most common etiologies. Traditionally, diagnostic efforts for mediastinal lymphadenopathy have relied heavily on imaging techniques such as chest radiography and computed tomography (CT) scans [9]. While these methods provide valuable insights, they fall short in terms of sensitivity, specificity, and the ability to perform real-time tissue analysis [9, 10]. Also, their limited guidance for fine-needle aspirations restricts their utility in obtaining cytological or histopathological samples, essential for definitive diagnoses. Recently, the advent of endobronchial ultrasound-guided transbronchial needle aspiration (EBUS-TBNA) has marked a paradigm shift in the diagnostic landscape of mediastinal lymphadenopathy in some studies (**Figure 1**) [11, 12]. However, there have been relatively fewer systemic reports into the efficacy of EBUS-TBNA in ML patients. Accordingly, the sensitivity of EBUS-TBNA was reported ranging from 83 to 91.8%, with a diagnostic accuracy of 87 to 91.5% [11–15]. EBUS-TBNA emerges as a minimally invasive technique that not only offers real-time imaging but also facilitates the procurement of tissue samples directly from the mediastinal structures [16, 17]. This ultrasound-based technology enables dynamic evaluations of lymph node characteristics, including vascularity, a feat that might be unachievable using conventional CT scans [18]. The incorporation of guided biopsies through EBUS significantly enhances diagnostic

Disease	n	%
Mycobacterial	1317	50.9
Confirmed tuberculosis	846	32.7
Probable tuberculosis	360	13.9
Non-tuberculosis mycobacterial lymphadenopathy	111	4.3
Malignancy	503	19.5
Adenocarcinoma	193	7.5
Small cell	109	4.2
Squamous cell	91	3.5
Hodgkin lymphoma	75	2.9
Other	35	1.3
Sarcoidosis	482	18.6
None-malignant reactive adenopathy	239	9.2
Inadequate sample	43	1.6

Table 1.
Final diagnosis of 2584 patients with mediastinal lymphadenopathy.

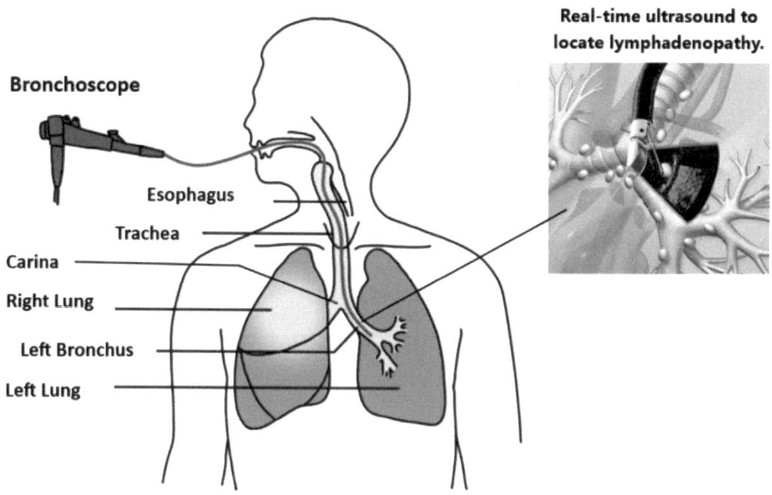

Figure 1.
Endobronchial ultrasound (EBUS)-guided transbronchial needle aspiration (TBNA).

accuracy while diminishing the need for more invasive surgical procedures [11]. The objective of this chapter is to evaluate the diagnostic performance of EBUS-TBNA and identify the underlying etiologies in patients who underwent this procedure for mediastinal lymphadenopathy (ML). This evaluation focuses on elucidating the operational benefits and challenges of EBUS. Furthermore, integrating EBUS with traditional diagnostic techniques such as CT scans provides a more holistic assessment by combining the advantages of each modality.

2. Methodology

This chapter incorporates a systematic review of the literature focusing on the diagnostic performance of EBUS and CT-guided mediastinal lymph node biopsies. The studies included were selected based on their relevance to assessing the sensitivity and specificity of these diagnostic tools for mediastinal lymphadenopathy (ML). A comprehensive search was conducted in multiple electronic databases including PubMed, MEDLINE, and EMBASE, covering publications from January 2000 to December 2023. The search terms used were "endobronchial ultrasound," "EBUS," "CT-guided biopsy," "mediastinal lymphadenopathy," and "diagnostic performance." Inclusion criteria for the studies were: (1) studies that directly compared the sensitivity and specificity of EBUS and CT-guided biopsies, (2) studies involving human subjects diagnosed with ML, and (3) studies published in English. Exclusion criteria included case reports, conference abstracts, and reviews. Data extraction was performed independently by two reviewers using a standardized data extraction form. The form captured details such as study author, publication year, study design, number of participants, diagnostic methods evaluated, sensitivity, specificity, and relative ratios. Any discrepancies between reviewers were resolved through discussion or by consulting a third reviewer. The quality of the included studies was assessed using the Quality Assessment of Diagnostic Accuracy Studies-2 (QUADAS-2) tool, which evaluates the risk of bias and applicability of the diagnostic accuracy studies across four domains: patient selection, index test, reference standard, and flow and timing. Meta-analytic techniques were used to combine the sensitivity and specificity data from the included studies to estimate pooled values for these parameters. Heterogeneity amongst studies was assessed using the I^2 statistic, which measures the percentage of total variation across studies due to heterogeneity rather than chance. An I^2 value greater than 50% was considered indicative of substantial heterogeneity, prompting the use of random-effect models to pool the data. The comparative effectiveness of EBUS and CT-guided biopsies was further analyzed using relative risk ratios for sensitivity and specificity.

3. Revolutionizing mediastinal lymphadenopathy diagnosis and management via EBUS

The diagnosis and management of mediastinal abnormalities, particularly lymphadenopathy, are crucial yet challenging aspects of pulmonary medicine. Traditional diagnostic methods have limitations, necessitating advancements in this field. The introduction of EBUS-TBNA represents a significant breakthrough, transforming the approach to these challenges. The transducer emits sound waves that bounce off bodily tissues, creating echoes that are then converted into detailed, live images. These images are crucial for guiding procedures such as needle aspirations, enhancing both the accuracy and safety of the process [19]. EBUS-TBNA offers several significant advantages over conventional imaging methods like CT scans and MRI. It provides real-time imaging and biopsy guidance, allowing for the direct visualization of lymph nodes and masses during biopsy procedures, which increases the accuracy and yield of the samples collected. Being minimally invasive, EBUS avoids the need for surgical incisions, reducing patient morbidity and speeding up recovery [20]. The high-resolution images obtained through EBUS enable the distinction between benign and malignant lesions based on size, shape, and internal structure, leading to improved diagnostic accuracy. In the context of lung cancer, EBUS is instrumental for staging, enabling the sampling of critical nodal stations to ascertain the extent of the disease [14]. Additionally, EBUS can be more cost-effective than more invasive diagnostic procedures, potentially reducing overall healthcare costs [19].

The EBUS-TBNA procedure is a comprehensive process that begins with the patient's preparation using local anesthesia and sedation to ensure comfort. The throat is numbed to suppress the gag reflex. The EBUS bronchoscope is then inserted through the mouth or nose and advanced into the trachea and bronchial passages. Once in position, the ultrasound is activated, and the operator assesses the airway walls and surrounding mediastinal structures [21]. Lymph nodes and masses are identified using ultrasound images, and a fine needle is passed through the bronchoscope into the target tissue under ultrasound guidance. Suction is applied, and samples are collected for cytological or histopathological examination. The collected samples are then prepared on glass slides for pathology, with additional samples possibly reserved for microbiological cultures. After the procedure, patients are monitored for complications and given post-procedure instructions [21].

EBUS-TBNA has established itself as a cornerstone in the diagnosis and staging of lung cancer, sarcoidosis, and other diseases associated with mediastinal lymphadenopathy in several studies [21–23]. It is also vital for investigating unexplained chest imaging findings, especially when malignancy is suspected. Looking ahead, the future of EBUS may include advancements like the integration of higher-resolution imaging, molecular testing of samples obtained, and the development of new ultrasound probes for better access and visualization. As technology progresses, the utility of EBUS is expected to expand, solidifying its role as an indispensable tool in pulmonary medicine.

3.1 Assessing EBUS and CT Scan efficacy in lymphadenopathy diagnosis

The diagnostic potential of endobronchial ultrasound (EBUS) in evaluating mediastinal and hilar lymph nodes has been suggested in various studies, indicating a trend toward high sensitivity, with figures often cited between 88 and 93%, for detecting malignancies [23]. Its specificity, while not universally consistent, is frequently reported to be high, sometimes reaching 100% in certain patient groups [24]. The positive predictive value (PPV) of EBUS often approaches or exceeds 90%, suggesting a likelihood of accurately identifying malignant lymph nodes. Similarly, its negative predictive value (NPV) is generally strong, typically above 80%, which points to its potential reliability in ruling out cancer when no malignant cells are detected [25].

Emerging research has begun to shed light on sonographic characteristics of lymph nodes that might indicate malignancy. These characteristics, such as a lymph node size greater than 1 cm, round shape, non-hilar vascular pattern, heterogeneous echogenicity, hyper echogenicity, distinct margins, and signs of necrosis, offer promising insights [13]. Moreover, previous analyses between EBUS and spiral chest CT scans have shown some level of congruence, though these findings are not conclusive. For instance, one study reported an 80.5% concordance rate between EBUS and CT scan findings [13]. In previous reports, five studies [15, 26–29] have prospectively examined the differences in sensitivity and specificity of CT-guided biopsy versus EBUS-TBN as depicted in **Tables 2** and **3**. Accordingly, the data indicate that EBUS generally shows high sensitivity, with most studies reporting values close to or at 1.00, suggesting excellent ability to correctly identify true positive cases. In contrast, the specificity of EBUS varies more widely, ranging from as low as 0.16 to perfect specificity, indicating some inconsistencies in correctly identifying true negative cases across different studies. CT-guided biopsies also demonstrate high sensitivity, comparable to EBUS in many instances, with several studies reporting perfect scores. However, the specificity of CT-guided procedures tends to be consistently higher than that of EBUS, as evidenced by fewer variations and generally higher-lower bounds in confidence intervals. Overall, while both biopsy techniques exhibit strong diagnostic capabilities, CT-guided biopsies may offer a slight advantage in specificity. This

Author	Number		Sensitivity		Relative Ratio
	EBUS	CT-guided	EBUS	CT-guided	
Gupta et al. 2014 [27]	62	68	0.75 (0.61–0.85)	0.48 (0.35–0.61)	7.63 (2.14–19.256)
Arslan et al. [26]	30	30	1.00 (0.81–1.00)	1.00 (0.66–1.00)	3.99 (1.18–9.63)
Tremblay et al. [29]	26	24	0.86 (0.66–0.97)	0.74 (0.49–0.91)	4.65 (2.00–15.96)
Herth et al. [28]	100	100	1.00 (0.95–1.00)	1.00 (0.94–1.00)	3.58 (1.66–7.85)
Haghi et al. [15]	40	40	1.00 (0.75–1.00)	1.00 (0.65–1.00)	4.99 (1.68–9.63)

Table 2.
Comparison of sensitivity amongst endobronchial ultrasonography biopsy versus CT-guided mediastinal lymph node biopsy.

Author	Number		Specificity		Relative Ratio
	EBUS	CT-guided	EBUS	CT-guided	
Gupta et al. [27]	62	68	1.00 (0.59–1.00)	1.00 (0.54–1.00)	0.93 (0.91–0.82)
Arslan et al. [26]	30	30	0.74 (.046–0.95)	0.95 (0.76–1.00)	0.89 (0.71–4.56)
Tremblay et al. [29]	26	24	1.00 (0.30–1.00)	1.00 (0.59–1.00)	0.95 (0.75–3.33)
Herth et al. [28]	100	100	0.65 (0.43–0.84)	0.92 (0.78–0.98)	0.75 (0.65–2.88)
Haghi et al. [15]	40	40	0.16 (0.11–0.75)	0.22 (0.17–0.85)	0.66 (0.31–0.82)

Table 3.
Comparison of specificity amongst endobronchial ultrasonography biopsy versus CT-guided mediastinal lymph node biopsy.

suggests that while EBUS is highly effective in ruling in diseases, CT-guided biopsies might be more reliable for ruling out conditions when mediastinal lymphadenopathy is suspected. The selection of a diagnostic approach should therefore consider the clinical context and the necessity for high precision in either detecting or excluding specific pathologies. These results suggest that both EBUS and CT scans have potential as highly sensitive tools for detecting infiltrating lymph nodes, yet their specificity and accuracy might be less optimal, particularly for CT scans. Therefore, they are often considered valuable screening tools that may benefit from additional confirmatory methods like pathology for a definitive diagnosis. Of note, the alignment between EBUS and CT scans suggests the potential benefits of a multi-modality approach in the diagnostic process. While EBUS offers real-time imaging and biopsy capabilities, CT scans provide a more comprehensive view of the chest, contributing to the overall clinical assessment [19]. This approach, which combines the strengths of both EBUS and CT scans, is seen as a hopeful strategy for a more thorough diagnosis of mediastinal lymphadenopathy, aiming to ensure optimal patient care by leveraging the unique capabilities of each modality.

3.2 Integrating EBUS and CT in lymph node analysis

EBUS and computed tomography CT-scans each play a vital role in the evaluation of mediastinal lymphadenopathy, offering unique and complementary insights. EBUS excels in providing real-time imaging and the opportunity for direct tissue sampling, making it invaluable for assessing the internal characteristics of lymph nodes. CT scans, on the other hand, offer a more comprehensive anatomical overview of the mediastinum and the entire thoracic cavity, excelling in initial assessments and identifying lymphadenopathy based on size and morphological features like enhancement patterns and calcifications. However, CT scans may not always reliably differentiate between benign and malignant lymphadenopathy [15].

Recent studies have further explored these differences. For instance, a study compared EBUS and contrast-enhanced computed tomography (CECT) in lung cancer evaluation, noting the distinct features of mediastinal lymph nodes on EBUS and CECT that aid in predicting metastatic disease. Another study focused on the diagnostic value of CT attenuation in mediastinal lymph node metastases, highlighting the usefulness of attenuation values on CT scans for diagnosing enlarged mediastinal lymph node metastases [15, 30]. Discrepancies between EBUS and CT findings can arise due to several factors. Small lymph nodes that may be overlooked on CT scans can be detected on EBUS, thanks to its superior resolution [30]. EBUS provides higher spatial resolution compared to CT scans, enabling the visualization of internal structures and vascularity of lymph nodes that CT scans might miss [31]. EBUS's functional imaging with Doppler assessment can detect increased vascularity within malignant nodes, a feature beyond the capabilities of CT imaging [32]. Additionally, while CT scans cannot provide tissue diagnosis, leading to potential misinterpretations, EBUS can directly sample lymph nodes, offering a more definitive diagnosis. In conclusion, EBUS and CT scans are indispensable yet complementary tools in thoracic medicine [30]. CT scans are crucial for initial evaluation and staging, while EBUS is essential for obtaining tissue diagnosis and evaluating lymph nodes that do not meet the size criteria for malignancy on CT. Understanding the strengths and limitations of each modality is key to ensuring accurate diagnosis and optimal patient management.

3.3 Emerging applications in thoracic disease diagnosis

EBUS is increasingly being recognized for its potential in the diagnostic evaluation of granulomatous diseases, including tuberculosis (TB), particularly in areas with a high prevalence of TB [16]. EBUS seems to allow for precise sampling of affected lymph nodes, which may lead to a more rapid diagnosis and the initiation of appropriate therapy. It shows promise in distinguishing between TB and other granulomatous conditions such as sarcoidosis by potentially identifying specific sonographic features indicative of TB, like necrotizing granulomas or calcifications, although these findings are not universally definitive [14, 16].

In the context of lung cancer, EBUS is emerging as a crucial tool in staging by providing a minimally invasive means to sample mediastinal lymph nodes. It appears to be becoming a key component in the lung cancer staging process, aiding in assessing lymph node involvement, which is vital for determining the stage of the disease, informing treatment options, and understanding prognostic implications. The use of EBUS-TBNA has been associated with a reduction in the need for mediastinoscopy, which was previously the standard procedure for mediastinal staging [25]. Additionally, EBUS seems to assist in differentiating primary tumors from metastatic disease, thereby guiding therapeutic decisions [24].

The real-time imaging capability of EBUS offers immediate feedback during procedures, allowing for adjustments in needle placement and ensuring adequate tissue sampling. This aspect of EBUS is thought to enhance the yield of diagnostic material and increase the safety of the procedure by helping to avoid vascular structures. However, EBUS is not without its limitations. The procedure demands specialized training and expertise for accurate interpretation of sonographic images and safe performance of needle aspirations. While EBUS is effective for sampling and evaluating lesions adjacent to the airways, its efficacy for peripheral lesions might be limited, with other modalities such as transthoracic needle aspiration or surgical biopsy potentially being more suitable.

In summary, EBUS is becoming increasingly important in the management of thoracic diseases, showing promise in diagnosing and staging lung cancer and in differentiating between various granulomatous diseases. Its real-time imaging capability is a significant advantage, yet it comes with certain limitations.

3.4 Enhancing diagnosis and treatment in thoracic medicine

Endobronchial ultrasound (EBUS) is increasingly recognized for its nuanced role in differentiating between benign and malignant mediastinal lymph nodes, enhancing clinical decision-making in thoracic disease management. Recent evidence suggests that EBUS's high-resolution imaging, combined with specific sonographic features, aids in this differentiation [30]. Malignant nodes often appear larger and more rounded compared to the oval or reniform shape of benign nodes. They tend to have irregular or spiculated margins, whereas benign nodes usually present smooth, well-defined borders. Heterogeneous echogenicity is more commonly associated with malignancy, in contrast to the homogeneous echogenicity of benign nodes. The presence of necrosis within a lymph node, appearing as a hypoechoic area without vascular signals on Doppler, is also suggestive of malignancy [30, 33]. Additionally, increased vascular signals or non-hilar blood flow patterns on Doppler can indicate malignancy. Recent advancements in EBUS elastography, measuring tissue stiffness, further contribute to distinguishing between benign and malignant nodes, as malignant tissues are typically stiffer.

EBUS-TBNA provides material for cytological and molecular analysis, crucial for managing patients with mediastinal lymphadenopathy. Diagnosing and staging lung cancer non-invasively with EBUS alters treatment pathways, enabling personalized and targeted therapies. Identifying lymph node metastases, for instance, can direct patients toward neoadjuvant therapy or systemic treatment rather than surgery. In benign conditions like sarcoidosis or TB, EBUS can confirm diagnoses without more invasive procedures, leading to appropriate medical therapy, preventing unnecessary surgeries, and reducing healthcare costs.

Recent studies have reinforced the value of EBUS in clinical decision-making. In cases with indeterminate EBUS findings, it helps identify patients who may need additional diagnostic procedures, such as mediastinoscopy or PET scans. This capability positions EBUS as a pivotal tool in patient management, guiding toward the most effective and least invasive treatment options, thereby significantly impacting patient prognosis and quality of care [30, 34].

To be more detailed, mediastinal lymph nodes, characterized by their distinct ultrasound features, are pivotal in the differential diagnosis of thoracic diseases. Endobronchial ultrasound (EBUS) plays an instrumental role in evaluating these features, offering detailed insights that, when correlated with pathological results, significantly enhance the accuracy of diagnoses. In the realm of EBUS evaluation, the size of a lymph node is a primary consideration. Nodes exceeding 1 cm in the short axis are often viewed with suspicion for malignancy. Complementing this, the shape of the nodes provides additional diagnostic clues; malignant nodes typically exhibit a round appearance, in contrast to the oval or triangular shape more commonly associated with benign nodes [30, 35]. Further, vascular patterns within lymph nodes, assessed using Doppler ultrasound in EBUS, offer further diagnostic insights. Malignant nodes may display non-hilar vascular patterns or increased vascular signals, which are indicative of neo angiogenesis. In contrast, benign nodes frequently exhibit a hilar vascular pattern or may even be avascular, underscoring the diversity in vascular presentation between benign and malignant conditions [36]. Another critical feature is echogenicity, which refers to the ability of lymph nodes to reflect ultrasound waves. Nodes that demonstrate heterogeneous echogenicity, suggesting the presence of varying densities, are often associated with malignancy [37]. Conversely, homogeneous echogenicity is more typical in benign conditions, providing a stark contrast in the ultrasound presentation of different types of nodes [37]. The margins of lymph nodes are also highly telling in this diagnostic process. Benign nodes generally present with sharp, well-defined margins, while malignant nodes may have blurred or irregular margins, a manifestation of invasive growth. Furthermore, the presence of necrosis, manifesting as hypoechoic or anechoic areas, or calcification, appearing as hyperechoic foci within lymph nodes, can be indicative of malignancy [38]. However, it's noteworthy that calcification can also be seen in benign conditions, such as granulomatous diseases, depending on its pattern and distribution within the node. The interpretation of these sonographic features requires a high level of expertise, and their integration with pathological data can lead to highly accurate diagnoses. For instance, a lymph node that is large and round, with heterogeneous echogenicity and a non-hilar blood flow pattern, if found to contain malignant cells upon EBUS-guided aspiration, would confirm the initial suspicion raised by the ultrasound characteristics. EBUS also facilitates real-time correlation of these sonographic features with cytological analysis, thereby enhancing the precision of the diagnostic process. For example, if sonographic features are suggestive of lymphoma and cytology reveals a monotonous population of lymphocytes, this concordance confirms the diagnosis. Similarly, the identification of granulomas on cytology, in conjunction with sonographic signs of calcification, can confirm the diagnosis of granulomatous diseases like sarcoidosis or TB [19, 33].

In summary, the ultrasound characteristics of mediastinal lymph nodes serve not merely as diagnostic tools but also as integral guides for pathologic evaluation. They often provide a provisional diagnosis even before the availability of pathology results, playing a crucial role in facilitating timely and accurate diagnosis and treatment planning in thoracic medicine.

4. The future horizons in EBUS technology

The potential for advancements in EBUS technology and techniques is substantial, with recent studies indicating various directions for future development. Innovations in transducer design are anticipated to provide higher resolution imaging, which could significantly improve the differentiation between benign and malignant nodal features [39]. The integration of three-dimensional (3D) ultrasound capabilities is expected to offer more comprehensive views of mediastinal structures, aiding in precise needle placement during transbronchial needle aspiration (TBNA) [16, 39]. Furthermore, the development of EBUS elastography, assessing tissue stiffness, may enhance the specificity in differentiating various pathologies [40].

Recent research has also explored the integration of artificial intelligence (AI) in interventional pulmonology, including EBUS [41, 42]. Some investigations also highlight the potential of AI, particularly deep learning, in analyzing endobronchial ultrasound images to distinguish between benign and malignant targets with high accuracy [42]. This advancement is facilitated by increased computational power and the use of large datasets, enabling more precise detections and predictions.

Another area of innovation is the use of image-guided navigation in surgical procedures. The integration of imaging modalities like CT, MRI, and ultrasound with surgical navigation systems, including in EBUS procedures, is enhancing surgeons' ability to navigate complex anatomical features and plan surgical paths with greater confidence [43].

Furthermore, the effectiveness of EBUS and endoscopic ultrasound (EUS) in cytomorphological verification of malignant processes has been evaluated in a study by Pavlyuk et al. The combination of EBUS and EUS with TBNA showed high effectiveness, with the sensitivity, specificity, and accuracy of cytologic analysis during EBUS and EUS with TBNA being significantly improved by rapid on-site evaluation

(ROSE) [18]. Additionally, deep learning applications in EBUS-TBNA image analysis, as explored by Wang et al., show promise in improving the overall diagnostic yield of sampling mediastinal lymphadenopathy. This research represents the first fully automated analysis of enlarged mediastinal lymph node using EBUS-TBNA cytological whole-slide images (WSIs), achieving high precision and sensitivity [44, 45].

In conclusion, the trajectory of EBUS technology is marked by ongoing research and technological innovation, with the integration of AI, advanced imaging techniques, and new diagnostic tools promising to make EBUS an even more indispensable tool in pulmonary medicine. These advancements are expected to significantly improve patient outcomes through early and accurate diagnosis, personalized treatment approaches, and minimally invasive therapeutic options.

5. Strengths and limitations

The current study highlights the operational, diagnostical, and technical benefits of EBUS, such as its minimally invasive nature and its ability to provide real-time imaging and tissue analysis. These features not only improve the safety and comfort of the patient but also increase the precision of the biopsy, which is critical for accurate diagnosis and staging of diseases. Also, the use of relative ratios to compare sensitivity and specificity between the two methods introduces a quantitative measure that can be directly applied in clinical practice to assess and choose the most appropriate diagnostic approach. This aspect of the study underscores its practical applicability and potential to impact patient care positively by guiding the selection of diagnostic techniques based on empirical evidence. The study examining the diagnostic performance of endobronchial ultrasound (EBUS) and CT-guided mediastinal lymph node biopsies presents several limitations that warrant consideration. First, the variability in EBUS specificity across different studies suggests potential inconsistencies in procedural execution or interpretation of results, which could affect the reliability of EBUS as a diagnostic tool. Additionally, the studies included in the analysis have a limited number of patients, which may not provide a comprehensive representation of the broader patient population and could affect the generalizability of the findings. Furthermore, the studies are retrospective in nature, which inherently includes biases related to case selection and data collection. The comparison between EBUS and CT-guided biopsies might also be influenced by technological differences and operator skill, which are not uniformly controlled across studies. These factors can introduce variability in sensitivity and specificity outcomes, potentially skewing the comparative effectiveness of these diagnostic methods. Lastly, while the data suggest EBUS has high diagnostic sensitivity, the lower specificity in some cases indicates a need for adjunctive diagnostic modalities to confirm EBUS findings. This dependence on additional testing could complicate the diagnostic process and impact the overall efficiency and cost-effectiveness of using EBUS in clinical settings. As such, further research involving larger, prospective studies is needed to validate these findings and improve the diagnostic algorithms that incorporate EBUS.

6. Summary

This chapter has highlighted the pivotal role of endobronchial ultrasound (EBUS) in the diagnosis and management of mediastinal lymphadenopathy. EBUS stands out for its minimally invasive approach, offering real-time, high-resolution imaging and guided biopsy capabilities, which surpass traditional methods like CT scans in sensitivity and specificity. Key to its utility is the sonographic features EBUS identifies, aiding in the differentiation of thoracic diseases and in the management of conditions like tuberculosis, sarcoidosis, and lung cancer. Looking forward, the potential for advancements in EBUS technology, including 3D imaging and molecular diagnostics, is promising. These innovations, alongside ongoing research, are expected to enhance the specificity and accuracy of EBUS, extending its applications and solidifying its role in pulmonary medicine and thoracic oncology. As we continue to evolve our understanding and improve the technology, EBUS has significantly advanced mediastinal lymphadenopathy diagnosis while facing challenges like limited accessibility and operator-dependence. Future advancements are anticipated to overcome these limitations, further enhancing EBUS's role in thoracic medicine.

Acknowledgements

The author acknowledges the usage of ChatGPT for language polishing and grammar correction of the manuscript.

Conflict of interest

The authors hereby declare that there are no conflicts of interest that could have influenced or biased the work presented. This declaration encompasses financial, personal, or professional relationships that could be perceived as potential sources of bias.

Acronyms and abbreviations

AI	artificial intelligence
CECT	contrast-enhanced computed tomography
CT	computed tomography
EBUS	endobronchial ultrasound
EUS	endoscopic ultrasound
MRI	magnetic resonance imaging
NPV	negative predictive value
PPV	positive predictive value
TB	tuberculosis
TBNA	transbronchial needle aspiration
WSIs	whole-slide images

Author details

Arda Kiani[1], Fatemehsadat Rahimi[2], Pegah Soltani[2], Siamak Afaghi[2], Mehdi Kazempour Dizaji[3] and Atefeh Abedini[2*]

1 Clinical Research Development Unit of Lung Tehran, Shahid Beheshti University of Medical Sciences, Tehran, Iran

2 Tracheal Disease Research Center, National Research Institute of Tuberculosis and Lung Diseases (NRITLD), Shahid Beheshti University of Medical Sciences, Tehran, Iran

3 Biostatistics Department, Mycobacteriology Research Centre, National Research Institute of Tuberculosis and and Lung Diseases, Shahid Beheshti University of Medical Sciences, Tehran, Iran

*Address all correspondence to: dr.abedini110@gmail.com

References

[1] Iyer H et al. Mediastinal lymphadenopathy: a practical approach. Expert Review of Respiratory Medicine. 2021;**15**(10):1317-1334

[2] Pathak V, Adhikari N, Conklin C. Management of isolated thoracic lymphadenopathy of unclear etiology: a survey of physicians and literature review. Cureus. 2023;**15**(7):e41867

[3] Faraz M, Rosado FGN. Reactive lymphadenopathies. Clinics in Laboratory Medicine. 2021;**41**(3): 433-451

[4] Slack GW. The pathology of reactive lymphadenopathies: a discussion of common reactive patterns and their malignant mimics. Archives of Pathology & Laboratory Medicine. 2016;**140**(9):881-892

[5] Nin CS et al. Thoracic lymphadenopathy in benign diseases: A state of the art review. Respiratory Medicine. 2016;**112**:10-17

[6] Sharma P et al. Clinicopathological analysis of mediastinal masses: a mixed bag of non-neoplastic and neoplastic etiologies. Türk Patoloji Dergisi. 2017;**33**(1):37-46

[7] Habermann TM, Steensma DP. Lymphadenopathy. Myoclinic Proceeding (Elsevier). 2000;**75**(7):723-732

[8] Porte H et al. The role of mediastinoscopy in the diagnosis of mediastinal lymphadenopathy. European Journal of Cardio-Thoracic Surgery. 1998;**13**(2):196-199

[9] Koda E et al. CT texture analysis of mediastinal lymphadenopathy: Combining with US-based elastographic parameter and discrimination between sarcoidosis and lymph node metastasis from small cell lung cancer. PLoS One. 2020;**15**(12):e0243181

[10] Zheng Y et al. Enlarged mediastinal lymph nodes in computed tomography are a valuable prognostic factor in non-small cell lung cancer patients with pathologically negative lymph nodes. Cancer Management and Research. 2020;**12**:10875-10886

[11] Gahlot T et al. Endobronchial ultrasound-guided transbronchial needle aspiration in diagnosing mediastinal lymphadenopathy. Lung India. 2017;**34**(3):241-246

[12] Pajares V et al. Diagnosis and invasive staging: Non-surgical invasive mediastinal staging. Endobronchial ultrasound. Journal of Clinical and Translational Research. 2020;**6**(4):121-126

[13] Abedini A et al. The utility of elastography during EBUS-TBNA in a population with a high prevalence of anthracosis. The Clinical Respiratory Journal. 2020;**14**(5):488-494

[14] Agrawal S et al. Diagnostic utility of endobronchial ultrasound (EBUS) features in differentiating malignant and benign lymph nodes-A systematic review and meta-analysis. Respiratory Medicine. 2020;**171**:106097

[15] Haghi S et al. The diagnostic accuracy of endobronchial ultrasound and spiral chest computed tomography scan in the prediction of infiltrating and non-infiltrating lymph nodes in patients undergoing endobronchial ultrasound. Polish Journal of Radiology. 2019;**84**:e565-e569

[16] Gupta N et al. Role of EBUS-TBNA in the diagnosis of tuberculosis and sarcoidosis. Journal of Cytology. 2019;**36**(2):128-130

[17] Gompelmann D, Eberhardt R, Herth FJ. Endobronchial ultrasound. Endoscopic Ultrasound. 2012;**1**(2):69-74

[18] Guarize J et al. Diagnostic performance and cell count of EBUS-TBNA needle gauges: a prospective trial. Journal of Clinical Medicine. 2023;**12**(12):4033

[19] Biondini D et al. Clinical applications of endobronchial ultrasound (EBUS) scope: challenges and opportunities. Diagnostics. 2023;**13**(15):2565

[20] Madan K et al. Efficacy and safety of EBUS-TBNA and EUS-B-FNA in children: A systematic review and meta-analysis. Pediatric Pulmonology. 2021;**56**(1):23-33

[21] Righi L et al. Endobronchial ultrasound-guided transbronchial needle aspiration (EBUS-TBNA)-from morphology to molecular testing. Journal of Thoracic Disease. 2017;**9**(Suppl. 5): S395-s404

[22] Jaliawala HA et al. Endobronchial ultrasound-guided transbronchial needle aspiration (EBUS-TBNA): Technical updates and pathological yield. Diagnostics (Basel). 2021;**11**(12):2331

[23] Jiang J et al. TBNA with and without EBUS: a comparative efficacy study for the diagnosis and staging of lung cancer. Journal of Thoracic Disease. 2014;**6**(5):416-420

[24] Muriana P, Rossetti F. The role of EBUS-TBNA in lung cancer restaging and mutation analysis. Media. 2020;**4**:23

[25] Haranguş A et al. EBUS in optimizing non-small cell lung cancer diagnosis and treatment. Medicine and Pharmacy Reports. 2021;**94**(2):176-184

[26] Arslan Z et al. Conventional vs. endobronchial ultrasound-guided transbronchial needle aspiration in the diagnosis of mediastinal lymphadenopathies. Tüberküloz ve Toraks. 2011;**59**(2):153-157

[27] Gupta D et al. Endobronchial ultrasound-guided transbronchial needle aspiration vs conventional transbronchial needle aspiration in the diagnosis of sarcoidosis. Chest. 2014;**146**(3):547-556

[28] Herth F, Becker HD, Ernst A. Conventional vs endobronchial ultrasound-guided transbronchial needle aspiration: a randomized trial. Chest. 2004;**125**(1):322-325

[29] Tremblay A et al. A randomized controlled trial of standard vs endobronchial ultrasonography-guided transbronchial needle aspiration in patients with suspected sarcoidosis. Chest. 2009;**136**(2):340-346

[30] Huang H et al. Effectiveness of the benign and malignant diagnosis of mediastinal and hilar lymph nodes by endobronchial ultrasound elastography. Journal of Cancer. 2017;**8**(10):1843-1848

[31] Yasufuku K et al. Comparison of endobronchial ultrasound, positron emission tomography, and CT for lymph node staging of lung cancer. Chest. 2006;**130**(3):710-718

[32] Fu YF et al. Endobronchial ultrasound-guided versus computed tomography-guided biopsy for peripheral pulmonary lesions: A meta-analysis. The Clinical Respiratory Journal. 2021;**15**(1):3-10

[33] Zhi X et al. Diagnostic value of endobronchial ultrasound image

features: A specialized review. Endoscopic Ultrasound. 2021;**10**(1):3-18

[34] Wang Y et al. Diagnostic value of endobronchial ultrasound elastography in differentiating between benign and malignant hilar and mediastinal lymph nodes: a retrospective study. Quantitative Imaging in Medicine and Surgery. 2023;**13**(7):4648-4662

[35] Pan F et al. Utility and safety of endobronchial ultrasound-guided transbronchial needle aspiration in the diagnosis of isolated mediastinal masses. Journal of Multidisciplinary Healthcare. 2021;**14**:2047-2052

[36] Yan Y et al. Endobronchial ultrasound-guided transbronchial needle aspiration in patients with previously treated malignancies: diagnostic performance and predictive value. BMC Pulmonary Medicine. 2022;**22**(1):470

[37] Sanz-Santos J et al. Endobronchial ultrasound-guided transbronchial needle aspiration in the diagnosis of intrathoracic lymph node metastases from extrathoracic malignancies. Clinical & Experimental Metastasis. 2013;**30**(4):521-528

[38] Sun X et al. All-shot aspirations in endobronchial ultrasound-guided transbronchial needle aspiration (EBUS-TBNA) are associated with malignancy. Technology in Cancer Research & Treatment. 2023;**22**:15330338231169881

[39] Piro R et al. Safety and diagnostic accuracy of the transnasal approach for endobronchial ultrasound-guided transbronchial needle aspiration (EBUS-TBNA). Diagnostics (Basel). 2023;**13**(8):1405

[40] Dietrich CF, Jenssen C, Herth FJ. Endobronchial ultrasound elastography. Endoscopic Ultrasound. 2016;**5**(4):233-238

[41] Liu E, Bhutani MS, Sun S. Artificial intelligence: The new wave of innovation in EUS. Endoscopic Ultrasound. 2021;**10**(2):79-83

[42] Li J et al. Deep learning with convex probe endobronchial ultrasound multimodal imaging: A validated tool for automated intrathoracic lymph nodes diagnosis. Endoscopic Ultrasound. 2021;**10**(5):361-371

[43] Pathak V, Shepherd RW. The utility of EBUS-guided transbronchial forceps biopsy with or without an electrocautery knife for the diagnosis of mediastinal and hilar lymphadenopathy. Cureus. 2023;**15**(6):e40684

[44] Davri A et al. Deep learning for lung cancer diagnosis, prognosis and prediction using histological and cytological images: a systematic review. Cancers (Basel). 2023;**15**(15):3981

[45] Mohan A et al. Guidelines for endobronchial ultrasound-transbronchial needle aspiration (EBUS-TBNA): Joint Indian Chest Society (ICS)/Indian Association for Bronchology (IAB) recommendations. Lung India. 2023;**40**(4):368-400

Chapter 9

Lung Ultrasound Findings in COVID-19 Patients, Patients Recovered from COVID-19, and Patients without Lung Disorders

Susana González Suárez

Abstract

The use of lung ultrasound progressively increased during the SARS-CoV-2 pandemic. The presence of a pulmonary interstitial pattern, consolidations, and pleural alterations, with a typically bilateral, predominantly peripheral, and patchy distribution, are common ultrasound findings in COVID-19 pneumonia. In asymptomatic patients recovered from SARS-CoV-2 infection, residual lung lesions were also detected by ultrasound. Ultrasound lung abnormalities have also been found in asymptomatic patients without baseline lung pathology and with some systemic disease. Therefore, although lung ultrasonography has demonstrated comparable sensitivity to other imaging techniques, its specificity is limited, especially compared to CT for the diagnosis of COVID-19. The real impact of the lesions caused by SARS-CoV-2 must be determined by integrating the ultrasound pattern with the clinical context and laboratory results. Lung ultrasound has not only contributed to the early identification of COVID-19 but is also a very useful tool in making decisions about hospital admission and therapeutic strategies.

Keywords: lung ultrasound, COVID-19, SARS-CoV-2 infection, post-COVID-19 patients, interstitial involvement, pleural alterations, lung consolidations

1. Introduction

Severe acute respiratory syndrome coronavirus 2 (SARS-CoV-2) was first detected in China in late 2019 and spread rapidly around the world [1]. As of mid-September 2022, the SARS-CoV-2 pandemic infected more than 600 million people, causing more than 6 million deaths worldwide. Most countries experienced five consecutive waves of the disease in their epidemiological curve. The severity of the epidemics in each country varied depending on multiple factors, viral, patient-related, and social [2], including behavioral restrictions and disease mitigation strategies [3].

Overall, COVID-19 deaths increased during the first three waves but decreased significantly during the next two [4]. Furthermore, mortality increased in those patients with COVID-19 who required surgery, especially in the context of ischemic phenomena (of the intestine, lower extremities). Increased mortality and pulmonary complications were also observed in patients undergoing surgery within 6 weeks of SARS-CoV-2 diagnosis. Therefore, it was indicated that surgery should be delayed for at least 7 weeks after infection, and even longer in those patients with persistent symptoms [5].

The early diagnosis of COVID-19 during the pandemic made it possible to establish appropriate patient management and isolation measures. Early lung ultrasound (LU) demonstrated good discrimination between COVID-19 patients who could be treated on an outpatient basis and those who required hospital admission [6].

This review article addresses the important role of LU in patients with coronavirus disease 2019 (COVID-19), the pulmonary sequelae produced, and the interpretation of the real impact of these lesions for the diagnosis and management of the disease. A bibliographic search was carried out in the PubMed and Google Scholar databases using the keywords "lung ultrasound", "COVID-19".

2. SARS-CoV2 infection

2.1 Imaging modalities in COVID-19

Chest imaging has been recommended for patients with COVID-19 to inform decisions regarding hospital admission (inpatient ward versus intensive care unit [ICU], as well as the decision to discharge home) [7].

At the beginning of the pandemic, the use of chest X-ray and chest computed tomography (CT) was more established than the use of LU. Chest radiography shows lower sensitivity and similar specificity to chest CT [8]. Additionally, chest radiography requires fewer resources and involves less exposure to ionizing radiation compared to chest CT.

The use of LU has increased significantly during the pandemic, particularly in the evaluation of acute or critical patients, and in the early identification of patients with symptoms suggestive of COVID-19 [9]. Furthermore, the rapid spread of LU is since it is a noninvasive, rapid, and reproducible procedure, which can be performed at the point of care and requires nonionizing radiation, allowing for repeated examinations.

2.2 Equipment of LU

Ultrasound machines are potentially portable, require little maintenance, and run on a standard power supply and/or batteries. Any commercially available portable ultrasound device with standard B-mode imaging could be sufficient for transthoracic ultrasound [10]. Both convex probes and high-resolution linear probes can be used. Phased array cardiac probes can be used to perform integrated lung-heart analysis [11]. Low-frequency phased arrays and convex transducers allow visualization of deeper structures such as consolidations and pleural effusions [11]. High-frequency and high-definition linear transducers are preferable for imaging superficial structures and abnormalities (pleural irregularities, small amounts of pleural effusion, pneumothorax, and subpleural consolidations). Microconvex (small surface) probes provide a magnified view of the pleural surface and deeper penetration [12]. The use of low-frequency probes allows visualization of more B lines compared to high-frequency probes [11].

Advanced ultrasound modes with processing techniques, tissue harmonic imaging, and interpolation algorithms should be disabled for better visualization of lung artifacts [11].

On the other hand, two advanced applications can be used in LU, which are contrast-enhanced ultrasound (CEUS) and shear wave elastography (SWE) [13]. It is necessary to define the role of both applications in the study of COVID-19 pneumonia. CEUS can detect peripheral areas of low perfusion and infarction in patients with COVID-19 [14]. It uses sulfur hexafluoride microbubbles as a contrast medium to detect perfusion changes at the capillary level. Ultrasound elastography provides a quantitative assessment of lung tissue elasticity by analyzing wave propagation in tissues [15]. In case of interstitial pulmonary edema, SWE demonstrated a decrease in the velocity of lung surface waves [16].

Although lack of knowledge of the benefits of ultrasound and lack of qualified personnel are often the main barriers to the utilization of ultrasound, some studies showed that completing 25 expert-supervised LU exams could be sufficient for inexperienced staff to gain proficiency [17].

2.3 Standardization of LU and scoring system

The examination should be performed systematically to produce information that is as reliable as possible. The exam begins with probe selection and image setup and then continues by dividing the surface of the chest to cover all lung areas. For patients in a sitting position, 14 thoracic evaluations have been proposed (three posterior, two lateral, and two anterior for each hemithorax). However a more simplified protocol with acquisition of 12 or even 10 zones is often used in patients in the supine position. Three longitudinal lines are drawn (parasternal, anterior, and posterior axillary) that delimit the anterolateral and posterior areas and a mammary line delimits the upper and lower areas of each hemithorax, resulting in six exploration areas per hemithorax. Anterosuperior and anteroinferior areas of the thorax correspond to areas 1 and 2, respectively; laterosuperior and lateroinferior thoracic areas correspond to areas 3 and 4, respectively, and areas 5 and 6 correspond to the posterosuperior and posteroinferior thoracic areas, respectively. Regions that are not explored by LU are the dorsal lung segments of the upper lobes, located behind the scapula. The probe is placed perpendicular to the ribs at a depth of approximately 9–12 cm to the hemithorax, with the focus placed at the pleural level. A longitudinal examination should be performed to allow correct identification of the pleura within the intercostal space ("bat sign") (**Figure 1**).

For each lung zone, a quantification of the loss of aeration is carried out; the most common uses four progressive steps, according to an ultrasound pattern where a higher score indicates less aeration (**Figure 2**). The score "zero" includes the presence of lung sliding with A lines or one or two isolated B-lines; the pleural line is continuous and regular. The score "one" includes the presence of three or more B lines with an obvious distance indicating a moderate loss of lung aeration; the pleural line may be indented. In the score "two," the pleural line may be broken, with subpleural consolidations, and the presence of a large area of coalescent, crowded B lines indicates severe loss of lung aeration. Finally, a score of "three" points refers to a white, dense lung with a tissue-like pattern (consolidation) and is characterized by a complete loss of lung aeration. The total score obtained ranges between 0 and 36 (for 12 lung areas). It must be considered that not only the degree of lung deaeration must be determined but also the qualitative pattern and distribution of the alterations.

The extent and degree of loss of lung aeration were related to the clinical outcome of the disease and its progression, anticipating a worsening or improvement of clinical symptoms [18].

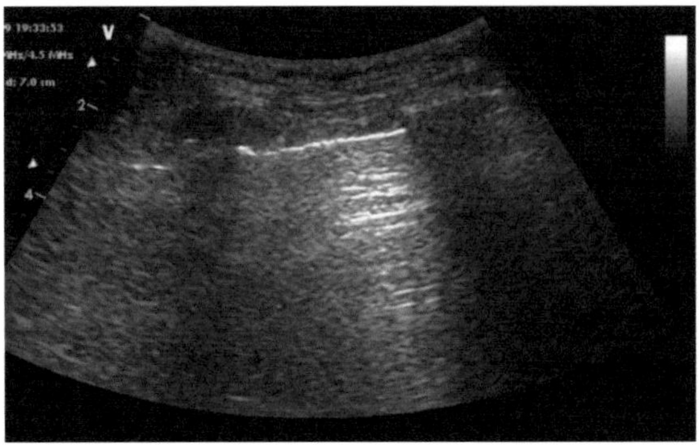

Figure 1.
The normal aerated lung ultrasound image. The outer periosteum of the ribs represents the bat´s wings, and the pleural line between two adjacent ribs represents the bat´s body. A-lines are horizontal lines below and parallel to the pleural line.

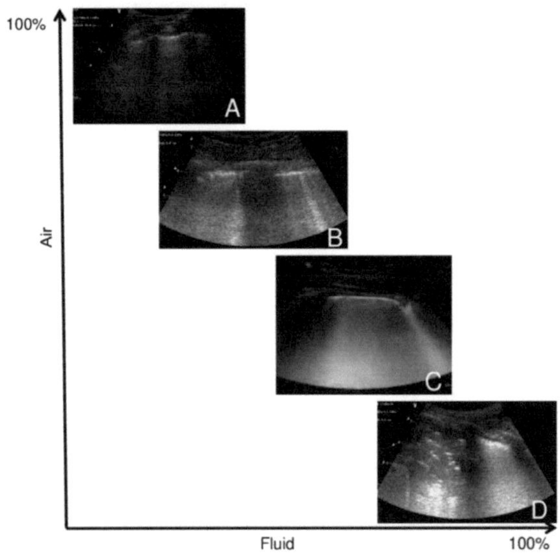

Figure 2.
Different degrees of lung aeration. From top to bottom, from more to less lung aeration. A: normal aeration, B: B-lines, C: confluent B-lines, D: consolidation.

On the other hand, in LU procedures, effective implementation of infection prevention and control measures is essential to prevent the spread of COVID-19 and ensure the safety of both patients and healthcare personnel. All exposed components of the machine and ultrasound probe must be disinfected. In addition, the use of portable equipment with a touch screen and single-use gel packs is recommended [19].

2.4 Clinical use of LU in COVID-19

2.4.1 Typical lung ultrasound findings in COVID-19

Lung ultrasound findings are mainly constituted by artifacts produced by air, lung parenchyma, chest wall, and pleura.

COVID-19 pneumonia is characterized by acute alveolar damage, typically bilateral, with peripheral and irregular distribution [8], and with clearly defined preserved areas [20]. When using LU, interstitial patterns (60–90% of patients), irregular pleural lines (59–78%), and subpleural consolidations (35–55%) are the most frequent findings in COVID-19 pneumonia [21–23]. At the beginning of the disease, pathological changes appear in the peripheral regions of the lungs, mainly in the lower lung lobes, progressing to the pulmonary center in more advanced stages. These peripheral findings allow LU to be a suitable tool for diagnosing COVID-19 pneumonia in the early stages. On ultrasound, focal B lines (affected segmental lung areas) appear as intermittent bright bands alternating with normal lung ("light beam" sign). Subsequently, focal B lines progress to confluent B lines with subpleural consolidations that may evolve into larger bilateral lung consolidations in multiple lung lobes and occasional air bronchogram. Typical LU findings in patients with COVID-19 pneumonia are shown in **Figure 3**.

2.4.1.1 Interstitial involvement

Lung ultrasound is predominantly artifact-based. Normal lung parenchyma cannot be visualized, and the pleura is seen as a hyperechoic line because LU is reflected from the pleura due to acoustic impedance mismatch at the air-tissue interface. In air-filled lungs or normal lungs, A lines can be seen. These lines are horizontal reverberation artifacts from the hyperechoic pleural line (**Figure 1**).

When the pulmonary interstitium is thickened (pulmonary edema, interstitial inflammation and/or infection, or pulmonary fibrosis), B lines appear replacing normal A lines. Thus, the ultrasound manifestation of interstitial syndrome consists

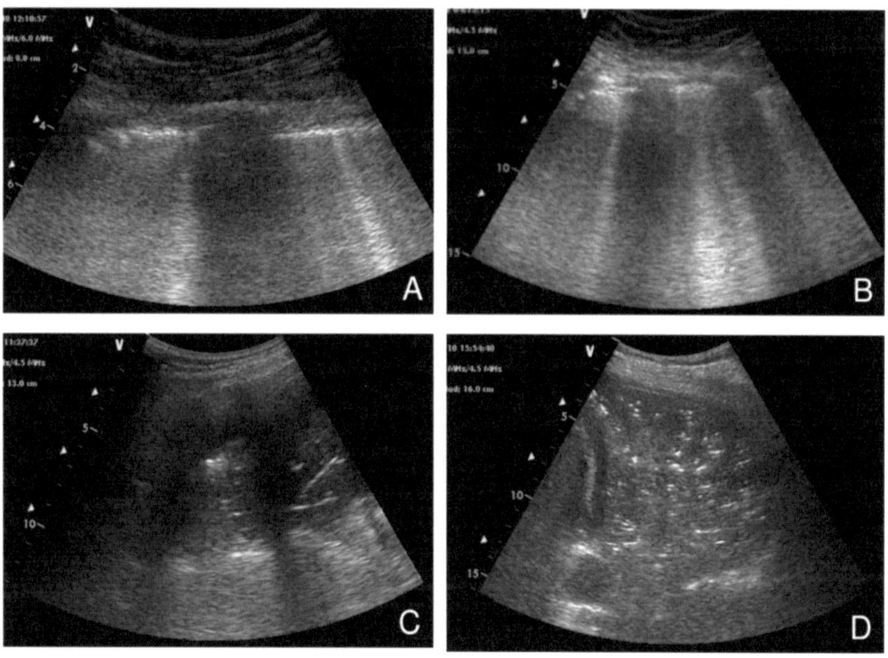

Figure 3.
Lung ultrasound findings in COVID-19. A and B: B-lines and alterations of the pleural line (thickened, fragmented and irregular). C and D: consolidations.

of the presence of three or more B lines between two ribs. These B-lines are vertical hyperechogenic artifacts, bilateral in distribution, that originate from the pleural line and usually reach the bottom of the screen and move synchronously with respiration. If the interstitial involvement is mild, a few scattered B-lines appear, while if the involvement is severe, the B lines are more frequent and convergent, giving a "white lung" pattern [24].

An artifact called a "light beam" has been described in patients with COVID-19 and could correspond to ground-glass opacities seen on CT during early active disease. This artifact consists of a large shining band-form B-line, arising from a portion of the normal pleural line, and appearing and disappearing frequently during the breathing.

2.4.1.2 Alterations of the pleural line

During respiration, sliding of the visceral and parietal pleura is visualized as a bright movement of the pleural line, known as pulmonary sliding. Lung ultrasound in COVID-19 shows a reduction or complete absence of normal pleural sliding in association with pleural alterations. The pleural line may be thickened, fragmented, or irregular in affected areas.

2.4.1.3 Lung consolidations

Consolidations occur when the air content in the lung tissue falls below 10% of normal lung aeration, altering the pleural line and eliminating the A-line artifact, allowing direct visualization of the lung parenchyma. Patients with COVID-19 pneumonia, consolidations appear mainly in the posterior and inferior regions of each hemithorax and may or may not present an air bronchogram and are usually multiple [25]. Lobar hepatization is not a frequent finding, however it usually appears in bacterial pneumonia.

A higher prevalence of pleural thickening and subpleural consolidations and a higher LU score were ultrasound findings predictive of clinical deterioration and mortality [26]. Also, these findings, along with the presence of multiple and coalescing B lines, were found in patients with refractory hypoxemia admitted to critical care units [27] and were associated with an increased need for mechanical ventilation and risk of death [28].

2.4.1.4 Pulmonary infarction and pulmonary embolism

Both venous and arterial thromboembolism are common in COVID-19, with rates of pulmonary embolism described between 1.6 and 36% in patients admitted to the ward and between 14 and 25% in hospitalized ICU patients [29]. Among the causes of the development of thromboembolism, hypoxia, excessive inflammation, diffuse intravascular coagulation, and immobilization have been described [30].

CT pulmonary angiography should be considered the imaging technique of choice in patients with suspected pulmonary thromboembolism, because it is difficult to diagnose using ultrasound [31]. Triangular or round pleural lesions seen on ultrasound examination, which characterize pulmonary embolism [32], are difficult to distinguish from other inflammatory abnormalities of COVID-19. In this case, CEUS may be useful to distinguish these lesions [33] along with the appearance of symptoms of dyspnea or respiratory failure or thrombi in the deep venous territory of the lower extremities.

2.4.2 Uncommon presentations of COVID-19

2.4.2.1 Pleural effusion

Pleural effusion is a rare finding in COVID-19 and usually arises from a concurrent condition (**Figure 4**) [34]. Ultrasound directly visualizes the pleural fluid, with simple effusions being visualized as anechoic fluid and more complex collections (malignant, chronic effusions, hemothorax, and empyema) with a more heterogeneous ultrasound appearance. It is a very reliable method in the detection, quantification, and monitoring of pleural effusion with better diagnostic accuracy than chest radiography [35]. Additionally, LU is useful for image-guided procedures such as pleural drainage or thoracentesis.

2.4.2.2 Pneumothorax

Spontaneous pneumothorax is rare, although it can be observed in severely ill patients with COVID-19 associated with a high mortality rate [36]. In pneumothorax, there is a separation between the visceral and parietal pleura, eliminating the normal sliding of the lung between these two layers. Thus, specific features of LU include the lack of lung sliding and the identification of a lung point (transition point between pneumothorax and normal lung), which is 100% specific for pneumothorax, and the absence of B lines.

Pneumothorax can also be identified on M-mode ultrasound. The M-mode LU pattern seen in a healthy lung is called the "seashore sign" because it represents the boundary between the stationary chest wall ("ocean") and the lung in motion ("sand"). The tissue superficial to the pleural line is visualized with horizontal lines, and below the pleural line, a granular or "sandy" pattern appears. In case of pneumothorax, the horizontal lines are uninterrupted, creating an image called "bar code sign" since the chest wall and the air deep in the pleura are stationary in pneumothorax (**Figure 5**).

Lung ultrasound for the detection and monitoring of pneumothorax is superior to chest radiography [37]. Lung ultrasound surpasses chest radiography in sensitivity

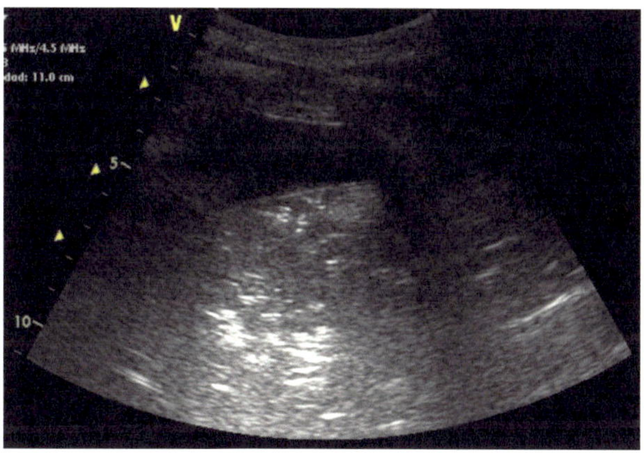

Figure 4.
Pleural effusion and consolidation.

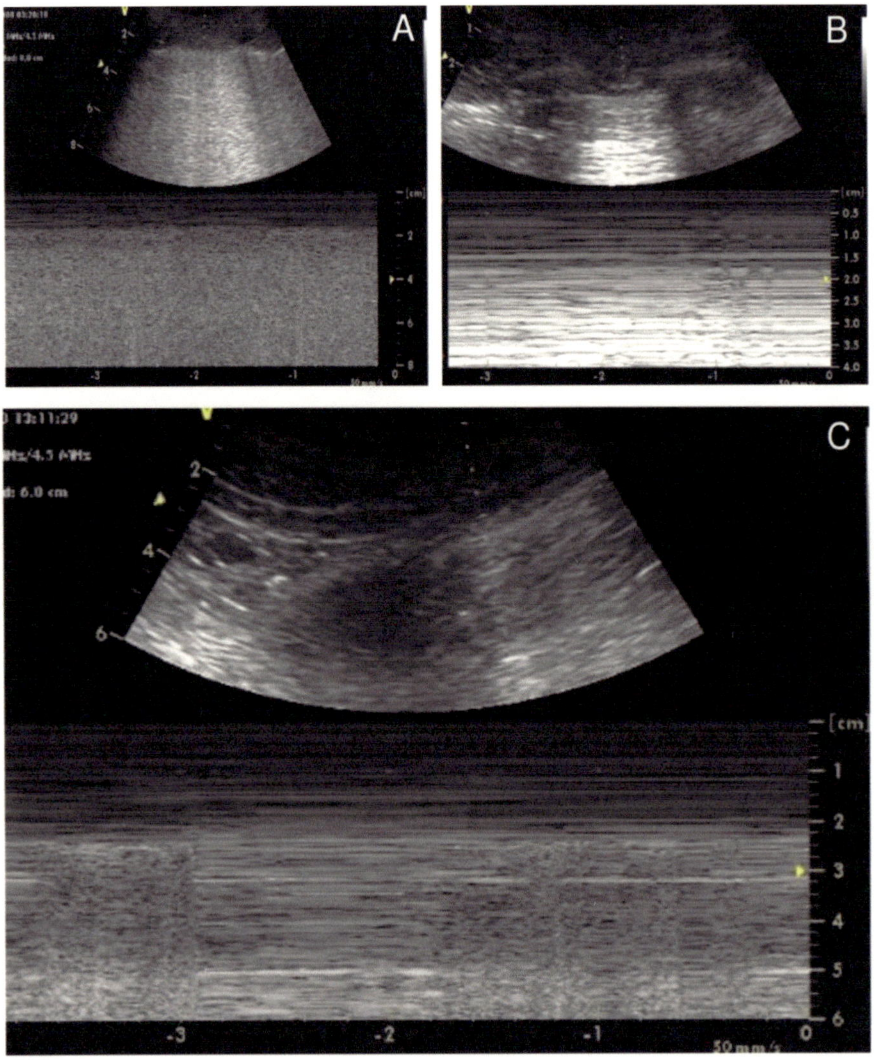

Figure 5.
A: the M-mode LU pattern seen in a healthy lung "seashore sign"; the tissue superficial to the pleural line is visualized with horizontal lines, and below the pleural line a granular or "sandy" pattern appears. B: M-mode LU pattern seen in pneumothorax "bar code sign"; below the pleural line horizontal lines appear. C: lung point M-mode (transition point between pneumothorax and normal lung); below the pleural line a granular pattern and horizontal lines appear.

for pneumothorax; thus, the sensitivity of ultrasound ranges between 78 and 90%, compared with 39–52% of chest radiography, while the specificity is >98% [37].

2.4.2.3 Diffuse and symmetrical B lines with a gravity-related

The presence of diffusely and symmetrically distributed B lines can be observed in pulmonary edema of cardiac origin, being rare in COVID-19 pneumonia. In these cases, making a good diagnosis includes performing an ultrasound of the heart, as well as the great vessels (inferior vena cava) and the deep veins of the lower extremities.

2.4.2.4 Subcutaneous emphysema

Subcutaneous emphysema is rare in patients with COVID-19 but may be found in patients with severe disease, undergoing mechanical ventilation, and associated with barotrauma, pneumothorax, or pneumomediastinum [38]. Subcutaneous gas bubbles produce many reverberation artifacts that prevent visualization of deeper structures such as the ribs or lungs.

2.5 Lung ultrasound in post-COVID-19 patients

Lung ultrasound was performed to determine the existence of residual lung lesions in asymptomatic patients who had suffered a SARS-CoV-2 infection [39]. The results showed that 24.27% of patients presented ≥3 B lines and 28% of patients presented pleural thickening. Furthermore, the pathological findings detected by lung ultrasound were associated with the severity of the infection suffered by SARS-CoV-2. Thus, patients with residual pleural thickening had a higher incidence of acute respiratory syndrome and pneumonia and required more vasoactive drugs and longer hospital stays during SARS-CoV-2 infection. Patients with ≥3 B lines required more days in an ICU and vasoactive drugs during SARS-CoV-2 infection. Other authors also demonstrated the presence of residual lung wounds due to SARS-CoV-2 infection [40].

But not all the ultrasound findings can be attributed to SARS-CoV-2 infection. The differential diagnosis with other viral lung infections is difficult since the LU findings (subpleural consolidations, white lung areas, abnormalities of the pleural lines and B lines) are similar in different viral pneumonias [41]. B lines are not specific to COVID-19 and can be observed in other pulmonary disorders with a reduced ratio between aerated and non-aerated lung spaces, and in interstitial lung disorders associated with pulmonary edema or fibrosis.

2.6 Diagnostic value of LU and CT in COVID-19

Computed tomography showed advantages in the diagnosis of COVID-19 at the time of hospital admission compared with LU (sensitivity and specificity for CT 90–95% and 43–70% vs. 94% and 7–30% for LU respectively) [42]. However, although CT was used in the early stages of the pandemic for the diagnosis of COVID-19 pneumonia, it required more resources and carried a risk of radiation exposure and nosocomial spread of infection. The American College of Radiology did not recommend it as a primary tool for the diagnosis of SARS-CoV-2 lung involvement [43]. The safety and accessibility of LU make it a widely accepted tool and an alternative to CT, with a good correlation between ultrasound findings and those obtained by CT [44]. Several studies found that LU in the diagnosis of interstitial syndrome is a very sensitive test [45]. Also, lung ultrasound was useful in excluding COVID-19 lung abnormalities, especially in patients with no medical history of cardiopulmonary disease (negative predictive value and sensitivity of 100%) [46], and in emergency departments in high-risk settings for SARS-CoV-2 prevalence. In any case, the low specificity of LU should be considered. To rule out COVID-19 pneumonia, the different patterns obtained from LU must be integrated with clinical and laboratory findings [47].

2.7 Lung ultrasound findings in patients without pulmonary pathology

Ultrasound lung abnormalities have also been found in asymptomatic patients without baseline lung pathology and with some systemic disease. In this context, 3.8% of patients presented pleural effusion of probable cardiogenic and/or renal etiology and 6.73% of patients presented B lines ≥3 [48]. ASA Physical Status Classification System is a tool that evaluates the patient's medical comorbidities prior to anesthesia. This classification system along with other factors (patient frailty, type, and severity of surgery) can predict perioperative risks. ASA grade I indicates a healthy patient with minimal risks and grade VI a brain-dead patient with organ donation plans. No pathological B lines were observed in ASA I patients, but ≥3 B lines could be observed in ASA II (mild systemic disease), ASA III (severe systemic disease), or ASA IV (severe health-threatening systemic disease) patients; the lung parenchyma, vasculature, pleural membranes, and respiratory muscles can be variably affected by systemic processes.

Other authors [49] also pointed out that it is possible to find B lines in volunteers without respiratory disease, but the "normal" number of B lines that can be observed in this context is unknown. It is possible that the existence of B lines in the laterobasal areas of the lung is a normal finding, and the appearance of ≥3 B lines has also been described in 34% of hospitalized patients [50].

3. Conclusion

Lung ultrasound contributes to the early identification of patients with COVID-19 and allows pulmonary monitoring of these patients, supporting therapeutic decisions. It offers different advantages such as avoiding exposure to ionizing radiation, and can be repeated on multiple occasions, especially in pregnant women and children. In addition, it can be performed in different clinical settings (including outpatient settings) when using portable devices.

A well-known limitation of LU is that it is highly operator-dependent and requires a standardized approach. Furthermore, although B-lines and pleural irregularities constitute the so-called ultrasound interstitial syndrome, we must consider that it is not specific and there may be ultrasound alterations in patients without lung pathology. The interpretation of the ultrasound pattern is always linked to the need to integrate all the available information considering the clinical context and laboratory results. Finally, although LU has shown comparable sensitivity to other imaging techniques, its specificity is limited, especially compared to CT for the diagnosis of COVID-19. However, the safety and accessibility of LU make it a widely accepted tool and an alternative to CT, with a good correlation between ultrasound findings and those obtained by CT.

Acknowledgements

I thank Lourdes Pérez Rodríguez for her teachings in lung ultrasound.

Conflict of interest

The author declares no conflict of interest.

Author details

Susana González Suárez[1,2]

1 Department of Surgery Autonomous University of Barcelona, Barcelona, Spain

2 Department of Anesthesiology, University Hospital Vall d'Hebron, Barcelona, Spain

*Address all correspondence to: susana.gonzalez@uab.cat;
susana.gonzalez@vallhebron.cat

References

[1] World Health Organization. Timeline: WHO's COVID-19 response 2021. Available from: https://www.who.int/emergencies/diseases/novel-coronavirus-2019/interactive-timeline

[2] Rosenbaum L. Facing Covid-19 in Italy: Ethics, logistics, and therapeutics on the epidemic's front line. The New England Journal of Medicine. 2020;**382**(20):1873-1875. DOI: 10.1056/NEJMp2005492

[3] Salyer SJ, Maeda J, Sembuche S, Kebede Y, Tshangela A, Moussif M, et al. The first and second waves of the COVID-19 pandemic in Africa: A cross sectional study. Lancet. 2021;**397**:1265-1275. DOI: 10.1016/S0140-6736(21)00632-2

[4] Madahar P, Wunsch H, Jha P, Slutsky AS, Brodie D. Trends in COVID-19-related in-hospital mortality: Lessons learned from nationwide samples. The Lancet Respiratory Medicine. 2021;**9**(4):322-324. DOI: 10.1016/S2213-2600(21)00080-1

[5] Nepogodiev D et al. COVIDSurg collaborative. Timing of surgery following SARS-CoV-2 infection: An international prospective cohort study. Anaesthesia. 2021;**76**(6):748-758. DOI: 10.11116anae.15458

[6] Brahier T, Meuwly JY, Pantet O, Brochu MJ, Donnet HG, Hartley MA, et al. Lung ultrasonography for risk stratification in patients with COVID-19: A prospective observational cohort study. Clinical Infectious Diseases. 2021;**73**(11):e4189-e4196. DOI: 10.1093/cid/ciaa1408

[7] Mozafari A, Miladinia M, Sabri A, Movaseghi F, Gholamzadeh B. The challenge of deciding between home-discharge versus hospitalization in COVID-19 patients: The role of initial imaging and clinic laboratory data. Clinical Epidemiology and Global Health. 2021;**10**:100673. DOI: 10.1016/j.cegh.2020.11.006

[8] Borakati A, Perera A, Johnson J, Sood T. Diagnostic accuracy of X-ray versus CT in COVID-19: A propensity-matched database study. BMJ Open. 2020;**10**(11):e042946. DOI: 10.1136/bmjopen-2020-042946

[9] Vetrugno L, Mojoli F, Boero E, Berchialla P, Bignami EG, Orso D, et al. Level of diffusion and training of lung ultrasound during the COVID-19 pandemic—A national online Italian survey (ITALUS) from the lung ultrasound working group of the Italian Society of Anesthesia, Analgesia, Resuscitation, and Intensive Care (SIAARTI). Ultraschall in der Medizin. 2022;**43**(5):464-472. DOI: 10.1055/a-1634-4710

[10] Güney T, Gürsel G, Özdemir U, Tekin O, Cimen M, Mamadova A, et al. Are pocket sized ultrasound devices sufficient in the evaluation of lung ultrasound patterns and aeration scoring in pulmonary ICU patients? Journal of Clinical Monitoring and Computing. 2021;**35**:1491-1499. DOI: 10.1007/s10877-020-00617-5

[11] Dietrich CF, Mathis G, Blaivas M, Volpicelli G, Seibel A, Wasti D, et al. Lung B-line artefacts and their use. Journal of Thoracic Disease. 2016;**8**(6):1356-1365. DOI: 10.21037/jtd.2016.04.55

[12] Lichtenstein D, Mézière G, Biderman P, Gepner A, Barré O. The

comet-tail artefact. An ultrasound sign of alveolar-interstitial syndrome. American Journal of Respiratory and Critical Care Medicine. 1997;**156**(5):1640-1646. DOI: 10.1164/ajrccm.1556.5.96-07096

[13] Tee A, Wong A, Yusuf GT, Rao D, Sidhu PS. Contrast-enhanced ultrasound (CEUS) of the lung reveals multiple areas of microthrombi in a COVID-19 patient. Intensive Care Medicine. 2020;**46**(8):1660-1662. DOI: 10.1007/s00134-020-06085-4

[14] Yusuf GT, Wong A, Rao D, Tee A, Fang C, Sidhu PS. The use of contrast-enhanced ultrasound in COVID-19 lung imaging. Journal of Ultrasound. 2022;**25**(2):319-323. DOI: 10.1007/s40477-020-00517-z

[15] Zhou B, Yang X, Zhang X, Curran WJ, Liu T. Ultrasound elastography for lung disease assessment. IEEE Transactions on Ultrasonics, Ferroelectrics, and Frequency Control. 2020;**67**(11):2249-2257. DOI: 10.1109/TUFFC.2020.3026536

[16] Zhang X, Zhou B, Osborn T, Bartholmai B, Kalra S. Lung ultrasound surface wave elastography for assessing interstitial lung disease. IEEE Transactions on Biomedical Engineering. 2019;**66**(5):1346-1352. DOI: 10.1109/TBME.2018.2872907

[17] Rouby JJ, Arbelot C, Gao Y, Zhang M, Lv J, An Y, et al. Training for lung ultrasound score measurement in critically ill patients. American Journal of Respiratory and Critical Care Medicine. 2018;**198**(3):398-401. DOI: 10.1164/rccm.201802-0227LE

[18] Vetrugno L, Sala A, Orso D, Meroi F, Fabbro S, Boero E, et al. Lung ultrasound signs and their correlation with clinical symptoms in COVID-19 pregnant women: The 'PINK-CO' observational study. Frontiers in Medicine. 2022;**8**:768261. DOI: 10.3389/fmed.2021.768261

[19] Kim DJ, Jelic T, Woo MY, Heslop C, Olszynski P. Just the facts: Recommendations on point-of-care ultrasound use and machine infection control during the coronavirus disease 2019 pandemic. CJEM. 2020;**22**(4):445-449. DOI: 10.1017/cem.2020.364

[20] Sorlini C, Femia M, Nattino G, Bellone P, Gesu E, Francione P, et al. The role of lung ultrasound as a frontline diagnostic tool in the era of COVID-19 outbreak. Internal and Emergency Medicine. 2021;**16**(3):749-756. DOI: 10.1007/s11739-020-02524-8

[21] Sahu AK, Mathew R, Bhoi S, Sinha TP, Nayer J, Aggarwal P, et al. Lung sonographic findings in COVID-19 patients. The American Journal of Emergency Medicine. 2021;**45**:324-328. DOI: 10.1016/j.ajem.2020.08.080

[22] Caroselli C, Blaivas M, Marcosignori M, Cheng YT, Falzetti S, Mariz J, et al. Early lung ultrasound findings in patients with COVID-19 pneumonia: A retrospective multicenter study of 479 patients. Journal of Ultrasound in Medicine. 2022;**41**:2547-2556. DOI: 10.1002/jum.15944

[23] Yasukawa K, Minami T, Boulware DR, Shimada A, Fischer EA, et al. Point-of-care lung ultrasound for COVID-19: Findings and prognostic implications from 105 consecutive patients. Journal of Intensive Care Medicine. 2021;**36**:334-342. DOI: 10.1177/0885066620988831

[24] Millington SJ, Koenig S, Mayo P, Volpicelli G. Lung ultrasound for patients with coronavirus disease 2019 pulmonary disease. Chest. 2021;**159**(1):205-211. DOI: 10.1016/j.chest.2020.08.2054

[25] Xing C, Li Q, Du H, Kang W, Lian J, Yuan L. Lung ultrasound findings in patients with COVID-19 pneumonia. Critical Care. 2020;**24**(1):174. DOI: 10.1186/s13054-020-02876-9

[26] Lichter Y, Topilsky Y, Taieb P, Banai A, Hochstadt A, Merdler L, et al. Lung ultrasound predicts clinical course and outcomes in COVID-19 patients. Intensive Care Medicine. 2020;**46**(10):1873-1883. DOI: 10.1007/s00134-020-06212-1

[27] Zhao L, Yu K, Zhao Q, Tian R, Xie H, Xie L, et al. Lung ultrasound score in evaluating the severity of coronavirus disease 2019 (COVID-19) pneumonia. Ultrasound in Medicine & Biology. 2020;**46**(11):2938-2944. DOI: 10.1016/j.ultrasmedbio.2020.07.024

[28] Gil-Rodríguez J, Pérez de Rojas J, Aranda-Laserna P, Benavente-Fernández A, Martos-Ruiz M, Peregrina-Rivas JA, et al. Ultrasound findings of lung ultrasonography in COVID-19: A systematic review. European Journal of Radiology. 2022;**148**:110156. DOI: 10.1016/j.ejrad.2022.110156

[29] Rodigiani C, Iapichino G, Carenzo L, Cecconi MI, Ferrazzi P, Sebastian T, et al. Venous and arterial thromboembolic complications in COVID-19 patients admitted to an academic hospital in Milan, Italy. Thrombosis Research. 2020;**191**:9-14. DOI: 10.1016/j.thromres.2020.04.024

[30] Klok FA, Kruip MJHA, van der Meer NJM, Arbous MS, Gommers DAMPJ, Kant KM, et al. Incidence of thrombotic complications in critically ill ICU patients with COVID-19. Thrombosis Research. 2020;**191**:145-147. DOI: 10.1016/j.thromres.2020.04.013

[31] Rubin GD, Ryerson CJ, Haramati LB, Sverzellati N, Kanne JP, Raoof S, et al. The role of chest imaging in patient management during the COVID-19 pandemic: A multinational consensus statement from the Fleischner society. Chest. 2020;**158**(1):106-116. DOI: 10.1016/j.chest.2020.04.003

[32] Mathis G, Blank W, Reissig A, Lechleitner P, Reuss J, Schuler A, et al. Thoracic ultrasound for diagnosing pulmonary embolism: A prospective multicenter study of 352 patients. Chest. 2005;**128**(3):1531-1538. DOI: 10.1378/chest.128.3.1531

[33] Bartelt S, Trenker C, Görg C, Neesse A. Contrast-enhanced ultrasound of embolic consolidations in patients with pulmonary embolism: A pilot study. Journal of Clinical Ultrasound. 2016;**44**(3):129-135. DOI: 10.1002/jcu.22313

[34] Casella F, Barchiesi M, Leidi F, Russo G, Casazza G, Valerio G, et al. Lung ultrasonography: A prognostic tool in non-ICU hospitalized patients with COVID-19 pneumonia. European Journal of Internal Medicine. 2021;**85**:34-40. DOI: 10.1016/j.ejim.2020.12.012

[35] Kocijancic I, Vidmar K, Ivanovi-Herceg Z. Chest sonography versus lateral decubitus radiography in the diagnosis of small pleural effusions. Journal of Clinical Ultrasound. 2003;**31**(2):69-74. DOI: 10.1002/jcu.10141

[36] Wang XH, Duan J, Han X, Liu X, Zhou J, Wang X, et al. High incidence and mortality of pneumothorax in critically ill patients with COVID-19. Heart & Lung. 2021;**50**(1):37-43. DOI: 10.1016/j.hrtlng.2020.10.002

[37] Alrajhi K, Woo MY, Vaillancourt C. Test characteristics of ultrasonography for the detection of pneumothorax: A systematic review and meta-analysis. Chest. 2012;**141**(3):703-708. DOI: 10.1378/chest.11-0131

[38] Manna S, Maron SZ, Cedillo MA, Voutsinas N, Toussie D, Finkelstein M, et al. Spontaneous subcutaneous emphysema and pneumomediastinum in non-intubated patients with COVID-19. Clinical Imaging. 2020;**67**:207-213. DOI: 10.1016/j.clinimag.2020.08.013

[39] González-Suárez S, Bárbara A, Caicedo M, Aznar M. Detection of residual pulmonary alterations with lung ultrasound and effects on postoperative pulmonary complications for patients with asymptomatic SARS-CoV-2 infection undergoing surgery. BMC Anesthesiology. 2022;**22**(1):186. DOI: 10.1186/s12871-022-01715-4

[40] Abdulrahman A, Abuhamdah M, Balhamar A, Faqihi F, Nasim N, Ahmad S, et al. Residual lung injury in patients recovering from COVID-19 critical illness: A prospective longitudinal point-of-care lung ultrasound study. Journal of Ultrasound in Medicine. 2020;**40**(9):1823-1838. DOI: 10.1002/jum.15563

[41] Vollmer I. Thoracic ultrasound in viral infections. Radiología. 2021;**63**(3):252-257. DOI: 10.1016/j.rx.2020.12.005

[42] Colombi D, Petrini M, Maffi G, Villani G, Bodini F, Morelli N, et al. Comparison of admission chest computed tomography and lung ultrasound performance for diagnosis of COVID-19 pneumonia in populations with different disease prevalence. European Journal of Radiology. 2020;**133**:109344. DOI: 10.1016/j.ejrad.2020.109344

[43] ACR Recommendations for the use of Chest Radiography and Computed Tomograghy (CT) for Suspected COVID-19 Infection. 2020. Available from: https://www.acr.org/Advocacy-and-Economics/ACR-Position-Statements/Recommendations-for-Chest-Radiography-and-CT-for-Suspected-COVID19-Infection

[44] Tung-Chen Y, Martí de la Gracia M, Díez-Tascón A, Alonso-González R, Agudo-Fernández S, Parra-Gordo ML. Correlation between chest computed tomography and lung ultrasound in patients with coronavirus disease. Ultrasound in Medicine & Biology. 2020;**46**:2918-2926. DOI: 10.1016/j.ultrasmedbio.2020.07.003

[45] Laursen CB, Clive A, Hallifax R, Pietersen PI, Asciak R, Davidsen JR, et al. European respiratory society statement on thoracic ultrasound. The European Respiratory Journal. 2021;**57**(3):2001519. DOI: 10.1183/13993003.01519-2020

[46] Haak SL, Renken IJ, Jager LC, Lameijer H, Van der Kolk BYM. Diagnostic accuracy of point-of-care lung ultrasound in COVID-19. Emergency Medicine Journal. 2021;**38**:94-99. DOI:10.1136/emermed-2020-210125

[47] Volpicelli G, Gargani L, Perlini S, Spinelli S, Barbieri G, Lanotte A, et al. Lung ultrasound for the early diagnosis of COVID-19 pneumonia: An international multicenter study. Intensive Care Medicine. 2021;**47**(4):444-454. DOI: 10.1007/s00134-021-06373-7

[48] González-Suárez S, Aznar M, Bárbara A, Caicedo M, Peláez EM, Blázquez J, et al. Lung ultrasound abnormalities in patients without pulmonary pathology prior to surgery. Anesthesia and Pain Medicine. 2023;**13**(3):e137900. DOI: 10.5812/aapm-137900

[49] Zoneff ER, Baker K, Sweeny A, Keijzers G, Sanderson J, Watkins S. The prevalence of lung surface abnormalities in a healthy population as detected by a screening lung ultrasound protocol:

Comparison between young and older volunteers. Australasian Journal of Ultrasound in Medicine. 2019;**22**(2): 129-137. DOI: 10.1002/ajum.12124

[50] Volpicelli G, Caramello V, Cardinale L, Mussa A, Bar F, Frascisco MF. Detection of sonographic B-lines in patients with normal lung or radiographic alveolar consolidation. Medical Science Monitor. 2008;**14**(3):CR122-8

Chapter 10

Lung Ultrasound in the Treatment of Pneumonia

Valentin Stoilov, Georgi Pavlov and Aleksandrina Topalova-Shishmanova

Abstract

Respiratory diseases have continuously been in the top five causes of death globally for the past century. Prompt and adequate diagnosis relies on imaging studies with high diagnostic accuracy. Chest radiography and computed tomography have been the method of choice. Lung ultrasound is a versatile new alternative that can be performed at the bedside, repeated when needed, and is not associated with radiation exposure. It can be used not only for diagnosis but also to distinguish between etiological reasons, monitor the progression of the disease, and guide respiratory therapy, mechanical ventilation, and the weaning process. Outpatients can also benefit from fast and accurate examination with simultaneous results. Training in lung ultrasound can be achieved through a variety of methods, each with its own strengths.

Keywords: lung ultrasound, thoracic sonography, BLUE protocol, consolidation, air bronchogram, recruitment, respiratory therapy, mechanical ventilation, weaning, simulation training

1. Introduction

According to the World Health Organization, pneumonia is the leading cause of infectious disease-related morbidity and mortality worldwide. Compromising normal gas exchange in the lungs can result in severe hypoxemia and tissue hypoxia, as well as sepsis, septic shock, and multiorgan dysfunction syndrome. Therefore, early diagnosis and prompt and adequate treatment of pneumonia could significantly improve outcomes.

Along with clinical presentation and laboratory results, imaging studies play a pivotal role in a convincing diagnosis of pneumonia by proving a new-onset pulmonary infiltrate. At present chest radiography is the most commonly used study in many settings to provide the information, while computed tomography is considered the golden standard. However, some limitations exist for their use.

Advances in diagnostic radiology provide a non-invasive, non-radiating, simple tool to improve the diagnosis of pneumonia through point-of-care lung ultrasound (LUS). The use of LUS has gained popularity in emergency departments (ED) and intensive care units (ICU) in the last decade and has become more widely accepted as a potentially useful diagnostic approach. LUS has recently been shown to be highly effective in the diagnosis, severity assessment, and progression monitoring of pneumonia. The aim of this chapter is to provide essential information on the application of LUS in the management of pneumonia.

2. Imaging studies

Lung diseases are one of the most commonly found pathologies in emergency and intensive care units. Even if not the primary reason for hospitalization, most patients are at risk of developing pneumonia during their stay. Acute respiratory failure affects up to 50% of ICU patients and has mortality as high as 30% [1]. The diagnosis, monitoring of the progression of the disease, and follow-up depend on imaging studies.

2.1 Chest radiography

X-ray is often done on a routine basis in critically ill patients in an effort to find a pathology that would otherwise be missed. Even protocols suggest daily chest radiography (CXR) for patients with acute respiratory and cardiac diseases and those on mechanical ventilation [2]. After a thorough investigation, this practice has been proven futile. It is expected that the findings from routine X-rays would be negligible and would not lead to significant changes in the clinical management of most critically ill patients [3].

The pitfalls of radiography include the overlay of soft tissues, bones, and lung parenchyma, invasive devices, endotracheal tubes, nasogastric tubes, thoracic drainage, catheters, etc. Patients who are uncooperative or unconscious are difficult to position, and technical equipment requires space, which is often scarce in emergency and intensive care departments. CXR is commonly acquired in the anteroposterior aspect, with rare cases of having another one in the lateral aspect [4]. This means that physicians manage a three-dimensional pathology based on a two-dimensional image.

It is necessary to highlight the fact that radiography comes with radiation exposure. Repeated X-rays lead to the accumulation of higher radiation doses. This is a problem, especially in the pediatric population. Based on studies showing an increased risk of developing cancer after exposure, the WHO has developed guidelines on performing imaging studies [5, 6].

In the early stages of pneumonia and in cases of small consolidation, an x-ray can be negative [7]. According to current studies, chest radiography is suboptimal in diagnosing lower respiratory tract infections with sensitivity of 75% (95% CI 54–88%) and specificity of 75% (95% CI 42–92%) [8].

2.2 Computed tomography

The golden standard in lung imaging is acquiring a detailed cross-sectional examination of the thoracic cavity and its organs with computed tomography (CT). However not all hospitals have access to CT. Transporting the patient to the imaging department is associated with increased risk when it comes to critically ill patients. Studies show up to 45% risk of adverse events during patient transport [9]. For unstable patients it is unreasonable to even consider transferring them for CT. Patients with lung pathology often require more than one imaging study. This is associated with increased cumulative doses and radiation-induced cancer risk [10].

2.3 Lung ultrasound

The need for a method that can be performed at the bedside of the patient without the need for transportation, repeated when necessary, and lacking radiation exposure has led to the development of thoracic sonography. Lung ultrasound (LUS) has been used to evaluate pleural effusion for over five decades [11]. After the publication of the BLUE protocol by Lichtenstein and colleagues, the method has gained more popularity in diagnosing and distinguishing different lung pathologies [12].

Lung ultrasound is not without its flaws. It cannot be performed in areas with dressings or subcutaneous emphysema. Acquiring the image of patients with obesity can be difficult, if not impossible. The uncooperative patient is another challenge. Performing examinations on the posterior regions requires placing the patient in a lateral or prone position, which cannot be done in some cases. With the continuing advances in the field, new artifacts are being found, and ongoing education is required. LUS is a highly operator-dependent skill that requires training.

3. Equipment

A vast choice of modern ultrasound machines exists. Most are sophisticated, with a lot of different filters, software enhancements, and options to choose from. Sizes range from small hand-held devices to bulky, heavy machines that hold multiple transducers. Having an ultrasound that can fit between beds and be transferred with ease is highly appreciated in emergency and intensive care departments. Ultrasound machines with smooth surfaces that can be properly cleaned are preferred due to the risk of cross-contamination between patients. LUS can be performed with different transducers. Three types show advantages over the others. Microconvex transducers have a small footprint that can be conveniently placed in the intercostal space. Convex transducers provide the ability to visualize larger pathologies with ease. Linear transducers can produce high-resolution and detailed images of the area around the pleural line.

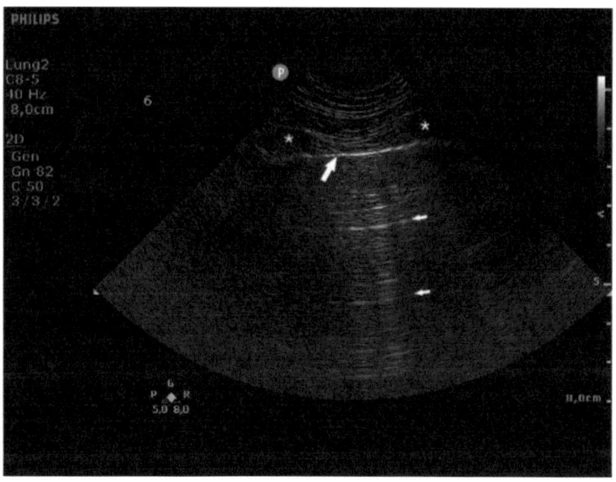

Figure 1.
*Pleural line; * - ribs, arrow - pleural line, small arrows – A-lines.*

3.1 Settings

Lung ultrasound is based on the interpretation of artifacts. With that in mind, we should note that there is no need for the image to be optimized, which also usually creates some lag between the movement of the operator's hand and the corresponding image. Turning on image harmonics or using software to smooth out the picture can even have a detrimental effect on interpretation. Since the study is done on anterior, lateral and posterior regions of the thorax the advisory depth in adults is around 10 cm (4inch). The gain of the image should be such that the pleural line stands out as hyperechoic from the rest of the structures, which should be darker (**Figure 1**).

4. Examination

4.1 Lung regions

For the purpose of organization and reproducibility of the gathered information, each hemithorax is divided into six regions. The parasternal, anterior, and posterior axillary line and paravertebral line distinguish anterior, lateral, and posterior zones, each divided into two by a perpendicular line at the fourth intercostal space (**Figure 2**). The corresponding regions in the left hemithorax are 5 and 6 in the anterior, 7 and 8 in the lateral, and the left upper and lower posterior in the posterior zone. There are studies that divide each hemithorax into 18 smaller areas, with a total of 36 for both lungs. It is important that no matter the number of regions, the gathering of information is consistent so that it can be easily explained, compared, and reproduced.

For patients who are cooperative, the examination can be done in both sitting and supine positions. The unconscious ICU patients, however, can be a challenge. Examining the lateral and posterior regions requires that someone lifts and keeps the ipsilateral arm out of the zones of interest. The posterior regions can be assessed by shifting the patient's position by 15^0 to the opposite side and setting the probe tightly against the mattress. Another option is to have the patient in a prone position, but this requires more staff to flip the patient and is a potential source of complications for the critically ill on mechanical ventilation.

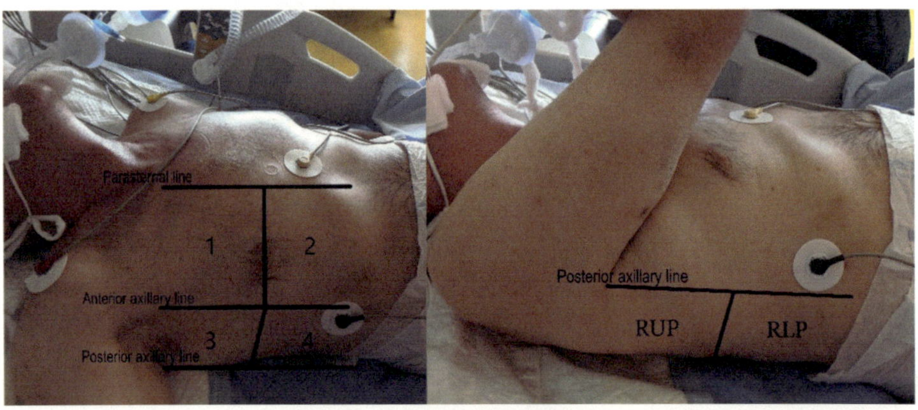

Figure 2.
Lung regions, RUP – right upper posterior, RLP - right lower posterior.

4.2 Lung ultrasound artifacts

There are 12 main artifacts on which pulmonary echography is based: Pleural line, A-lines, Lung sliding, Quad sign, Sinusoid sign, Shred sign, Tissue-like sign, Lung rockets, Abolished lung sliding, Lung point, Air bronchogram, Lung pulse.

Physiologically, the visceral and parietal pleura are in constant contact with only a minimal amount of fluid between them. Sonographically, they make up the pleural line which is the main hyperechoic horizontal artifact. In most adults, it is situated approximately a centimeter below the rib line. The A-lines are reverberations of the pleural line, which are also hyperechoic, have the same curvature, and are placed between themselves and the pleural line in distance equal to the one between the skin and the pleural line (**Figure 1**).

Lung sliding is a fundamental phenomenon in the BLUE protocol. It is created by the constant movement of the visceral pleura on top of the parietal and is seen as a shining phenomenon in ultrasonography. In physiological conditions in M-mode, the space below the pleural line, the Merlin space, resembles a grainy image and is called a seashore sign. In cases of single lung ventilation atelectasis or massive consolidation, the pulmonary parenchyma conveys the heart beats leading to the so-called Lung pulse phenomenon Video 1, https://youtu.be/TS0AU7CUjJU.

The B-lines are comet-tail artifacts that arise from the pleural line, and they are hyperechoic like the pleural line, move with lung sliding, are well-defined, erase the A-lines, and reach the end of the image (**Figure 3**) [13]. B-lines are considered as pathology and interstitial syndrome when there are three or more in the same inter-coastal space and resemble lung rockets.

The absence of lung sliding on its own has low sensitivity and specificity in ruling out pneumothorax. It can be seen in pleural adhesions, severe pneumonia with consolidation, acute respiratory distress syndrome (ARDS), massive fibrosis, and other pathologies. The combination of the absence of sliding and B-lines increases the specificity. The lung point is a pathognomonic ultrasound sign of pneumothorax. This is the place where the parietal and the visceral pleura make contact in cases of partial pneumothorax. It is a combination of the stratosphere and seashore sign in M-mode (**Figure 4**), Video 2, https://youtu.be/1xCFjCHCfD4.

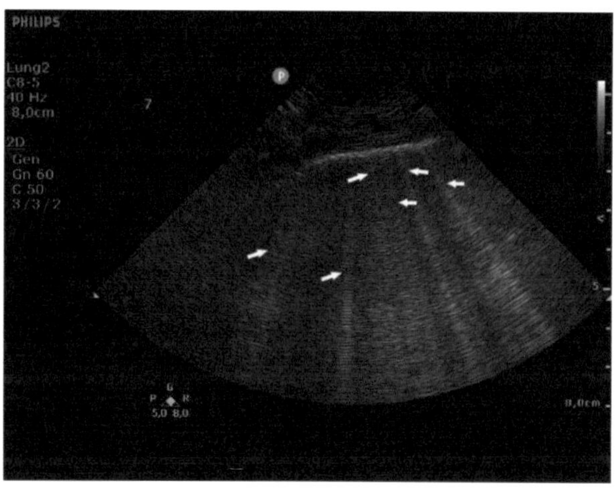

Figure 3.
B-lines.

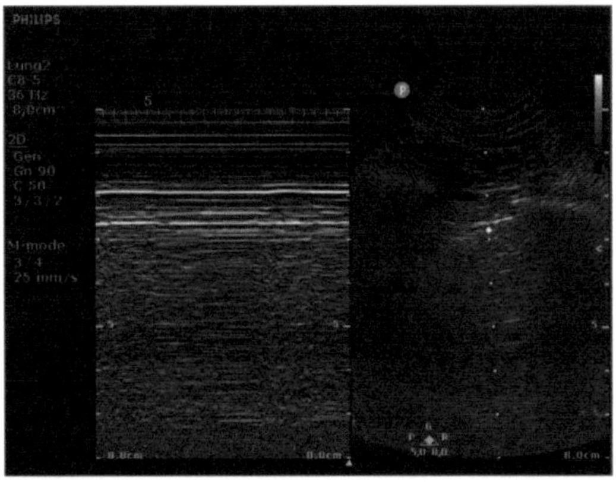

Figure 4.
Lung point.

From a pathophysiological point of view, the reasons that lead to pleural effusion can cause pulmonary consolidation as well. Acute pulmonary edema, pneumonia, and pulmonary embolism are examples of the two pathologies coexisting. Pleural effusions are positioned almost always in the dependent regions, while consolidations can be observed in non-dependent regions, such as in cases of bacterial pneumonia. On sonography, the pleural effusion is located between the borders of the upper and lower ribs, as well as the visceral and parietal pleura, and is called the Quad sign. Due to the movement of the lung, the effusion compresses and decompresses during the respiratory cycle. In M-mode, it is called the Sinusoid sign (**Figure 5**).

Pulmonary consolidation is a pathology in which the alveoli are filled with fluid – transudate, exudate, blood, or aspirate. The reasons can be hydrostatic, infectious, and mechanical. Consolidations can be seen in pulmonary edema, pneumonia, ARDS, pulmonary embolism, and tumors. The Shred sign is a consolidation with distinct borders from the still-aerated lung parenchyma. In massive consolidation, when the pathology passes the border of the interlobular septa and becomes translobar the image resembles liver tissue and is called tissue-like sign (**Figure 6**).

The BLUE protocol is based on combining the ultrasound artifacts into profiles and reaching a clinical decision [14]. In four cases, the end-point is pneumonia.

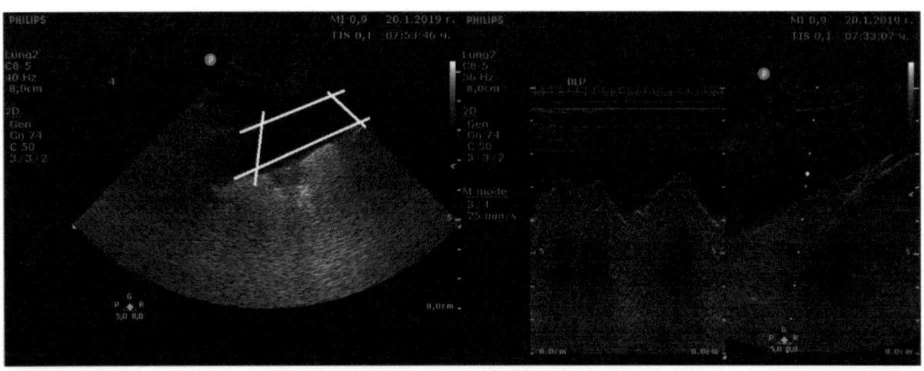

Figure 5.
Quad sign and Sinusoid sign.

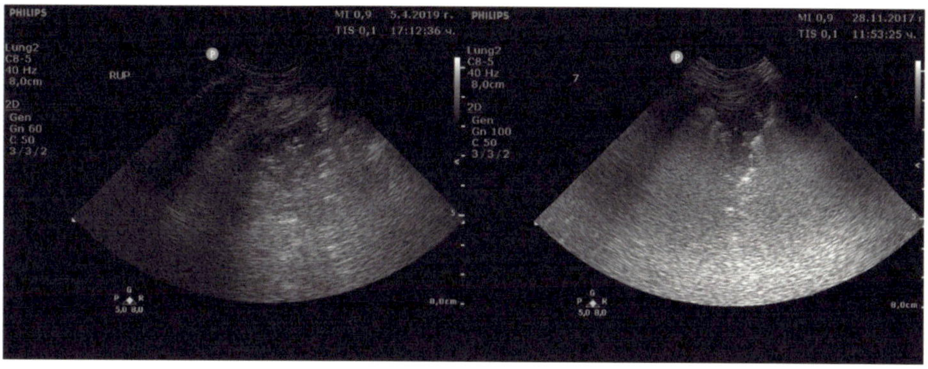

Figure 6.
Tissue-like sign and Shred sign.

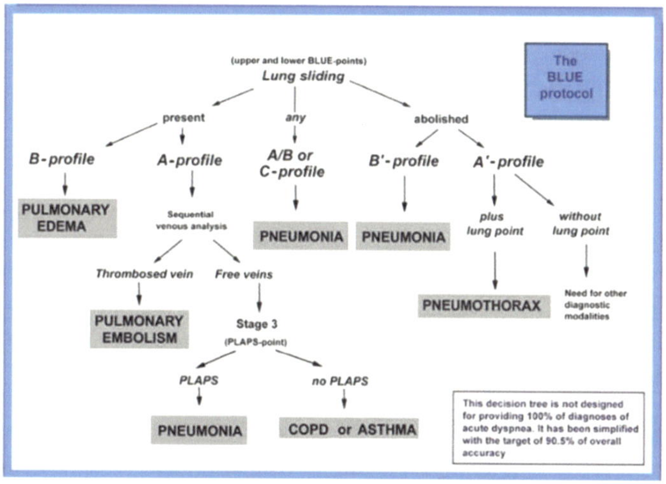

Figure 7.
The BLUE protocol [14].

A-noV-PLAPS-profile is normal lung sliding, without B-lines, and deep venous thrombosis but minimal reactive effusion or consolidation – posterolateral alveolar and/or pleural syndrome (PLAPS) in the dependent regions. The combination of regions with A-lines and other regions with more than three B-lines is called the A/B-profile. According to the BLUE protocol anterior lung consolidations or C-profiles, as well as abolished lung sliding with B-lines present, are specific to pneumonia (**Figure 7**).

5. Pneumonia

5.1 Pathophysiology

Pneumonia is the result of host defense mechanisms being overwhelmed by an infectious pathogen. This may occur because of an inadequate patient's immune response or a large inoculum of particularly virulent microorganisms to which the patient has no preexisting immunity or is unable to form an adequate acute immune response. Studies have shown that in most patients with unilateral pneumonia, the inflammatory response is limited to the site of infection. It has been found that in patients with localized pneumonia, tumor necrosis factor-alpha (TNF-α), interleukin (IL)-6, and IL-8 levels were increased in the pneumonic lung and generally not increased in the uninvolved lung and in the serum. By contrast, in patients with bilateral pneumonia, the immune response is characterized by a "spillover" of the inflammatory response into the systemic circulation and increases in serum levels of TNF-α and IL-6. It remains unclear why localization does not occur in all individuals and why some patients develop diffuse lung injury.

The infectious process resulting from the invasion and overgrowth of pathogenic microorganisms in the lung parenchyma, combined with the breaking down of local defense mechanisms and the production of intra-alveolar exudates, gives a basic definition of pneumonia. Typically, the alveoli in intensely inflamed areas are filled with inflammatory fluid or pus, and this is known as consolidation. Depending on the host response, the virulence of the microorganism, disease severity, and progression, the changes in the lungs may be interstitial, patchy, lobar, or widespread.

Ultrasound can detect the pulmonary changes associated with pneumonia as long as the process involves some of the outer (non-mediastinal) pleural surface of the lungs – as it almost always does. Pneumonia progresses through stages, which can create some distinct patterns on LUS depending on the degree and extent of the pathology as follows:

- Lung interstitial syndrome. In early pneumonia, inflammatory fluid fills only some of the alveoli or the interstitial space. Where fluid-filled pulmonary interstitium and subpleural alveoli are surrounded by air-filled lung, laser-like vertical hyperechoic artifacts arising from the pleural line can be seen, called B-lines (also "comet tails"). They are a sign of lung interstitial syndrome.

- Non-translobar consolidation. With the progression of the disease, consolidations advance. More commonly, smaller areas of lobular consolidations occur. Where these are about the pleural surface, they are linear, but their deeper borders usually demonstrate an irregular interface with the underlying aerated lung. This irregular junction between consolidated and aerated lung in LUS is known as the Shred sign. If there is lobar consolidation, the borders of the consolidated areas will be linear and well-defined – as consolidated and aerated lung lie adjacent on opposite sides of the linear pleural fissures.

- Translobar consolidation (hepatization): in these cases, the inflammatory process goes beyond the borders of a pulmonary lobe and involves two or three adjacent lobes. The ultrasound image bears a resemblance to ultrasound imaging of the liver. The "hepatized" lung is tissue visible due to the absence of air, creating a texture similar to organ tissue. Translobar consolidations are often linked to pneumonia or atelectasis.

5.2 Sonographic patterns of pneumonia

The proper interpretation of the B-lines is a fundamental part of the BLUE protocol. B-lines can be observed in cardiogenic pulmonary edema, interstitial diseases, pneumonia, ARDS. In order to be considered pathological, there should be more than three B-lines in one intercoastal space. Multiple well-defined B-lines, more than

7 mm apart, are reflections of the thickening of the interlobular septa (**Figure 3**). Abbuting(coalescent) B-lines, with less than 3 mm between them, represent alveolar interstitial syndrome with further impairment of alveolocapillary gas exchange and worsening of the condition [15]. Subpleural consolidations on ultrasound are the equivalent of the pathology passing the borders of the interlobular septa (**Figure 8**). With further progression of the disease and loss of lung aeration from lobar pneumonia, it becomes translobar. Lung ultrasound shows a heterogeneous image with punctiform and linear hyperechoic shadows that represent the terminal airways and resembles liver pattern – the so-called hepatization of the lung. The total loss of lung aeration is visualized as a tissue-like sign (**Figure 6**).

The inflammation of the lung tissue is commonly accompanied by reactive pleural effusion. While in the beginning, the effusion usually tends to be small and does not lead to sufficient pressure on the parenchyma, there is the risk of an increase in volume and further complications arising. Large pleural effusions compress the lung and lead to atelectasis and reduction in lung aeration. Ultrasound is a known method with excellent sensitivity and specificity in diagnosing pleural effusion [4]. It can even provide information on the approximate size of the pathology. With the patient in a supine position, the distance between the diaphragm and the lung is measured in mm, and this distance is multiplied by 10 [16]. There are at least four more formulas for calculating effusion volume without a clear consensus on which to use. Not only can we roughly estimate the volume, but we can also distinguish between different fluid characteristics based on the ultrasound pattern. Transudate, exudate, and blood have different consistency which is seen on sonography [17–19]. This is of paramount importance when considering that reactive effusion can get complicated by fibrin deposition, which can further progress to fibrous adhesions, septation of the effusion, and even empyema (**Figure 9**), Video 3, https://youtu.be/tJI5xw2Yfvw. The early detection of such pathology will not only lead to a change in therapy but might even require surgical placement of thoracic drainage or video-assisted thoracoscopic surgery with pleurodesis.

The worsening of arterial oxygenation can be a result of increased intrapulmonary shunting as a consequence of atelectasis or consolidation. Atelectasis is the result of obstruction of the airways or external pressure on the lung. Lung inflammation leads to the accumulation of exudate in the airways, thickening of the parenchyma, and progressive loss of aeration. CXR has low sensitivity, specificity, and diagnostic accuracy in distinguishing between these pathologies [20, 21]. The loss of aeration of

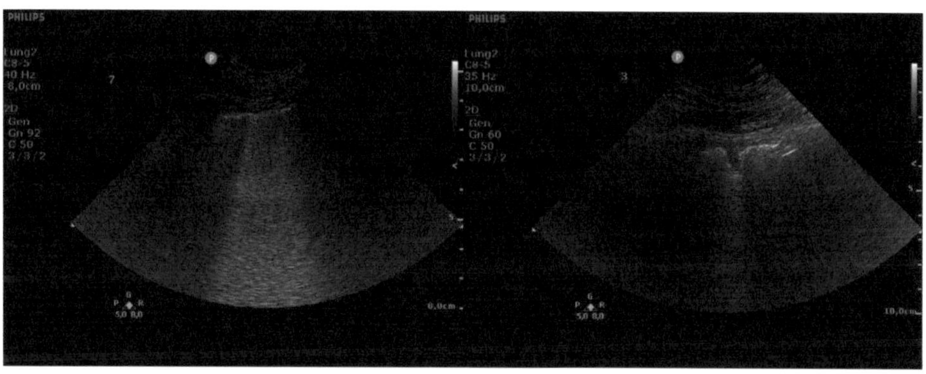

Figure 8.
Abbuting(coalescent) B-lines and Subpleural consolidation.

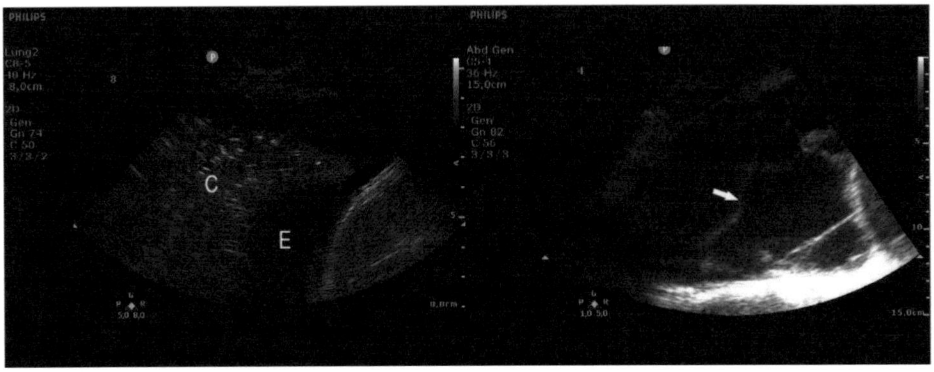

Figure 9.
Effusion and Septated effusion, C- consolidation, E – effusion, arrow – Septated effusion.

the lung conveys the heart rhythm more easily and is represented by the lung pulse phenomenon. While this can be observed in both atelectasis and consolidation, there is an ultrasound method to distinguish between them. The hepatization of the lung is associated with visualizing the terminal airways – air bronchograms. When visualized in cross-plane sections, they are punctiform, and in longitudinal sections – they linear. Closely observing linear bronchograms shows two different artifacts. Static air bronchograms lack any movement and are observed in cases of total obstruction or compression of the parenchyma. When air passes through the terminal airways, it leads to a centrifugal phenomenon during inspiration which is called dynamic air bronchogram Video 4, https://youtu.be/UFHwSgA7pFY. Static air bronchograms can be observed in consolidation but are most commonly found in atelectasis. Dynamic air bronchograms, however, are highly specific in cases of consolidation. Multiple studies suggest that using dynamic air bronchograms in both adult and pediatric populations increases diagnostic accuracy in pneumonia [22–26]. Using color Doppler to measure intrapulmonary flow is another method that increases lung ultrasound accuracy in diagnosing pneumonia [26].

5.3 Differential diagnosis

Proper and timely treatment have crucial role in managing pneumonia. Antimicrobial resistance has been steadily rising in past decades despite different strategies and is now a leading problem in the medical field. Inappropriate antibiotic use has led to the development of many resistant bacterial strains which are associated with longer hospital stay, higher costs and increased morbidity and mortality. Distinguishing between different etiologies is of paramount importance when initiating therapy. Imaging studies, biomarkers, and microbiological results all have an important role in differential diagnosis.

According to meta-analysis, LUS shows over 93% sensitivity and specificity in diagnosing pneumonia in both adult and pediatric population [27, 28]. A recent study by Buonsenso and colleagues has shown that based on LUS artifacts, a differentiation could be made between bacterial, viral and atypical pneumonia [29]. Small, multiple consolidations are more common in viral etiology, while larger consolidations are observed with bacterial infection. Superficial dynamic air bronchograms suggest atypical pneumonia, while deep dynamic air bronchogram are usually of bacterial origin. Static air bronchograms are more common in viral infections.

White blood cell (WBC), C-reactive protein (CRP), and procalcitonin (PCT) levels are widely used in the attempt to separate viral from bacterial infections and predict disease outcomes. Recent studies have implemented biomarkers and imaging studies in the diagnosis of pneumonia. LUS shows better results than conventional CXR in both sensitivity and specificity. This has been proven in both community-acquired pneumonia (CAP) and hospital-acquired pneumonia (HAP). Clinical pulmonary infection score is widely used in the diagnosis of HAP. Modifying the protocol by using LUS instead of CXR leads to higher sensitivity and specificity in diagnosing pneumonia and reduced radiation exposure. Lung ultrasound pattern of consolidation with dynamic air bronchograms and PCT > 1 ng/ml suggest bacterial pneumonia. The PROLUSP study (PROcalcitonin and Lung UltraSound algorithm to diagnose severe pneumonia in critical pediatric patients) proves that using LUS and PCT to guide pneumonia diagnosis and treatment leads to better diagnostic accuracy and less use of antibiotics [25, 26].

5.4 Nosocomial pneumonia

Pneumonia can be separated into subgroups based on place of acquisition – community-acquired pneumonia (CAP), healthcare-associated pneumonia (HCAP), nosocomial or hospital-acquired pneumonia (HAP), and in the case of patients on mechanical ventilation longer than 48 hours – ventilator-associated pneumonia (VAP). Nosocomial pneumonia is the second most commonly acquired hospital infection, with the highest mortality rate [30]. Early, accurate diagnosis is a mainstay in treatment. The classical diagnostic approach is based on a combination of clinical signs – tachypnea, fever, rales on auscultation; laboratory results – increased inflammatory markers, microbiological isolates, and imaging studies. Monitoring the progress of the disease relies heavily on visualizing the lung parenchyma. CXR is the most commonly used study to provide the information while CT is the golden standard. LUS has been showing promising results in diagnosing both CAP and HAP [23, 31–36]. VAP is associated with a significant increase in morbidity and mortality, days on mechanical ventilation, use of antibiotics, and a raise in drug-resistant microorganisms, as well as treatment costs. Studies have proven that adding LUS to the classically used CPIS score or substituting CXR with LUS increases sensitivity and specificity. New models for diagnosing VAP include the VAP LUS score (VPLUS), lung ultrasound simplified clinical pulmonary score (LUS-sCPIS), and Chest Echography and Procalcitonin Pulmonary Infection Score (CEPPIS). Studies show 85% sensitivity and 83% specificity over 81% compared to 80% sensitivity and 40% specificity for CPIS [26, 37, 38].

5.5 Monitoring pneumonia

LUS not only provides rapid and accurate diagnosis but also the ability to monitor the patient's lung whenever needed without exposing them to any radiation or complications associated with transportation. Sonographic artifacts accurately represent the progression of the pathology. A couple of well-separated B-lines become multiple B-lines or abbuting(coalescent) B-lines as interstitial syndrome worsens. Lobar infiltrations pass the interlobular septa with an image of subpleural consolidations, become translobar with a tissue-like sign, and show air bronchogram patterns. LUS provides the ability to grade the pathology based on the acquired image – 0 points for less than 3 B-lines, 1 point for 3 ≤ B-lines, 2 points for multiple, abbuting B-lines

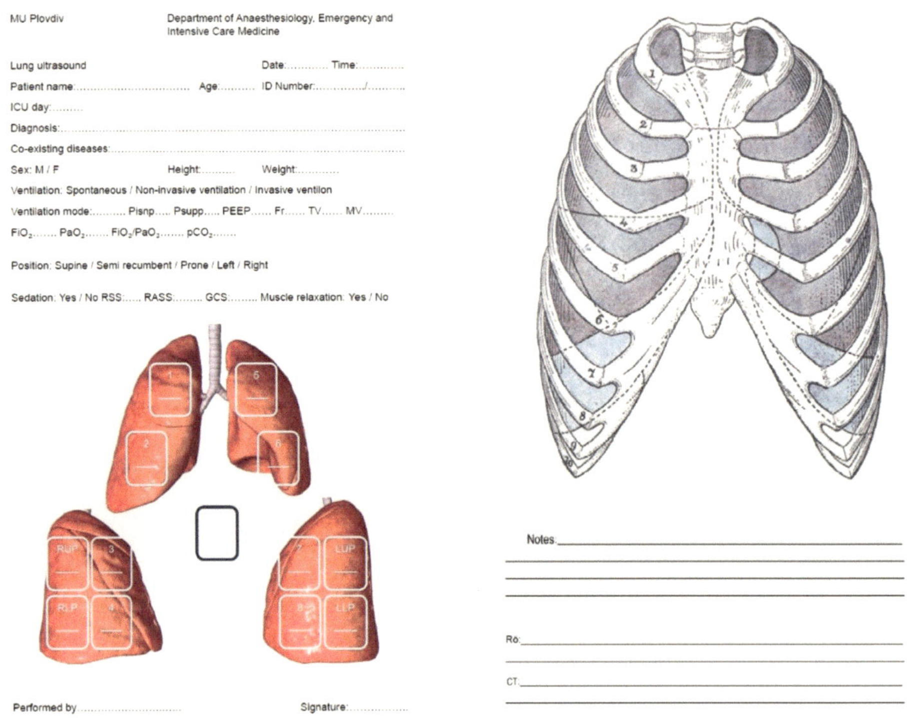
MU Plovdiv — Department of Anaesthesiology, Emergency and Intensive Care Medicine

Lung ultrasound — Date:........... Time:............

Patient name:................................ Age:.......... ID Number:............../..........

ICU day:........

Diagnosis:..

Co-existing diseases:...

Sex: M / F — Height:......... Weight:...........

Ventilation: Spontaneous / Non-invasive ventilation / Invasive ventilon

Ventilation mode:......... Pisnp.... Psupp.... PEEP..... Fr..... TV..... MV........

FiO_2...... PaO_2...... FiO_2/PaO_2...... pCO_2......

Position: Supine / Semi recumbent / Prone / Left / Right

Sedation: Yes / No RSS:..... RASS:........ GCS:........ Muscle relaxation: Yes / No

Performed by.............................. Signature:................

Notes:

Ro:

CT:

Figure 10.
Lung ultrasound examination – Front and back side.

or subpleural consolidation, and 3 points for consolidation. With a total of 12 lung regions, this leads to a maximal score of 36. Based on the scoring system, LUS provides not only regional but also cumulative representation of the condition's severity. By daily monitoring of the patient the physician can quickly assess the effect of the therapy. For the purpose of comparability it is important to systematically keep track of information (**Figure 10**).

5.6 Recruitment

The filling of the alveoli with fluid – transudate, exudate, or blood or their collapse leads to hypoxic respiratory failure. In cases of severe pneumonia and ARDS, patients suffer from hypoxemia due to increased intrapulmonary shunt. The main compensatory mechanism – hypoxic vasoconstriction is suppressed due to the infection, medication, and mechanical ventilation. One of the main strategies in patients on mechanical ventilation due to increased intrapulmonary shunt is increasing the volume of aerated lung tissue and protecting the alveoli from collapsing again. Mechanical ventilation leads to four main types of ventilator-induced lung injury (VILI) – volutrauma, barotrauma, atelectotrauma, and biotrauma. Selecting the proper mode of mechanical ventilation and its setting is of great importance in the treatment of pneumonia. The primary goal is to recruit the consolidated lung tissue and to maintain its ventilation. Using higher positive end-expiratory pressure (PEEP) is the most common way to achieve that.

The inflamed lung tissue is heterogeneous. There are areas that are normally aerated, others that have reduced ventilation, and still others that are consolidated and have no ventilation. The parts without pathology have normal compliance and resistance, inflamed regions have lower compliance, and the ones that are not ventilated due to consolidations have compliance close to zero. Keeping that in mind and the fact that the main strategy in lung recruitment is increasing PEEP, it should be considered that this pressure is not equally distributed in all regions. The compliant regions will receive most of the volume while the collapsed ones might still be left with no ventilation. In this case, the overdistention will lead to further trauma on the lung tissue. Selecting the proper PEEP level is very important when managing patients with pneumonia. Electrical impedance tomography (EIT) could guide PEEP level selection based on the optimal balance between overdistention and recruitment [39, 40]. The equipment, however, is not as widely distributed as ultrasound machines.

Thoracic sonography provides the ability to monitor ventilation changes at the bedside of the patient in real time. Both short- and long-term changes in the distribution of mechanical ventilation can be monitored in this way. Alveolar recruitment can be observed with shift in lung artifacts – consolidation starting to show a change in dynamic air bronchograms pattern, abbuting B-lines becoming multiple B-lines with space between them, and reduction of the number of B-lines. Overinflation cannot be directly observed with LUS, but the absence of B-lines in regions that previously had few B-lines is an indirect indicator of excess distention of lung tissue. The lung ultrasound scoring system provides the opportunity for fast and easy evaluation of changes in both regional and cumulative levels. By monitoring patterns and comparing results from different mode settings, lung ultrasound can be used to assess the adequacy of the changes in mechanical ventilation [41].

5.7 Weaning

Prolonged ICU treatment of pneumonia is associated with more complications, increased morbidity and mortality, longer hospitalization, and higher treatment costs. Ventilator-associated pneumonia is a nosocomial infection specific to critically ill patients who are on mechanical ventilation for longer than 48 hrs. Studies suggest that VAP on its own increases mortality rate by up to 13% and at even higher rates in surgical patients [42]. Unsuccessful weaning and reintubation represent other significant risk factors with unfavorable outcomes.

Assessing diaphragm dysfunction, thickness, and excursion with sonography can predict unsuccessful spontaneous breathing trials (SBT) [43–46]. LUS evaluation of aeration can also be used for weaning evaluation. LUS <11 is associated with a higher success rate of weaning while>15 with expected failure [47]. Combining diaphragm and lung evaluation increases prediction accuracy in the weaning process [48, 49]. EIT is another alternative for anticipating an extubation success rate [40].

5.8 Physiotherapy

Respiratory therapy aims to remove retained secretions, improve airway clearance, increase lung compliance, and promote lung recruitment, thus optimizing the ventilation/perfusion ratio. Physiotherapists use a variety of methods to achieve this goal – manual therapy, specific positioning of the patient, aspiration of secretions, hyperinflation techniques, and multiple mechanical and electronic devices. Selecting the appropriate mean depends on the specific pathology of the current patient. Auscultation and X-rays are suboptimal in achieving this task. LUS, on the other hand, is non-invasive, radiation-free, and readily available at the bedside of the patient. Providing accurate regional and global evaluation of the lung function at the time of examination gives the ability to choose the right method for improving pulmonary aeration. Meta-analysis shows that by utilizing lung and diaphragm sonography, respiratory diagnosis is changed in 63,9% of cases, which alters physiotherapy management in 16,8% of cases and treatment in 48,4% of cases [50].

5.9 Follow-up

Acute respiratory distress syndrome is the most severe form of lung inflammation. Pathophysiologically, it is divided into three stages – exudative, fibroproliferative, and resolution. Most of the patients that survive have severe pulmonary fibrosis that can take more than a year to recover. It is common for them to have depression, reduced physical activity, dyspnea, and other complications. It is important to be able to distinguish between the patient's complaints, assess his physical status, and monitor not only the progression of the disease but also the healing process in order to choose the proper outpatient treatment. LUS can be done in less than 10 minutes, depending on operator skills, with real-time results, comparability and repeatability without radiation exposure. It can detect parapneumonic effusions and intrapulmonary abscesses with excellent sensitivity and specificity and monitor their progression [51–53]. Providing rapid and accurate diagnosis, it is an excellent addition to the decision-making process regarding the treatment of outpatients.

6. Training

Lung ultrasound is an invaluable tool in managing respiratory failure at the bedside of the patient. In the past decade, discussions have been considering implementing it in the medical curriculum. LUS is a technical skill that relies on interaction with the machine and interpretation of artifacts. This provides the opportunity for a wide variety of learning techniques – web-based, hands-on, phantom models, animal models, volunteers, patients, and simulation training. There is not an agreement on which is the best method, with all of them having benefits and pitfalls [54]. It is generally accepted that LUS has a steep learning curve with a short time needed to obtain knowledge for proper baseline interpretation of the artifacts – less than 10 hrs, and trainees require minimal assistance during examination after just 6 scans [55, 56]. Simulation-based training is an excellent alternative to acquiring the fundamentals in diagnosing severe lung diseases in a controlled and calm environment [57]. With interobserver agreement ranging from fair to excellent, it is obvious that acquiring master skills will take dedication, but being able to distinguish between life-threatening respiratory pathologies with less than a week's training makes learning LUS worthwhile.

7. Conclusion

Early and accurate pneumonia diagnosis is the mainstay in timely and proper treatment. Lunt ultrasound is a versatile tool that can be successfully implemented in the management of respiratory failure. The addition of an imaging study that can readily be performed at the bedside, repeated when necessary, and compared with previous examinations without radiation exposure is an excellent addition to the personalized approach toward the patient. The ability to combine ultrasound and biomarkers to distinguish between different etiologies and select the appropriate treatment is of great importance, especially considering the ongoing antibiotic crisis. Being able to easily monitor the progression of the disease during the hospital stay can change the course of therapy and improve the overall outcome. Sonographic evaluation of outpatients is another useful addition to the arsenal of the physician. The modality has its limitations when it comes to obese patients, ones with dressings or subcutaneous emphysema, and does require extra training. Learning the required skills needed for performing the examination can be obtained with a variety of methods, each having its advantages. In conclusion, lung ultrasound is a pragmatic tool that can benefit the holistic approach to the treatment of pneumonia.

Conflict of interest

The authors declare no conflict of interest.

Author details

Valentin Stoilov[1*], Georgi Pavlov[1] and Aleksandrina Topalova-Shishmanova[2]

1 Department of Anaesthesiology, Emergency and Intensive Care Medicine, Medical University of Plovdiv, Plovdiv, Bulgaria

2 Department of Otorhinolaryngology, Medical University of Plovdiv, Bulgaria

*Address all correspondence to: valentin.stoilov@mu-plovdiv.bg

References

[1] Mac SR, McAuley DF, Matthay MA. Acute lung failure. Seminars in Respiratory and Critical Care Medicine. 2011;**32**(5):607-625

[2] Amorosa JK, Bramwit MP, Mohammed TLH, Reddy GP, Brown K, Dyer DS, et al. ACR appropriateness criteria routine chest radiographs in intensive care unit patients. Journal of the American College of Radiology [Internet]. 2013;**10**(3):170-174. Available from: http://linkinghub.elsevier.com/retrieve/pii/S1546144012007107

[3] Meta-analysis CU. Abandoning daily routine chest radiography in the intensive purpose: Methods: Results. Radiology. 2010;**255**:2. Available from: https://pubs.rsna.org/doi/10.1148/radiol.10090946?url_ver=Z39.88-2003&rfr_id=ori:rid:crossref.org&rfr_dat=cr_pub%20%200pubmed

[4] Xirouchaki N, Magkanas E, Vaporidi K, Kondili E, Plataki M, Patrianakos A, et al. Lung ultrasound in critically ill patients: Comparison with bedside chest radiography. Intensive Care Medicine. 2011;**37**(9):1488-1493

[5] Brenner DJ, Doll R, Goodhead DT, Hall EJ, Land CE, Little JB, et al. Cancer Risks Attributable to Low Doses of Ionizing Radiation: Assessing What we Really Know. 2003. Available from: www.pnas.orgcgidoi10.1073pnas.2235592100

[6] Communicating Radiation Risks in Paediatric Imaging: Information to Support Healthcare Discussions about Benefit and Risk [Internet]. Available from: https://www.who.int/publications/i/item/978924151034

[7] Hayden GE, Wrenn KW. Chest radiograph vs. computed tomography scan in the evaluation for pneumonia. Journal of Emergency Medicine [Internet]. 2009;**36**(3):266-270. Available from: http://linkinghub.elsevier.com/retrieve/pii/S0736467908001017

[8] Gentilotti E, De Nardo P, Cremonini E, Górska A, Mazzaferri F, Canziani LM, et al. Diagnostic accuracy of point-of-care tests in acute community-acquired lower respiratory tract infections. A systematic review and meta-analysis. Clinical Microbiology and Infection. Elsevier B.V. 2022;**28**:13-22

[9] Parmentier-decrucq E, Poissy J, Favory R, Nseir S, Onimus T, Guerry MJ, et al. Adverse events during intrahospital transport of critically ill patients: Incidence and risk factors. Annals of Intensive Care. 2013;**3**:1-10

[10] Sodickson A, Baeyens PF, Andriole KP, Prevedello LM, Nawfel RD, Hanson R, et al. Recurrent CT, cumulative radiation exposure, and associated radiation-induced cancer risks from CT of adults. Radiology [Internet]. 2009;**251**(1):175-184 Available from: http://pubs.rsna.org/doi/abs/10.1148/radiol.2511081296

[11] Joyner CR, Herman RJ, Reid JM. Reflected ultrasound in the detection and localization of pleural effusion. JAMA [Internet]. 1967;**200**(5):399-402. Available from: http://www.ncbi.nlm.nih.gov/pubmed/6071511

[12] Lichtenstein DA, Mezière GA. Relevance of lung ultrasound in the diagnosis of acute respiratory failure the BLUE protocol. Chest. 2008;**134**(1):117-125

[13] Lichtenstein DA. Lung Ultrasound in the Critically Ill: The Blue Protocol.

Switzerland: Springer International Publishing; 2016. p. 1. Available from: https://link.springer.com/book/10.1007/978-3-319-15371-1

[14] Lichtenstein DA, Access O. Lung ultrasound in the critically ill. Annals of Intensive Care [Internet]. 2014;**4**(1):1. Available from: http://www.pubmedcentral.nih.gov/articlerender.fcgi?artid=3895677&tool=pmcentrez&rendertype=abstract

[15] Bouhemad B, Liu ZHH, Arbelot C, Zhang M, Ferarri F, Le-Guen M, et al. Ultrasound assessment of antibiotic-induced pulmonary reaeration in ventilator-associated pneumonia. Critical Care Medicine [Internet]. 2010;**38**(1):84-92. Available from: http://www.ncbi.nlm.nih.gov/pubmed/19633538

[16] Remérand F, Dellamonica J, Mao Z, Ferrari F, Bouhemad B, Jianxin Y, et al. Multiplane ultrasound approach to quantify pleural effusion at the bedside. Intensive Care Medicine. 2010;**36**(4):656-664

[17] Tu CY, Hsu WH, Hsia TC, Chen HJ, Tsai KD, Hung CW, et al. Pleural effusions in fibrile medical ICU patients: Chest ultrasound study. Chest. 2004;**126**(4):1274-1280

[18] Yang PC. Value of Sonography in Determining the Nature of Pleural. American Journal of Roentgenology. Leesburg, VA USA; 2005. pp. 1-5. Available from: https://www.ajronline.org/doi/10.2214/ajr.159.1.1609716

[19] Sajadieh H, Afzali F, Sajadieh V, Sajadieh A. Ultrasound as an alternative to aspiration for determining the nature of pleural effusion, especially in older people. Annals of the New York Academy of Sciences. 2004;**1019**:585-592

[20] Ellis SM. Interpreting Chest x-Rays. Oxfordshire, UK: Scion Pub; 2010. 246 p

[21] Sk J. Textbook of Pulmonary and Critical Care Medicine Vols 1 &Amp; 2 [Internet]. Daryaganj, New Delhi, India: Jaypee Brothers Medical Publishers (P) Ltd.; 2011. Available from: http://www.jaypeedigital.com/bookdetails.aspx?id=9789350250730&sr=1

[22] Shah A, Oliva C, Stem C, Cummings EQ. Application of dynamic air bronchograms on lung ultrasound to diagnose pneumonia in undifferentiated respiratory distress. Respiratory Medicine Case Reports. 2022;**39**:2-3

[23] Reissig A, Copetti R. Lung ultrasound in community-acquired pneumonia and in interstitial lung diseases. Respiration. 2014;**87**(3):179-189

[24] Abid I, Qureshi N, Lategan N, Williams S, Shahid S. Point-of-care lung ultrasound in detecting pneumonia: A systematic review. Canadian Journal of Respiratory Therapy. Canadian Society of Respiratory Therapists. 2024;**60**:37-48

[25] Guitart C, Bobillo-Perez S, Rodríguez-Fanjul J, Carrasco JL, Brotons P, López-Ramos MG, et al. Lung ultrasound and procalcitonin, improving antibiotic management and avoiding radiation exposure in pediatric critical patients with bacterial pneumonia: A randomized clinical trial. European Journal of Medical Research. 2024;**29**(1):8-10

[26] Pasqueron J, Dureau P, Arcile G, Duceau B, Hariri G, Lepère V, et al. Usefulness of lung ultrasound for early detection of hospital-acquired pneumonia in cardiac critically ill patients on venoarterial extracorporeal membrane oxygenation. Annals of Intensive Care. 2022;**12**(1):4-8

[27] Chavez MA, Shams N, Ellington LE, Naithani N, Gilman RH, Steinhoff MC, et al. Lung ultrasound for the diagnosis of pneumonia in adults: A systematic review and meta-analysis. Respiratory Research [Internet]. 2014;**15**(1):7. Available from: https://pubmed.ncbi.nlm.nih.gov/24758612/

[28] Pereda MA, Chavez MA, Hooper-Miele CC, Gilman RH, Steinhoff MC, Ellington LE, et al. Lung ultrasound for the diagnosis of pneumonia in children: A meta-analysis. Pediatrics [Internet]. 2015;**135**(4):714-722 Available from: https://pubmed.ncbi.nlm.nih.gov/25780071/

[29] Buonsenso D, Musolino A, Ferro V, De Rose C, Morello R, Ventola C, et al. Role of lung ultrasound for the etiological diagnosis of acute lower respiratory tract infection (ALRTI) in children: A prospective study. Journal of Ultrasound. 2022;**25**(2):185-197

[30] Vincent JL, Rello J, Marshall J, Silva E, Anzueto A, Martin CD, et al. International study of the prevalence and outcomes of infection in intensive care units. JAMA [Internet]. 2009;**302**(21):2323. Available from: http://www.ncbi.nlm.nih.gov/pubmed/19952319

[31] Liu XL, Lian R, Tao YK, Gu CD, Zhang GQ. Lung ultrasonography: An effective way to diagnose community-acquired pneumonia. In: Liu X-lei, et al. Emergency Medicine Journal [Internet]. 2015;**32**:433-438. DOI: 10.1136/emermed-2013-203039

[32] Chalmers JD. The Modern Diagnostic Approach to Community-Acquired Pneumonia in Adults. New York, NY, USA: Thieme Medical Publishers; 2016. Available from: https://www.thieme-connect.com/products/ejournals/abstract/10.1055/s-0036-1592125

[33] Gupta A, Lessing A, Gada KD, Ahmad S. The use of bedside ultrasound IN the management of community-acquired pneumonia. Chest. 2023;**164**(4):A4078-A4079

[34] Bourcier JE, Braga S, Garnier D. Lung ultrasound will soon replace chest radiography in the diagnosis of acute community-acquired pneumonia. Current Infectious Disease Reports [Internet]. 2016;**18**(12):3-4. Available from:. DOI: 10.1007/s11908-016-0550-9

[35] Corradi F, Brusasco C, Garlaschi A, Paparo F, Ball L, Santori G, et al. Quantitative analysis of lung ultrasonography for the detection of community-acquired pneumonia: A pilot study. BioMed Research International. 2015;**2015**:4-7

[36] Boursiani C, Tsolia M, Koumanidou C, Malagari A, Vakaki M, Karapostolakis G, et al. Lung ultrasound as first-line examination for the diagnosis of community-acquired pneumonia in children. Pediatric Emergency Care. 2017;**33**(1):63-65

[37] Xu E, Pérez-Torres D, Fragkou PC, Zahar JR, Koulenti D. Nosocomial pneumonia in the era of multidrug-resistance: Updates in diagnosis and management. Microorganisms. 2021;**9**:6. DOI: 10.3390/microorganisms9030534

[38] Scopus Preview - Scopus - Document Details - Lung Ultrasound in Evaluation of Ventilator- a Ssociated Pneumonia [Internet]. Available from: https://www.scopus.com/record/display.uri?eid=2-s2.0-85107763201&origin=inward&txGid=3c546dbcc49632f39d9d0892afa872f7

[39] Tomicic V, Cornejo R. Lung monitoring with electrical impedance tomography: Technical considerations and clinical applications. Journal of

Thoracic Disease. AME Publishing Company. 2019;**11**:3122-3135

[40] Joussellin V, Bonny V, Spadaro S, Clerc S, Parfait M, Ferioli M, et al. Lung aeration estimated by chest electrical impedance tomography and lung ultrasound during extubation. Annals of Intensive Care. 2023;**13**(1):5-10

[41] Bouhemad B, Mongodi S, Via G, Rouquette I. Ultrasound for "lung monitoring" of ventilated patients. Anesthesiology [Internet]. 2015;**122**(2):437-447. Available from: http://content.wkhealth.com/linkback/openurl?sid=WKPTLP:landingpage&an=00000542-201502000-00034

[42] Melsen WG, Rovers MM, Groenwold RH, Bergmans DC, Camus C, Bauer TT, et al. Attributable mortality of ventilator-associated pneumonia: A meta-analysis of individual patient data from randomised prevention studies. The Lancet Infectious Diseases [Internet]. 2013;**13**(8):665-671. Available from: http://www.ncbi.nlm.nih.gov/pubmed/23622939

[43] Matamis D, Soilemezi E, Tsagourias M, Akoumianaki E, Dimassi S, Boroli F, et al. Sonographic evaluation of the diaphragm in critically ill patients. Technique and clinical applications. Intensive Care Medicine. 2013;**39**(5):801-810

[44] Zambon M, Greco M, Bocchino S, Cabrini L, Beccaria PF, Zangrillo A. Assessment of diaphragmatic dysfunction in the critically ill patient with ultrasound: A systematic review. Intensive Care Medicine. 2017;**43**(1):29-38

[45] Dennis DEGEJSJMM. Diaphragm ultrasound as a new index of discontinuation from mechanical ventilation. Thorax [Internet]. 2014;**69**(5):431-435. Available from: http://www.pubmedcentral.nih.gov/articlerender.fcgi?artid=4057909&tool=pmcentrez&rendertype=abstract

[46] Spadaro S, Grasso S, Mauri T, Dalla Corte F, Alvisi V, Ragazzi R, et al. Can diaphragmatic ultrasonography performed during the T-tube trial predict weaning failure? The role of diaphragmatic rapid shallow breathing index. Critical Care [Internet]. 2016;**20**(1):305. Available from: http://www.ncbi.nlm.nih.gov/pubmed/27677861%5Cnhttp://www.pubmedcentral.nih.gov/articlerender.fcgi?artid=PMC5039882

[47] Blanco JB, Esquinas A. Diaphragm evaluation and lung ultrasound score during weaning. Indian Journal of Critical Care Medicine [Internet]. 2022;**26**(9):1054. Available from: /pmc/articles/PMC9492736/

[48] Amara V, Vishwas P, Maddani SS, Natarajan S, Chaudhuri S. Evaluation of abdominal expiratory muscle thickness pattern, diaphragmatic excursion, and lung ultrasound score in critically ill patients and their association with weaning patterns: A prospective observational study. Indian Journal of Critical Care Medicine [Internet]. 2022;**26**(3):307-313. Available from: https://pubmed.ncbi.nlm.nih.gov/35519926/

[49] Tenza-Lozano E, Llamas-Alvarez A, Jaimez-Navarro E, Fernández-Sánchez J. Lung and diaphragm ultrasound as predictors of success in weaning from mechanical ventilation. Critical Ultrasound Journal [Internet]. 2018;**10**(1):12. Available from: /pmc/articles/PMC6004341/

[50] Lockstone J, Love A, Hung Lau Y, Hansell L, Ntoumenopoulos G. The use

of diaphragm and lung ultrasound in acute respiratory physiotherapy practice and the impact on clinical decision-making: A systematic review and meta-analysis. Australian Critical Care. Elsevier Ireland Ltd. 2024;**37**:176-184

[51] Pallarés JP, Bernal FL, Cabello Jabalquinto MDR, Jiménez Romero AA. Usefulness of thoracic ultrasound for diagnosis and follow-up of pneumonia. Revista Espanola de Quimioterapia [Internet]. 2022;**35**(Suppl 1(Suppl 1)):21-24. Available from: https://pubmed.ncbi.nlm.nih.gov/35488819/

[52] Reissig A, Gramegna A, Aliberti S. The role of lung ultrasound in the diagnosis and follow-up of community-acquired pneumonia. European Journal of Internal Medicine. Elsevier B.V. 2012;**23**:391-397

[53] Eman G, Synn S, Galen B, Shah R, Nauka P, Hope AA, et al. Thoracic ultrasound in COVID-19: Use of lung and diaphragm ultrasound in evaluating Dyspnea in survivors of acute respiratory distress syndrome from COVID-19 pneumonia in a post-ICU clinic. Lung. 2023;**201**(2):149-157

[54] Pietersen PI, Madsen KR, Graumann O, Konge L, Nielsen BU, Laursen CB. Lung ultrasound training: A systematic review of published literature in clinical lung ultrasound training. Critical Ultrasound Journal. Springer-Verlag Italia s.r.l. 2018;**10**:10-13

[55] Mozzini C, Fratta Pasini AM, Garbin U, Cominacini L. Lung ultrasound in internal medicine: Training and clinical practice. Critical Ultrasound Journal. 2016;**8**(1):3-6

[56] See KC, Ong V, Wong SH, Leanda R, Santos J, Taculod J, et al. Lung ultrasound training: Curriculum implementation and learning trajectory among respiratory therapists. Intensive Care Medicine. 2016;**42**(1):63-71

[57] Wolstenhulme S, Mclaughlan JR. Lung ultrasound education: Simulation and hands-on. The British Journal of Radiology. 2021;**94**:2-3

Chapter 11

Perspective Chapter: Bedside Lung Ultrasound Scan in Critically Ill – Uses and Techniques

Kingsley Ufuoma Tobi and Aderonke Adesiyan

Abstract

Bedside ultrasound has become integral to managing critically ill patients in critical care settings, including the emergency and intensive care units. It is highly sensitive and specific and has the advantage of being at the patient's bedside, real-time investigations, with reduced space requirements. Lung ultrasound, in particular, can promptly diagnose common causes of respiratory distress in critically ill patients, such as pulmonary oedema, pneumothorax, pleural effusion, acute respiratory distress syndrome and pneumonia. Therefore, acquiring skills in lung ultrasound is critical for all clinicians working in the intensive care unit to diagnose and manage common causes of respiratory distress in critically ill patients. This chapter thus deals with the technique of lung ultrasound and the ultrasonographic features of these lung pathologies.

Keywords: bedside, lung ultrasound, pneumothorax, pulmonary oedema, pleural effusion, intensive care unit

1. Introduction

Lung ultrasound scan has emerged as an important tool in the management of critically ill patients in the intensive care unit (ICU). Its use include prompt diagnosis of common causes of respiratory distress in critically ill patients, such as pulmonary oedema, pneumothorax, pleural effusion, acute respiratory distress syndrome and pneumonia.

Some of the advantages of lung ultrasound scan (USS) include: it is non-invasive, radiation-free, can be performed at the bedside, reproducible and relatively cheap and available even in resource-challenged environments.

Therefore, it is critical for clinicians caring for critically ill patients in the ICU to acquire skills in lung ultrasound. It is a necessary tool to diagnose and manage otherwise life-threatening lung pathologies accurately and promptly.

2. Overview

One of the most applied areas of bedside ultrasound (USS) in managing critically ill patients is lung ultrasonography. Bedside lung ultrasound plays a critical role in promptly diagnosing and managing patients with respiratory distress and other pulmonary conditions. Studies have also shown that lung USS has a higher sensitivity than chest X-ray in detecting pneumothorax, pulmonary oedema, pleural effusion and pneumonia [1]. This chapter thus explores the clinical applications and practical considerations of bedside lung ultrasound in the critically ill.

Tobi et al. [2] published a case series involving four patients with different clinical indications, such as confirmation of central line placement, confirmation of pneumothorax and diagnosis of haemoperitoneum. The authors highlighted how bedside ultrasound scans in the intensive care unit positively influenced the management of these patients. This report is a testament to the versatility of bedside USS, even in low-resource centres, offering hope for improved patient care.

Performing a bedside USS requires adequate knowledge of the USS machine, approach to the patient and patient-to-screen orientation. Sound waves travel from the machine as echoes to produce an image. The speed of ultrasound through tissues depends on the tissues' density and content. Absorption of ultrasound by the tissues also depends on the density; for example, denser tissues absorb sound waves better to produce white/bright images. For example, bone and the diaphragm appear bright on the USS, while fluid appears black.

Different probes are employed during bedside USS. These could be high or low-frequency probes. High-frequency probes, for example, linear probes, produce high resolution and low penetration, while low-frequency probes produce low resolution and high penetration. Note that frequency and resolution are inversely related to penetration (high-frequency probes for high (superficial) structures while low-frequency probes for lower (deeper) structures).

Linear probes, with a frequency of 5–15 MHz, are preferred for lung ultrasound scans because of their high resolution, which makes them suitable for examining the lungs and other superficial structures [3].

3. Technique of lung USS

A linear probe is applied to the anterior chest perpendicular to the ribs and between two ribs at eight quadrants: three anterior, three posterior and two lateral quadrants. During lung USS, the heart is usually avoided by using the Bedside Lung Ultrasound in Emergency (BLUE) hand manoeuvre, a technique that involves the use of the upper and lower blue hands to ensure accurate and safe scanning [4].

Another important consideration during lung USS is the location of the PLAPS (Posterior-Lateral Alveolar and Pleural Syndrome) point, which refers to the point of intersection between a transverse line drawn from the lower BLUE point to the posterior axillary line [5]. This point is crucial for identifying specific lung pathologies.

4. Normal lung USS features

It is essential to familiarise oneself with the features of a normal lung on ultrasound in order to recognise diseased lungs. The features of a normal lung include the following [6]

- Lung sliding refers to a shimmering movement of the pleural line.
- A-line: hyperechoic horizontal artefacts which arise from the pleural line and are equidistant.

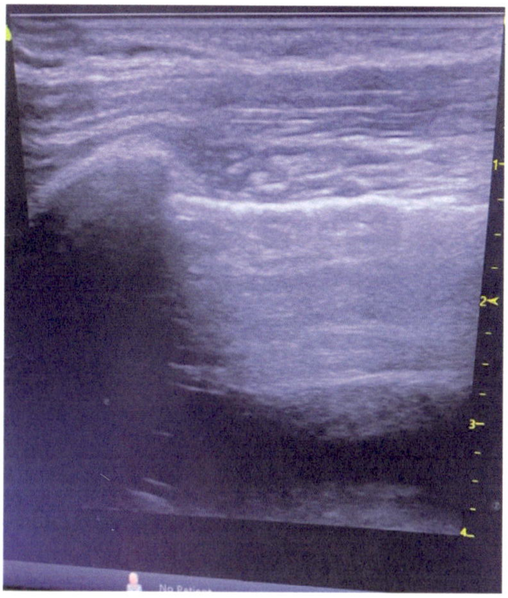

Figure 1.
A normal lung on USS showing horizontal hyperechoic A-lines.

- A-line signifies air.
- Seashore sign on M-mode: The pleural line appears continuous and smooth, with horizontal lines representing A-lines. It is seen as Sky = Skin/Subcutaneous Tissue, Ocean Muscle, Beach = Lung sliding motion (sandy appearance).

Thus, any deviation from these features represents lung pathology (**Figure 1**).

5. Common lung pathologies on lung USS

5.1 Pneumothorax

Pneumothorax is a common emergency in the ICU, characterised by the presence of air in the pleural space, resulting in lung collapse. The degree of collapse determines the clinical presentation of pneumothorax [7].

Signs and symptoms of pneumothorax include chest pain, dyspnoea, decreased breathing sounds and respiratory distress. It is crucial to promptly diagnose a pneumothorax to facilitate prompt management. This includes needle aspiration at the second intercostal space, mid-clavicular line, chest tube insertion into the pleural space connected to a one-way flow and thoracostomy with a small-bore catheter 7-14FG or a larger 28FG [8].

To identify a pneumothorax on lung USS: [9].

Place the probe first to the midclavicular line (MCL) to access apices of the lungs, then medial to the nipple to locate the middle base and then the AAL/PAL for the lower lung bases. Observe the following:

- absent lung sliding,

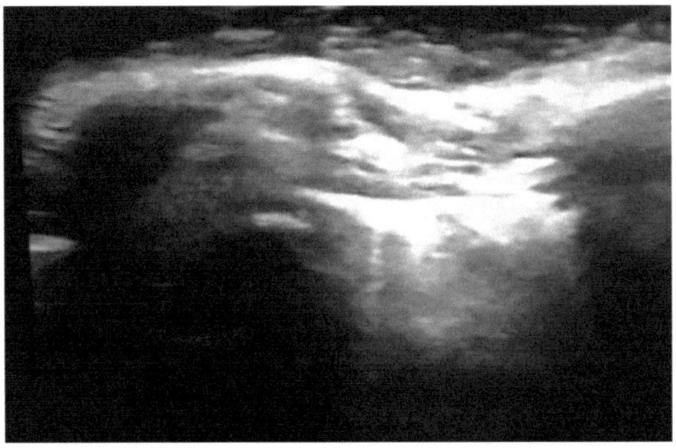

Figure 2.
Features of pneumothorax with absent lung sliding and presence of lung point in a 28-year-old male patient with polytrauma.

- no B-lines,
- barcode sign on M-mode,
- Lung point sign: the junction between lung sliding and absent Lung sliding. It refers to the point where the visceral begins to separate from the parietal pleural (**Figure 2**).

5.2 Pulmonary oedema

Pulmonary oedema results from an abnormal accumulation of extravascular fluid in the lung parenchyma, leading to diminished gas exchange at the alveolar level, progressing to potentially causing respiratory failure. It is usually classified into cardiogenic and non-cardiogenic.

Common causes of pulmonary oedema in the ICU include fluid overload, air embolism, sepsis and multiple blood transfusions. Clinical features include progressive worsening dyspnoea and worsening hypoxia, making an urgent diagnosis and management very crucial by the bedside using lung USS [10].

Diagnosis of pulmonary oedema with lung USS: [11].

- Presence of B-lines, which are comet-tail artefacts arising from the pleural line with a well-defined laser ray. It is hyperechoic and long, and it moves with lung sliding.
- > 3 B-lines = Lung rocket
- > 5 B-lines = ground glass rockets
- Diuretic challenge will reduce comet tails (**Figure 3**).

5.3 Pneumonia

Pneumonia is an infection of the lung parenchyma caused by various organisms, resulting in varied manifestations and sequelae [12]. Pneumonia can be classified

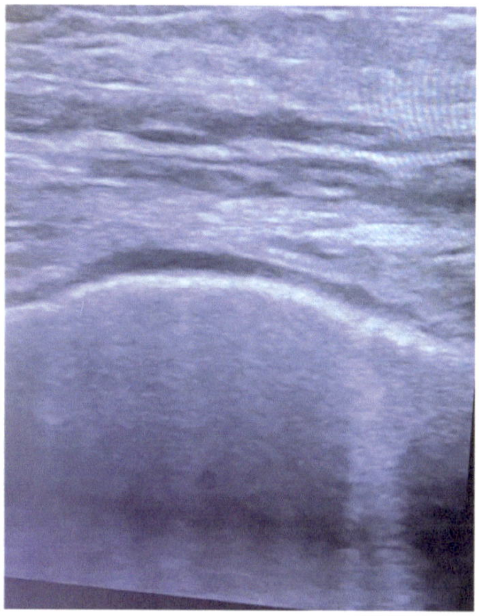

Figure 3.
B-lines, vertical hyperechoic arising from the pleural line in a 28-year-old male patient.

as Community-Acquired Pneumonia (CAP), referring to any pneumonia acquired outside a hospital in a community setting [13]. Hospital-acquired pneumonia (HAP), pneumonia acquired 48 hours after being admitted in an inpatient setting such as a hospital and not incubating at the time of admission, is considered as HAP [14]. and Ventilator-Associated Pneumonia (VAP), pneumonia acquired 48 hours after endotracheal intubation is considered as VAP [15].

Clinical features of pneumonia include tachypnoea, tachycardia, decreased or bronchial breath sounds and respiratory distress.

Diagnosis of Pneumonia with lung USS: [16].

- presence of bumping pleural lines, aka "Shred sign,"
- absent B-lines,
- presence of lung sliding,
- lung hepatisation lung looks like the liver, aka "tissue-like sign" (**Figure 4**).

5.4 Acute respiratory distress syndrome (ARDS)

Acute respiratory distress syndrome (ARDS) is a life-threatening condition characterised by fever, tachypnoea, poor oxygenation and pulmonary infiltrates, developing after 24 hours of an inciting process.

Common causes of ARDS include aspiration pneumonitis, respiratory infections and sepsis. The cornerstone of management is supportive care, which revolves around reducing shunt fraction, increasing oxygen delivery, decreasing oxygen consumption and avoiding further injury [17].

USS diagnosis of ARDS:

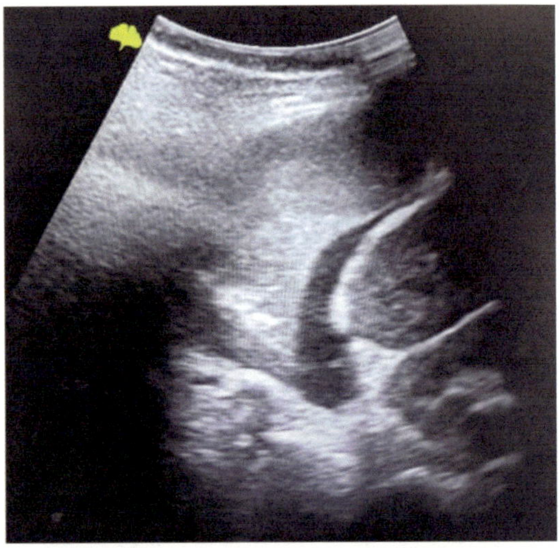

Figure 4.
This image shows a hepatisation of the lung shredded lower border, which is the shred sign, indicative of pneumonic consolidation.

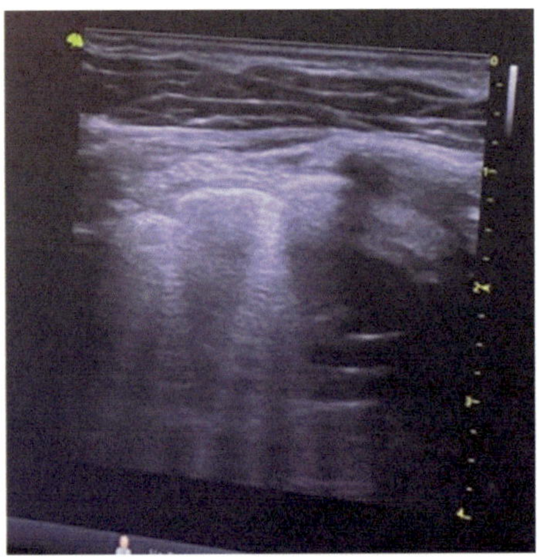

Figure 5.
Features of ARDS in a 28-year-old male patient with polytrauma.

- presence of diffuse bilateral comet tails pattern (B-lines), and
- diuretic challenge does not reduce the number of comet tails (**Figure 5**),

5.5 Pleural effusion

Pleural effusion is defined as fluid accumulation between the parietal and visceral pleura. It can be spontaneous or secondary to infection, malignancy or other inflammatory conditions [18].

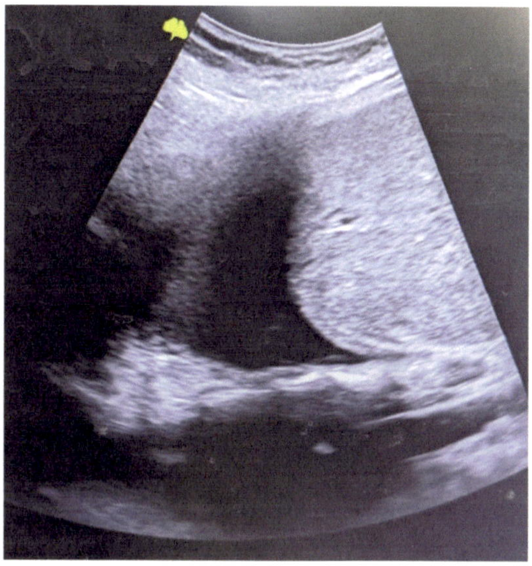

Figure 6.
Pleura effusion in a 33-year-old female patient with severe preeclampsia.

Pleural fluid is classified as a transudate or exudate. Signs and symptoms of symptomatic pleural effusion include exertional breathlessness, sharp, severe, localised crescendo/decrescendo pain with breathing or a cough [19].

Treatment usually includes chest tube drainage, usually with antibiotics. Small-bore drains (10 G to 14 G) are equally effective as large-bore drains, so thoracoscopic decortication or debridement may be necessary if there is no significant improvement.

USS diagnosis of pleural effusion: [20, 21].

- Spine sign (visualisation of vertebral bodies above the diaphragm)
- Loss of mirror image in the RUQ
- The Quad sign on B-mode and the Sinusoid sign on M-mode (**Figure 6**)

6. Discussion

Traditionally, the diagnosis of respiratory distress in the ICU has been made clinically by obtaining chest X-ray and computed tomography (CT) scans. Recently, lung USS has emerged as a valuable tool in this context, offering several advantages over traditional methods. As with all other clinical conditions, clinical examination is the initial step in evaluating a patient with respiratory distress. This includes a thorough history, and physical examination, including chest auscultation and assessment of vital signs. While clinical examination is essential, it is often impossible to obtain history from patients in the ICU who are sedated and requiring respiratory support. In addition, clinical examination such as chest auscultation is insufficient to diagnose specific pulmonary conditions accurately [22].

Chest radiography (CXR) is a widely used diagnostic tool in the ICU for evaluating respiratory distress. It is readily available and can identify causes of respiratory distress such as pneumothorax, pleural effusion, pulmonary oedema and consolidation. However, CXR has limitations, including radiation exposures and lower sensitivity and specificity compared to lung USS, particularly in critically ill patients who may have complex, overlapping pathologies [23, 24]. Furthermore, the unavailability of portable X-ray machines in most resource-limited environments necessitates transporting unstable patients to the radiological suite.

Computed tomography (CT) scans, on the other hand, offer detailed imaging and high diagnostic accuracy, making them the gold standard for many pulmonary conditions. Studies have shown that CT findings of causes of respiratory distress compare favourably well with lung USS. Moreover, CT scans have some disadvantages which include the need for patient transport, higher radiation exposure and a longer time to obtain results, which can be critical in an ICU setting [25, 26].

The appeal of lung USS in promptly diagnosing lung pathologies stems from its high sensitivity and specificity. It has been shown that lung USS has a sensitivity of 88% and a specificity of 99% for detecting pneumothorax, outperforming CXR, which has a sensitivity of around 75–85% and a specificity of 98% [27]. This makes the use of lung USS in diagnosing pneumothorax very high, making it a reliable tool for immediate bedside assessment and management.

For pleural effusion, lung USS has a sensitivity of 93% and specificity of 96%, significantly higher than CXR, which has a sensitivity of about 50–70% [28]. Lung USS also allows precise quantification of pleural fluid and can guide thoracentesis, increasing its clinical utility. Lung USS can detect pneumonic consolidation with, a sensitivity ranging from 80 to 90% and specificity from 90 to 95%, compared to CXR's sensitivity of 60–70% and specificity of 80–90% [29].

Nevertheless, false-positive results may arise with lung USS, including misinterpretation of ultrasound artefacts or normal anatomical structures as pathological findings. For instance, Z-lines can be mistaken for B-lines, leading to a false diagnosis of interstitial syndrome. Misidentification of pleural thickening as pneumothorax is another potential source of false positives. Some studies have reported several false-positive results with the use of lung USS in patients with neoplasia, atelectasis, pulmonary infarction and fibrotic band [25, 30].

False-negative results in lung USS can also occur due to operator inexperience, suboptimal scanning techniques or atypical presentations of diseases. For example, small pneumothoraces or early pneumonia might be missed if the examination is not thorough. Additionally, underlying conditions like severe subcutaneous emphysema can hinder ultrasound penetration, leading to false negatives.

Therefore, to limit false-negative results, ensuring proper training and regular practice for ICU clinicians to enhance their proficiency in lung USS interpretation is recommended. Furthermore, it is crucial to adopt a systematic approach to scanning, covering all lung zones to minimise missed diagnoses. Understanding and distinguishing between true pathological findings and artefacts such as A-lines, B-lines and Z-lines, and employing standard protocols like the BLUE (Bedside Lung Ultrasound in Emergency) protocol to guide diagnostic evaluation should be emphasised. Integrating lung USS findings with clinical assessment and other diagnostic tools helps to enhance overall diagnostic accuracy.

7. Conclusion

Bedside lung ultrasound in the critically ill is an important diagnostic tool with diverse applications in assessing various pulmonary conditions. Lung USS offers superior sensitivity, specificity and accuracy compared to traditional methods like clinical examination and CXR. While CT remains the gold standard for certain conditions, the advantages of lung USS, including bedside availability, rapidity and lack of radiation exposure, make it invaluable in the critical care setting. Awareness of potential false-negative and false-positive results and adherence to best practices can further enhance the utility of lung USS, ultimately improving patient outcomes in the ICU.

Author details

Kingsley Ufuoma Tobi[1*] and Aderonke Adesiyan[2]

1 Department of Anaesthesia and Intensive Care Unit, University Teaching Hospital, Kigali/University of Rwanda, Rwanda

2 Department of Anaesthesia and Intensive Care, Kibungo Referral Hospital/African Health Sciences University, Rwanda

*Address all correspondence to: tobikingsley265@gmail.com; tobikingsley@yahoo.com

References

[1] Tobi KU, Umuhire OF, Mumporese L, Uwamahoro L, Mbanjumucyo G, Banguti PR. Bedside ultrasound scan in the intensive care unit of a referral hospital in Kigali, Rwanda: Case reports and a review of the literature-case series. Rwanda Medical Journal. 2020;**77**(2):1-5

[2] Ebrahimi A, Yousefifard M, Mohammad Kazemi H, et al. Diagnostic accuracy of chest ultrasonography versus chest radiography for identification of pneumothorax: A systematic review and meta-analysis. Tanaffos. 2014;**13**(4):29-40

[3] Marini TJ, Rubens DJ, Zhao YT, Weis J, O'Connor TP, Novak WH, et al. Lung ultrasound: The essentials. Radiology: Cardiothoracic Imaging. 2021;**3**(2):1-5

[4] Lichtenstein D, Meziere G. The BLUE-points: Three standardized points used in the BLUE-protocol for ultrasound assessment of the lung in acute respiratory failure. Critical Ultrasound Journal. 2014;**3**:109-110

[5] Lichtenstein DA. Lung ultrasound in the critically ill. Annals of Intensive Care. 2014;**4**(1):1-12

[6] Miller A. Practical approach to lung ultrasound. BJA Education. 2016;**16**(2):39-45

[7] McKnight CL, Burns B. Pneumothorax. In: StatPearls [Internet]. Treasure Island (FL): StatPearls Publishing; 2023

[8] Mandt MJ, Hayes K, Severyn F, Adelgais K. Appropriate needle length for emergent pediatric needle thoracostomy utilizing computed tomography. Prehospital Emergency Care. Sep-Oct 2019;**23**(5):663-671. DOI: 10.1080/10903127.2019.1566422. Epub 2019 Feb 4. PMID: 30624127

[9] Rippey J. Lung ultrasound: Pneumothorax. Life in the Fastlane. 2022

[10] Murray JF. Pulmonary edema: Pathophysiology and diagnosis. The International Journal of Tuberculosis and Lung Disease. 2011;**15**(2):155-160

[11] Soldati G, Demi M, Demi L. Ultrasound patterns of pulmonary edema. Annals of Translational Medicine. Mar 2019;**7**(Suppl 1):S16. DOI: 10.21037/atm.2019.01.49. PMID: 31032297; PMCID: PMC6462619

[12] Mackenzie G. The definition and classification of pneumonia. Pneumonia (Nathan). 2016;**8**:14

[13] Mandell LA, Wunderink RG, Anzueto A, Bartlett JG, Campbell GD, Dean NC, et al. Infectious Diseases Society of America/American Thoracic Society consensus guidelines on the management of community-acquired pneumonia in adults. Clinical Infectious Diseases. 1 Mar 2007;**44**(Suppl 2):S27-72. DOI: 10.1086/511159. PMID: 17278083; PMCID: PMC7107997

[14] Kalil AC, Metersky ML, Klompas M, Muscedere J, Sweeney DA, Palmer LB, et al. Executive summary: Management of adults with hospital-acquired and ventilator-associated pneumonia: 2016 clinical practice guidelines by the Infectious Diseases Society of America and the American Thoracic Society. Clinical Infectious Diseases. 2016;**63**(5):575-582

[15] Canadian Critical Care Trials Group. A randomized trial of diagnostic techniques for ventilator-associated pneumonia. The New England Journal of Medicine. 2006;**355**(25):2619-2630

[16] Venkatesh M, Deng F, Gaillard F, et al. Shred Sign (Lungs). Reference Article, Radiopaedia.org. DOI: 10.53347/rID-30808 [Accessed: 19 January 2024]

[17] Diamond M, Peniston HL, Sanghavi DK, Mahapatra S. Acute respiratory distress syndrome. In: StatPearls [Internet]. Treasure Island (FL): StatPearls Publishing; 2023

[18] Kugasia IAR, Kumar A, Khatri A, Saeed F, Islam H, Epelbaum O. Primary effusion lymphoma of the pleural space: Report of a rare complication of cardiac transplant with review of the literature. Transplant Infectious Disease. Feb 2019;**21**(1):e13005. DOI: 10.1111/tid.13005. Epub 2018 Oct 30. PMID: 30276937

[19] Krishna R, Antoine MH, Rudrappa M. Pleural effusion. In: StatPearls [Internet]. Treasure Island (FL): StatPearls Publishing; 2023

[20] Soni NJ, Franco R, Velez MI, Schnobrich D, Dancel R, Restrepo MI, et al. Ultrasound in the diagnosis & management of pleural effusions. Journal of Hospital Medicine. 2015;**10**(12):811

[21] Carroll D, Knipe H, Sharma R, et al. Pleural effusion volume (ultrasound). Reference article, Radiopaedia.org. DOI: 10.53347/rID-63392 [Accessed: August 31, 2024]

[22] Lichtenstein D, Goldstein I, Mourgeon E, Cluzel P, Grenier P, Rouby JJ. Comparative diagnostic performances of auscultation, chest radiography, and lung ultrasonography in acute respiratory distress syndrome. Anesthesiology. 2004;**100**:9-15

[23] Fox JC, Irwin Z. Emergency and critical care imaging. Emergency Medicine Clinics of North America. 2008;**26**:787-812

[24] Chiumello D, Sferrazza Papa GF, Artigas A, et al. ERS statement on chest imaging in acute respiratory failure. The European Respiratory Journal. 2019;**54**:1900435

[25] Nazerian P, Volpicelli G, Vanni S, et al. Accuracy of lung ultrasound for the diagnosis of consolidations when compared to chest computed tomography. The American Journal of Emergency Medicine. 2015;**33**:620-625

[26] Raptis CA, Hammer MM, Short RG, et al. Chest CT and coronavirus disease (COVID-19): A critical review of the literature to date. AJR. American Journal of Roentgenology. 2020;**215**:839-842

[27] Ding W, Shen Y, Yang J, He X, Zhang M. Diagnosis of pneumothorax by radiography and ultrasonography. Chest. 2011;**140**(4):859-866. DOI: 10.1378/chest.10-2946

[28] Rocco M, Carbone I, Morelli A, et al. Diagnostic accuracy of bedside ultrasonography in the ICU: Feasibility of detecting pulmonary effusion and lung contusion in patients on respiratory support after severe blunt thoracic trauma. Acta Anaesthesiologica Scandinavica. 2008;**52**(6):776-784

[29] Lichtenstein DA, Meziere GA. Relevance of lung ultrasound in the diagnosis of acute respiratory failure: The BLUE protocol. Chest. 2008;**134**:117-125

[30] Ticinesi A, Lauretani F, Nouvenne A, et al. Lung ultrasound and chest x-ray for detecting pneumonia in an acute geriatric ward. Medicine. 2016;**95**:e4153

Section 5

Abdomen

Chapter 12

Perspective Chapter: Multiparametric Ultrasound in the Evaluation of Fatty Liver Disease

Ioan Sporea, Alexandru Popa and Alina Popescu

Abstract

Conventional ultrasound is an imaging technique that is both useful for screening and for the diagnosis of abdominal diseases. It is an effective method for diagnosing liver steatosis but cannot objectively assess the severity of fatty infiltration or the impact and prognosis of the disease. These limitations of conventional ultrasound have been overcome by the development of different ultrasound applications, namely ultrasound-based elastography and ultrasound-based fat quantification techniques. These advancements have led to the possibility of conducting a comprehensive ultrasound evaluation of the liver in the presence of diffuse changes—referred to as a multiparametric ultrasound evaluation (MPUS).

Keywords: multiparametric ultrasound (MPUS), fatty liver disease, ultrasound-based elastography, metabolic dysfunction-associated steatotic liver disease (MASLD), point of care ultrasound (POCUS)

1. Introduction

Fatty liver disease is currently the most common pathological condition encountered by hepatologists. While scientific focus once centered on the treatment of chronic viral diseases such as HBV, HCV, and HDV, the landscape has shifted. With the advent of highly effective treatments for HCV, which can eradicate the virus with oral medication within 8–12 weeks, and the availability of drugs that control HBV viral replication, like Entecavir or Tenofovir (one tablet daily), research emphasis has moved to areas where staging and treatment are imperative. Despite the high prevalence of alcoholic liver disease (ALD), it receives disproportionately low investment in terms of energy and resources. By contrast, in recent years, fatty liver disease has surged to the forefront in medical publications as a primary pathological concern.

Examining the prevalence of fatty liver in the general population, a recent epidemiological study by Younossi et al. indicates that approximately 30% of the general population is affected by this condition [1]. According to the study, Europe has the lowest prevalence at 25%, whereas South America has a prevalence of 44% and South Asia 34%. These figures represent an increase from previous studies which reported prevalence of 30.4% in South America and 23.7% in Europe [2]. It is also crucial to monitor the prevalence among specific populations, such as patients with type 2 diabetes mellitus (T2DM), where fatty liver is exceedingly common. An epidemiological review by Younossi et al. found a global prevalence of 55.5% among T2DM patients, with Europe reporting a rate of 68% [3]. More recently, a meta-analysis by Cho et al. included over 1.8 million patients with T2DM and revealed prevalence rates of fatty liver and steatohepatitis (NASH) at 65.0 and 31.5%, respectively. The study also found that 35.5% of T2DM patients with NAFLD had clinically significant fibrosis (F2-F4), and 14.9% had advanced fibrosis (F3-F4) [4].

Regarding the terminology for fatty liver, the term non-alcoholic fatty liver disease (NAFLD) was used for a long time. Recently, this term was modified to metabolically associated fatty liver disease (MAFLD) as proposed by Eslam et al., in the International Consensus Panel's publication: "MAFLD: A Consensus-Driven Proposed Nomenclature for Metabolically Associated Fatty Liver Disease" [5]. However, in 2023, a group of experts decided to change the nomenclature to metabolic dysfunction associated steatotic liver disease (MASLD), as detailed in the multisociety Delphi consensus statement on new fatty liver disease nomenclature by Rinella et al., published in Hepatology on June 24, 2023 [6].

Risk factors for MASLD, such as obesity, T2DM, and metabolic syndrome, are well-established. Given the high prevalence of MASLD, the challenge lies in how to detect this condition in the general population efficiently in a short time and cost-effectively. This is where Multiparametric Ultrasound (MPUS) comes into play. MPUS is a commonly used diagnostic tool that is integrated into ultrasound machines, providing a variety of parameters within minutes. The concept of "Point of Care Ultrasound" (POCUS) has gained traction in recent years, especially as more clinicians are performing ultrasound procedures themselves. This means that an ultrasound system in the consultation room allows for an immediate ultrasound examination following a clinical evaluation, which can then be extended to include a comprehensive MPUS assessment.

What does MPUS mean? MPUS stands for multiparametric ultrasound. It is the combination of multiple ultrasound techniques that allows the comprehensive assessment of various tissue parameters using a single ultrasound machine. In the context of patients with metabolic associated steatotic liver disease (MASLD), MPUS provides valuable insights into liver health. MPUS can provide comprehensive information about the liver, including the degree of steatosis (fat accumulation) and fibrosis (scarring). More recently, it has been used to evaluate shear wave dispersion (viscosity), which is presumed to be a marker of liver inflammation. This technique enables a rapid and non-invasive evaluation of these liver conditions, which is valuable in the diagnosis and management of MASLD [7].

Which is the definition of fatty liver? Fatty liver is defined as a condition where there is an excessive accumulation of fat in the liver cells, or hepatocytes. Specifically, it is characterized by more than 5% of hepatocytes containing fat droplets. While liver biopsy remains the gold standard for morphological evaluation and diagnosis, numerous non-invasive methods have been developed for diagnosing fatty liver. Among imaging techniques, ultrasound is widely used due to its safety and accessibility. However, computed tomography (CT), while effective, exposes patients to ionizing radiation, magnetic resonance imaging (MRI) provides excellent detail but is often more expensive and less accessible, making them less ideal for routine fatty liver screening. Although MR proton density fat fraction (PDFF) is the recommended reference standard by several guidelines for the quantification of liver fat content, its high cost and limited accessibility make it less feasible for routine use.

We propose ultrasound as the method of choice for assessing fatty liver infiltration. Ultrasound offers an economical and accessible solution, suitable for point-of-care settings, and it can be easily repeated over time to monitor changes. With MPUS, we can quickly diagnose fatty liver, assess liver stiffness, and presumably evaluate inflammation, all within a short timeframe.

2. Evaluation of steatosis using ultrasound

a. *Conventional ultrasound* has long been recognized as an effective method for assessing liver steatosis. Classic and simple indicators such as a "bright liver," "posterior attenuation," and an increased "hepato-renal index" facilitate a semi-quantitative evaluation of fatty infiltration in the liver. These signs allow for the subjective categorization of steatosis as mild, moderate, or severe. In addition to these, other practical scoring systems have been introduced, such as the Hamaguchi score. This score is based on four ultrasound signs: hepato-renal index, liver brightness, deep attenuation, and vessel blurring (the clarity of liver vessel borders and luminal narrowing). Hamaguchi et al. highlighted that the severity of ultrasonographic findings in nonalcoholic fatty liver disease is indicative of the metabolic syndrome and visceral fat accumulation (**Figures 1** and **2**) [8].

Although these ultrasonographic signs are simple and somewhat subjective, numerous studies have demonstrated their significant value in assessing the severity of liver steatosis. In a comprehensive meta-analysis by Hernaez et al., which included 49 studies and 4720 subjects, ultrasonography was compared with liver biopsy. The sensitivity of ultrasound for detecting moderate and severe steatosis was 84.8% (95% CI: 79.5–88.9%), with a specificity of 93.6% (95% CI: 87.2–97.0%) [9]. From a clinical standpoint, moderate steatosis and severe steatosis are of particular interest due to their implications. However, critical considerations in this type of evaluation include its

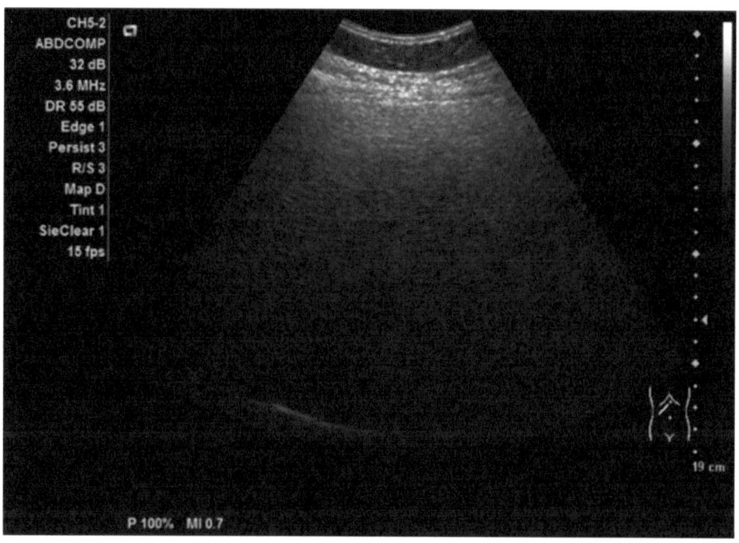

Figure 1.
Bright liver with posterior attenuation.

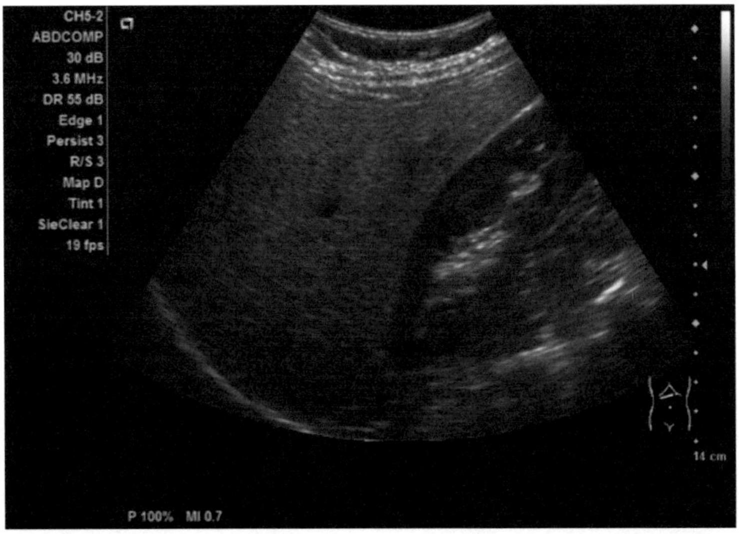

Figure 2.
Increased hepato-renal index.

subjective nature, the potential variability in interpretation, differences in ultrasound machine quality, and challenges in monitoring progression or regression over time.

b. Consequently, there is a need for more objective systems to quantify fatty infiltration. The advent of the FibroScan machine (Echosens, Paris, France) has enabled quantification of steatosis through its *Controlled Attenuation Parameter (CAP) module*, used alongside Vibration-Controlled Transient Elastography (VCTE) for stiffness evaluation. The CAP software, integrated into the FibroScan device since 2010, measures the attenuation of the ultrasound beam, which is directly related to the fat content in the liver. Results are reported in decibels per meter (dB/m), ranging from 100 to 400 dB/m, providing a quantitative assessment of liver steatosis (**Figure 3**) [10].

Numerous studies and meta-analyses have been conducted to evaluate the effectiveness of the CAP method, particularly in comparison with liver biopsy. The Area Under the Receiver Operating Characteristic curves (AUROCs) of CAP for the quantification of fatty infiltration in the liver have been found to range between 0.823 (95% CI: 0.809–0.837) and 0.865 (95% CI: 0.850–0.880) [11, 12]. Furthermore, a meta-analysis by Shi KQ, which included data from 11 patient cohorts, reported that the AUROCs for CAP were 0.85 (95% CI: 0.81–0.88) for ≥ S1 steatosis, 0.88 (95% CI: 0.85–0.91) for ≥ S2, and 0.87 (95% CI: 0.84–0.90) for ≥ S3 [13].

The cutoff values for assessing the severity of liver steatosis vary among different etiologies and authors. In the context of MASLD, the most reliable cutoff values were proposed by Eddowes et al. established using liver biopsy as the reference standard [14]: for S1 (mild)—294 dB/m, for S2 (moderate)—310 dB/m, and for S3 (severe)—331 dB/m. For ease of recall, these can be approximated to 290, 310, and 330 dB/m, respectively.

The CAP can be measured using either the M or XL probe, with the latter being particularly suitable for obese patients. This raises an important question: Should

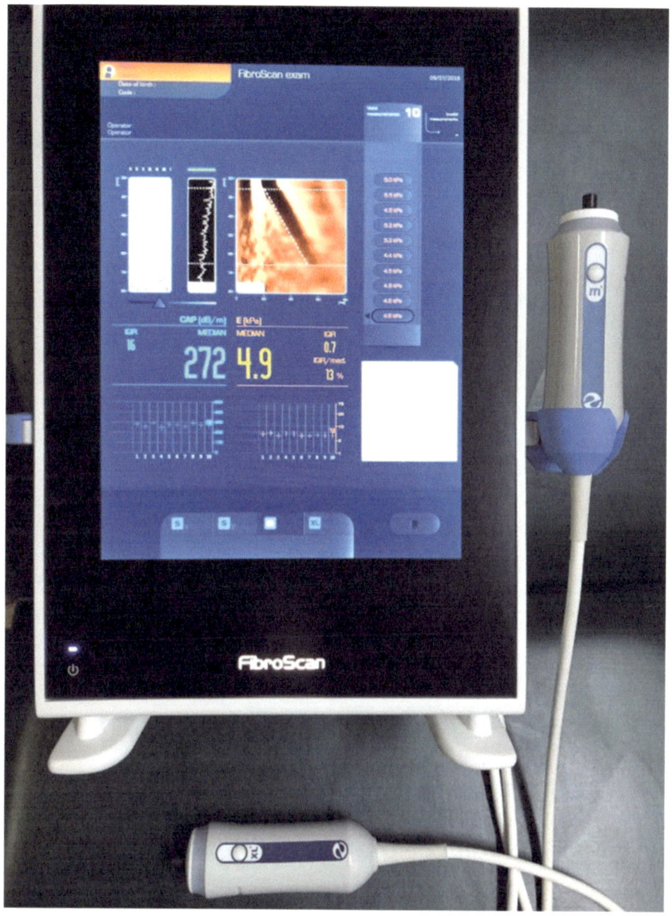

Figure 3.
FibroScan with CAP (CAP values are in light blue) with M and XL probes.

different cutoff values be applied for these two probes? A study by Chan et al., which involved 180 patients with fatty liver disease, that included evaluations using both M and XL probes and liver biopsy as reference method, found that the same CAP cutoff values could be applied for both probes in diagnosing the grade of hepatic steatosis [15]. This finding was corroborated by another study conducted by Eddowes et al. [14].

Steatosis quantification can also be performed using the FibroTouch system (iLivTouch), which employs the Ultrasound Attenuation Parameter (UAP) as described by Qu et al. [16]. In a prospective study involving 237 patients who underwent both FibroTouch and liver biopsy, the FibroTouch examination boasted a high success rate of 96.5%. The AUROC curve for UAP in diagnosing steatosis grades ≥S1, ≥S2, and S3 were 0.88, 0.93, and 0.88, respectively, with corresponding cutoff values of 244, 269, and 296 dB/m. A notable advantage of the FibroTouch system is its use of a single probe for all patients, along with a standard ultrasound probe for initial liver assessment before quantitative analysis. Similar to FibroScan, FibroTouch evaluates liver steatosis, stiffness, and more recently, liver inflammation (**Figure 4**) [16].

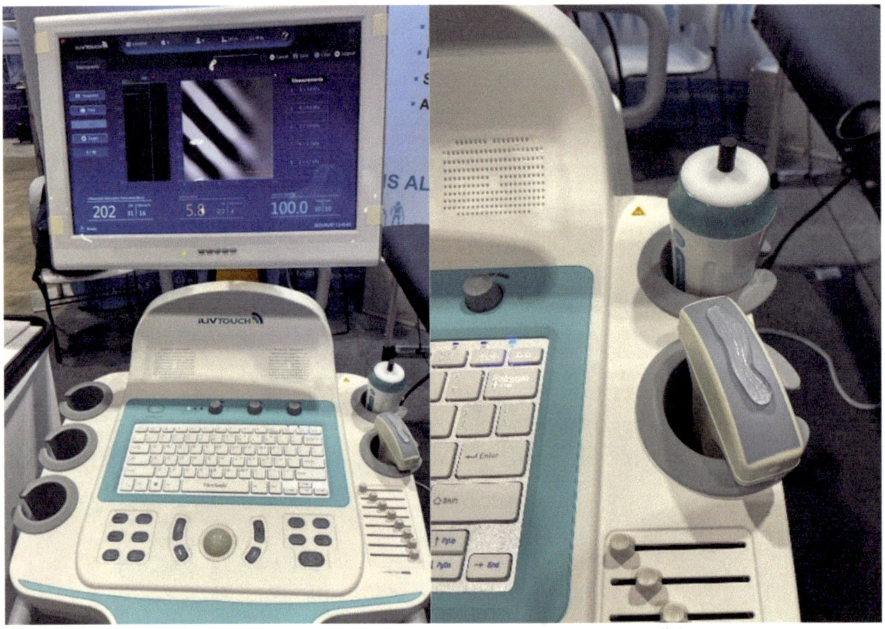

(a) (b)

Figure 4.
a-b. The iLivTouch system in a clinical setting, showcasing its user interface.

2.1 Quantitative ultrasound (QUS)

In the recent years, quantitative ultrasound (QUS) has emerged as a new and developing technique in the field for the objective assessment of fatty liver. Various companies have adopted different approaches for QUS, utilizing parameters such as attenuation, backscattering, or speed of sound. Some companies even combine these parameters to quantitatively measure steatosis. This technique, as detailed by Park et al., is remarkably straightforward and quick, offering the added benefit of being a point-of-care method (**Figure 5**) [17].

When patients undergo abdominal ultrasound and the conventional imaging reveals a fatty liver, a QUS evaluation can be immediately conducted to objectively measure steatosis. This method is also advantageous for patient follow-up, allowing for comparison of current results with previous ones. The subsequent images will showcase various QUS types from different manufacturers (**Figures 6–11**). The results in QUS can be expressed in units like dB/m, similar to CAP evaluation, or in dB/cm/MHz.

The validation of these QUS techniques has been supported by studies utilizing liver biopsy as the gold standard, with some of them also employing Proton Density Fat Fraction MRI (PDFF) for comparison. The favorable results obtained by many such systems render QUS as an appealing choice for the initial assessment of patients with MASLD and for subsequent follow-ups.

In the case of ATI, a study involving 114 subjects at potential risk of steatosis and 15 healthy controls compared ATI results with CAP, using MRI-PDFF as the reference. This study, conducted by Ferraioli et al., found ATI to have a higher correlation with MRI-PDFF ($r = 0.81$) than CAP ($r = 0.65$) [18]. Another study by Bae et al., which used liver histology as the standard of reference and included 108 subjects, reported AUROCs for ATI ranging from 0.84 to 0.93 [19].

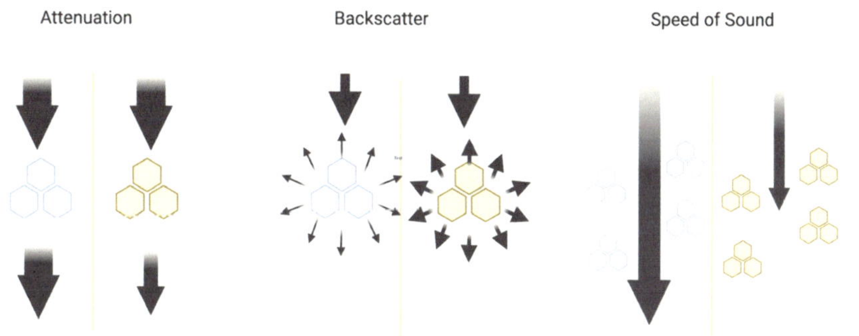

Figure 5.
Illustration of quantitative ultrasound parameters. (A) Attenuation—where the ultrasound wave's diminution is visualized as it passes through different tissues; (B) backscatter—depicting the reflection of ultrasound waves back to the transducer from the tissue interfaces; (C) speed of sound—representing the rate at which sound waves travel through various tissue densities.

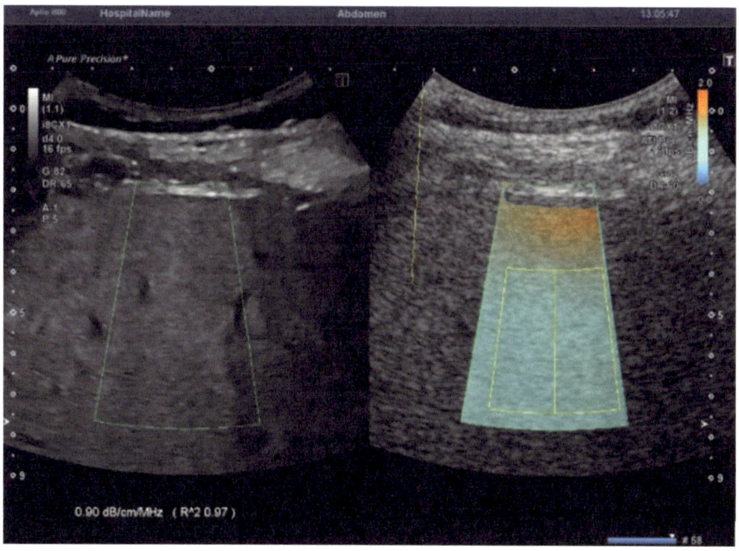

Figure 6.
Attenuation Imaging (ATI) from Canon™.

For Ultrasound Guided Attenuation Parameter (UGAP), Fujiwara et al. conducted a study that included 163 patients with chronic liver diseases. UGAP, CAP, and liver biopsies were conducted simultaneously. The AUROCs for UGAP in identifying steatosis grades >S1, >S2, and S3 were 0.900, 0.953, and 0.959, respectively. These figures were notably superior to those obtained with CAP [20]. A separate study by Imajo, encompassing 1010 patients from six Japanese liver centers, also examined UGAP alongside MRI-PDFF. The UGAP values demonstrated a significant correlation with MRI-PDFF, with an intraclass correlation coefficient of 0.768. Furthermore, the AUROCs for UGAP in distinguishing steatosis grades of ≥1 (MRI-PDFF>5.2%), ≥2 (MRI-PDFF>11.3%), and 3 (MRI-PDFF>17.1%) were consistently high, at 0.91 for grades ≥1 and ≥ 2, and 0.89 for grade 3, showcasing UGAP's diagnostic accuracy [21].

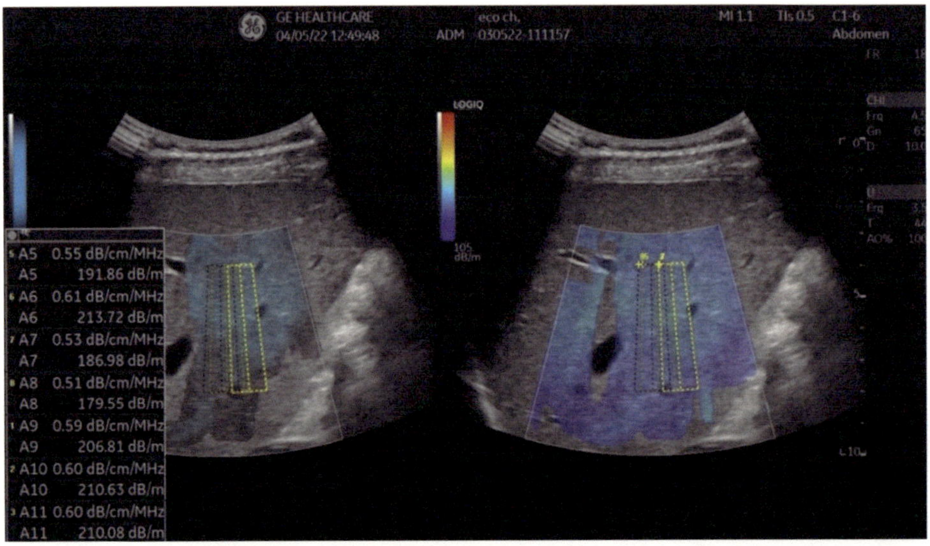

Figure 7.
Ultrasound-Guided Attenuation Parameter (UGAP) from General Electric™.

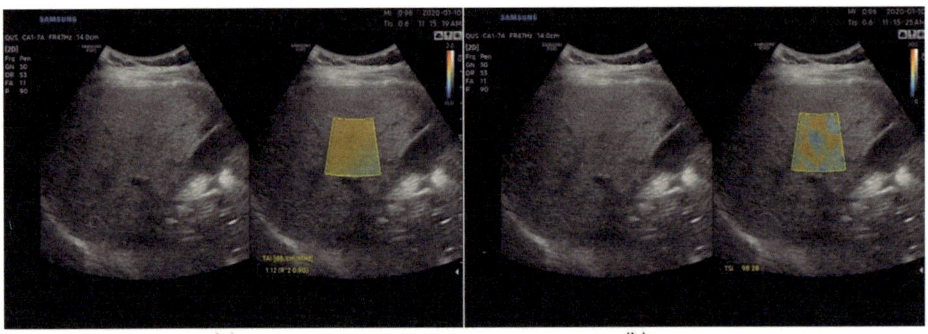

Figure 8.
a-b. Tissue Attenuation Imaging (TAI) and Tissue Scatter distribution Imaging (TSI) from Samsung™.

In a study conducted on 120 patients with clinically suspected NAFLD, Jeon et al. investigated the efficacy of the Samsung system's QUS techniques. The study compared MRI-PDFF with Attenuation Coefficient (AC) obtained from Tissue Attenuation Imaging (TAI) and Tissue Scatter-distribution Imaging (TSI). The findings revealed significant correlations between TAI and TSI with MRI-PDFF, with correlation coefficients of 0.659 and 0.727, respectively ($p < 0.001$ for both). When assessing for hepatic fat content thresholds of ≥5% and ≥ 10% in PDFF, the AUROC scores for TAI were 0.861 and 0.835, while TSI demonstrated superior AUROC scores of 0.964 and 0.935, respectively. These results underscore the potential of TAI and TSI in the non-invasive quantification of hepatic steatosis [22].

As observed in several previously published studies, a comparative analysis conducted between QUS and CAP, using PDFF as the reference method, has provided insightful results. Jung et al. examined a cohort of 123 participants. Their study demonstrated that QUS had a significantly higher AUROC for the diagnosis of NAFLD compared to CAP, with scores of 0.92 versus 0.79, respectively ($p = 0.03$) [23].

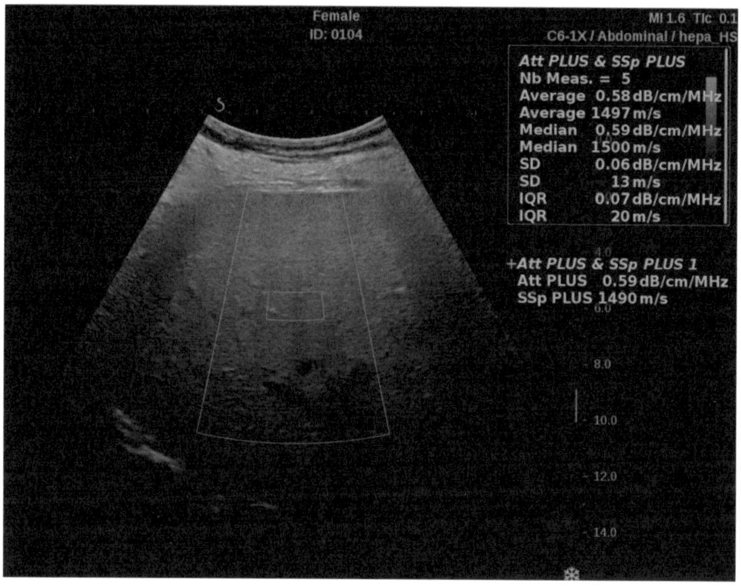

Figure 9.
Speed of Sound estimation (Att Plus and SSp Plus) from Aixplorer (Hologic™).

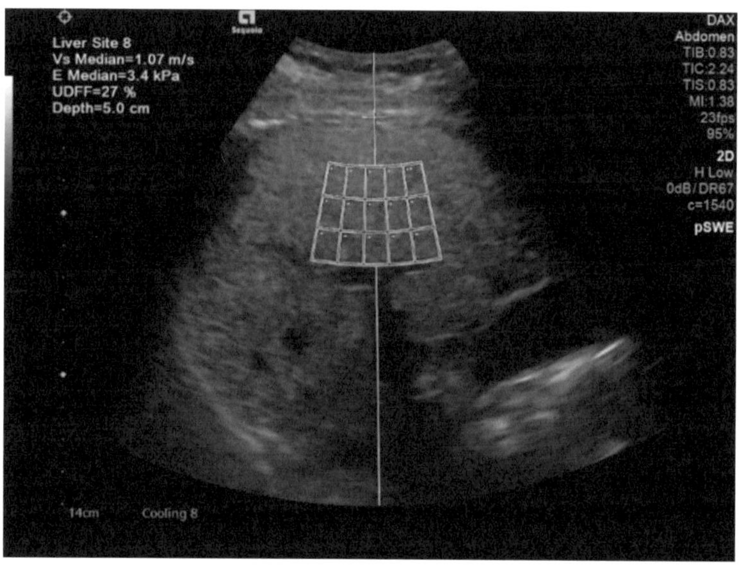

Figure 10.
Ultrasound Derived Fat Fraction (UDFF) from Siemens™, this method expresses fatty infiltration in %.

More and more papers are published regarding the clinical use of QUS in MASLD patients. These studies frequently demonstrate a strong correlation with histological findings and, more recently, with PDFF. Recent publications have found a depth dependence of the attenuation coefficient (AC) and that the size of the region of interest (ROI) affects results. Ferraioli et al. demonstrated that AC values decrease with increasing depth across different ultrasound systems (Canon, Philips, and Siemens) and that AC values with a 1 cm ROI were significantly higher than those

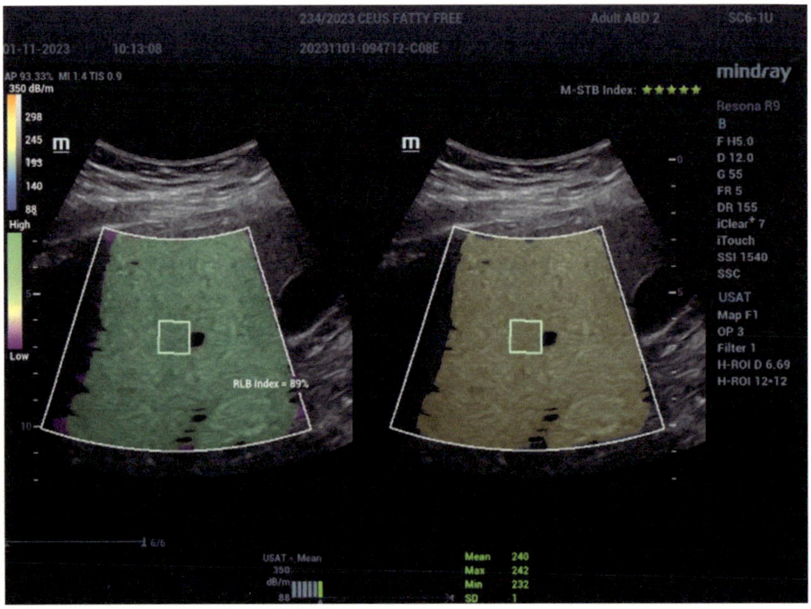

Figure 11.
UltraSound Attenuation Analysis (USAT) from Mindray™.

obtained with a 3 cm ROI at all depths. These issues emphasize the necessity of a standardized protocol to ensure consistent results. Therefore, there is an ongoing pursuit to determine precise cutoff values for various QUS systems, with continuous evaluations and developments [24, 25].

3. Liver stiffness evaluation using ultrasound

After assessing liver steatosis *via* ultrasound, patients with clinically significant steatosis can have their liver stiffness evaluated immediately during MPUS. Liver stiffness is an indicator of liver fibrosis; however, confounding factors such as fasting state, elevated aminotransferases, extrahepatic cholestasis, or right heart failure may influence stiffness measurements. Therefore, we advocate that this assessment should be conducted by trained individuals who are well-versed in the patient's history, ensuring that results are considered within the appropriate clinical context.

Initially, evaluations of liver stiffness were performed in comparison with liver biopsy, with subsequent comparisons made across various degrees of fibrosis, typically classified using the METAVIR score (F1, F2, F3, F4). However, more recently, this method of differentiation has been set aside in favor of new terminology that uses the term cACLD (compensated Advanced Chronic Liver Disease), as introduced in the Baveno VI consensus [26]. The advantage of this updated terminology is that it shifts the focus away from the need to distinguish absent or mild fibrosis (F0 and F1) and emphasizes the differentiation between significant fibrosis, advanced fibrosis, and cirrhosis.

In practice, the ultrasound-based elastographic methods used for liver stiffness evaluation are the Shear Wave Elastographic methods (SWE), as outlined in the EFSUMB Guidelines [27, 28]. These methods can be divided into *Vibration-Controlled*

Transient Elastography (VCTE), which applies a brief mechanical push to the skin's surface at a low frequency with a specific force, and *Acoustic Radiation Force Impulse (ARFI) techniques*, where the ultrasound probe itself produces the acoustic stimulus. ARFI techniques are further subdivided into point SWE (pSWE) and bidimensional SWE (2D-SWE). Results for VCTE are expressed in kilopascals (kPa), while for ARFI, they can be expressed in meters per second (m/s) or kPa [29].

Studies have shown high feasibility, usually over 90%, for all ultrasound-based elastographic methods. VCTE requires two different probes: an M probe and an XL probe for obese individuals. A notable limitation of VCTE is its inapplicability in cases of ascites, and the need for periodic probe calibration, which incurs additional costs. For all elastographic techniques, a crucial qualitative parameter is the IQR/median (interquartile range/median), which should be below 30%. For 2D-SWE, each system incorporates qualitative criteria to assess the quality of acquisition. Currently, all ultrasound companies on the market offer SWE elastographic modules within their systems, with some providing both pSWE and 2D-SWE (e.g., Samsung, Mindray). Why is better to have two elastography modules inside the system? Having dual elastographic modules is an advantage: If feasibility is compromised with one method, such as 2D-SWE, the alternative, pSWE, often yields correct values, allowing patients to leave with a valid result.

VCTE system is featured in both FibroScan and FibroTouch devices, as illustrated in the earlier images. Comparative studies, such as one by Xu et al., have shown similar results between these two machines. In a prospective study of a cohort of 435 patients with chronic liver disease, who also underwent liver biopsy, the AUROC for FibroTouch was comparable to that of FibroScan in diagnosing significant fibrosis, severe fibrosis, or cirrhosis. There was a strong correlation ($r = 0.85$, $p < 0.001$) between FibroTouch and FibroScan readings for liver stiffness. Additionally, no significant differences were found between FibroTouch and FibroScan in terms of sensitivity, specificity, negative predictive value, positive predictive value, and overall accuracy.

Numerous publications and meta-analyses have suggested various cutoff values for liver stiffness measurement using VCTE (FibroScan), taking into account different disease etiologies. More recently, the Baveno VI consensus and subsequently Baveno VII have endorsed the so-called "rule of 5"—a simplified approach to classifying stiffness values (**Figure 12**) [26, 30].

Liver stiffness measurement scale: Depicting cutoff values for the classification of liver stiffness as per Baveno VI and VII consensuses including the "rule of 5" for assessing the risk of liver decompensation and liver-related mortality, with specific thresholds for excluding or assuming cACLD and clinically significant portal hypertension (CSPH) across different liver diseases.

This "rule of 5" offers a straightforward and user-friendly framework: Less than 5 kPa indicates a normal liver; under 10 kPa rules out cACLD; over 15 kPa suggests the presence of cACLD; and values above 25 kPa denote CSPH. In clinical practice, these guidelines allow for the efficient use of elastography for various purposes, such as fibrosis assessment and the determination of cACLD or significant portal hypertension. By using the FibroScan system, firstly, CAP is used to stratify the severity of steatosis, while VCTE quickly confirms or excludes significant fibrosis in a very short time.

ARFI methods have the advantage of integration within a standard ultrasound system, enabling conventional ultrasound assessments, Doppler studies, fat quantification, and stiffness measurement. Additionally, when a focal liver lesion (FLL) is detected, a Contrast Enhanced Ultrasound (CEUS) can be immediately conducted. This comprehensive capability culminates in a truly MPUS approach. Despite the

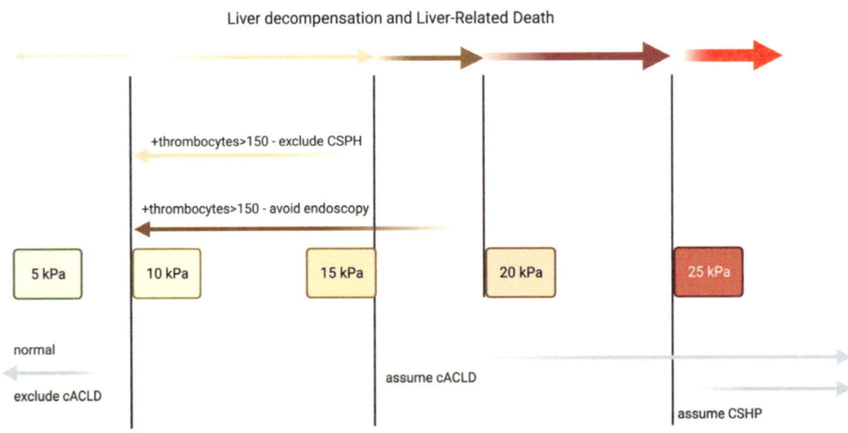

Figure 12.
Liver stiffness measurement scale (adapted after Baveno VII consensus).

varying implementations, all ARFI methods share a common principle where the probe induces tissue excitation. The following images provide examples of pSWE and 2D-SWE (**Figures 13–18**).

From a technical standpoint, the SWE-ARFI methods are straightforward to perform. The patient lies supine with their right arm in maximum abduction, similar to the positioning for VCTE. The ultrasound probe is positioned intercostally to capture the clearest liver image possible. In pSWE, a small measurement box measuring 10 by 5 mm is placed 1–2 cm beneath the liver capsule, ensuring an optimal section of the liver selection while avoiding blood vessels. The patient is then asked to hold his breath in a neutral position, and upon activation, the system takes 5 to 10 measurements, with the median value subsequently displayed. For 2D-SWE, which provides a color-coded and numerical assessment, a larger box around 3 by 2 cm is positioned in a similar manner beneath the liver capsule. Multiple loops are recorded, and a region

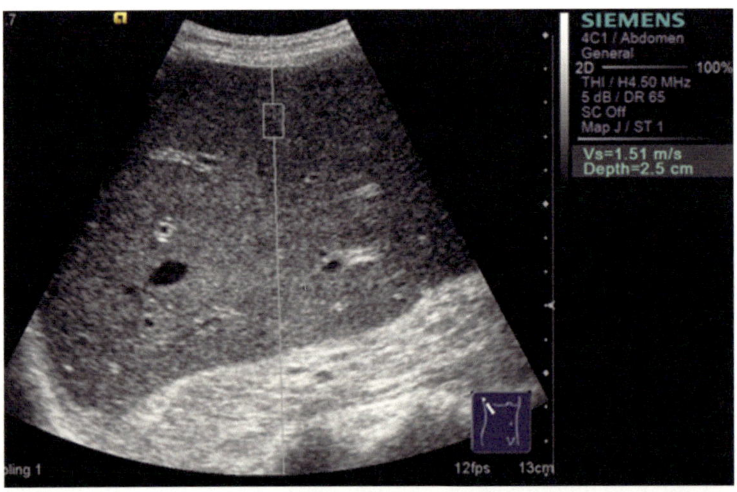

Figure 13.
pSWE-VTQ from Siemens™.

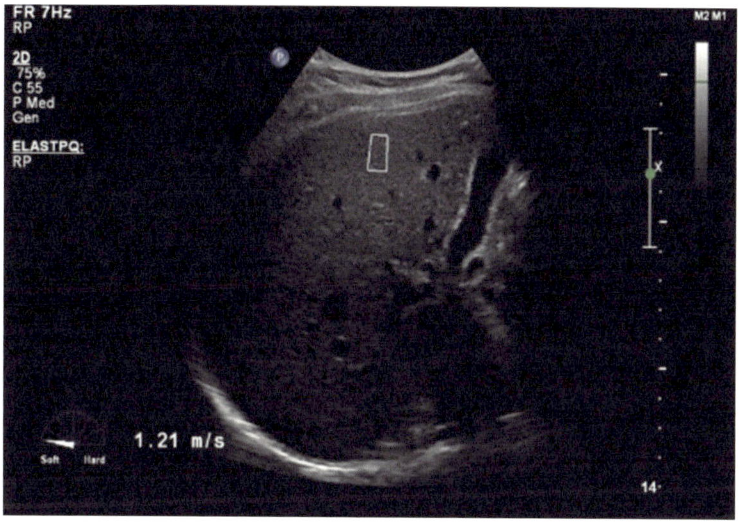

Figure 14.
pSWE-ElastPQ from Philips™.

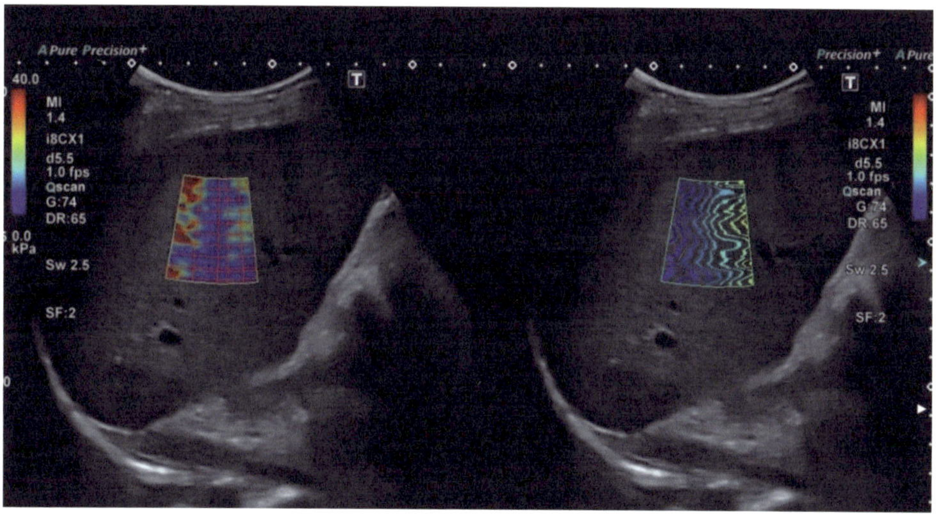

Figure 15.
2D-SWE from Canon™ with quality control.

of interest (ROI) is placed in each frame, to make the assessment. About 3 to 5 measurements are enough, and the system calculates and presents the median value [27].

In the past, every company proposed its own cutoff values, making it quite difficult to apply these in practice. In 2020, a simplified algorithm known as the "Rule of 4" was proposed by Barr in Radiology, facilitating easier application in clinical settings [31]. The recommendations for interpreting liver stiffness values obtained with ARFI techniques in patients with viral hepatitis and NAFLD:

- A stiffness value of ≤5 kPa (1.3 m/sec) suggests a high probability of the liver being normal.

- A value of <9 kPa (1.7 m/sec) in the absence of other known clinical signs indicates that cACLD is unlikely. If there are known clinical signs, further testing may be needed for confirmation.
- A value between 9 and 13 kPa (1.7–2.1 m/sec) is indicative of possible cACLD but requires additional tests for confirmation.
- A value >13 kPa (2.1 m/sec) rules in cACLD.
- A value >17 kPa (2.4 m/sec) is suggestive of CSPH.

The practical utility of SWE for assessing liver stiffness is well-supported in the literature. Numerous papers, including meta-analyses and prospective studies—most

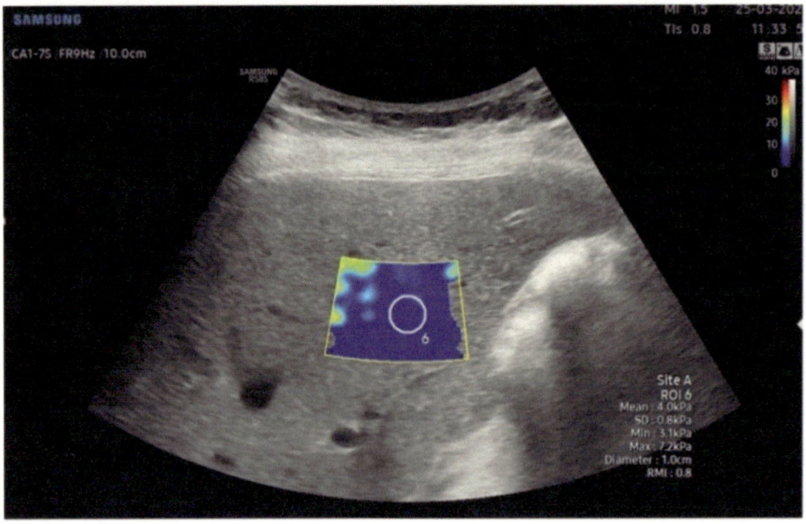

Figure 16.
2D-SWE from Samsung™.

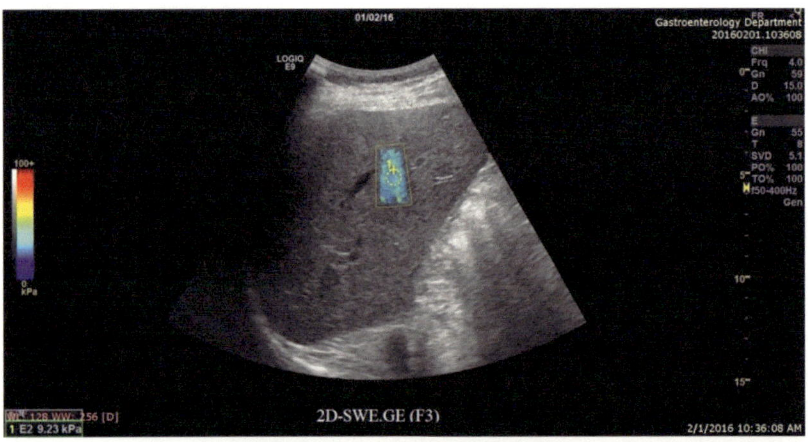

Figure 17.
2D-SWE from General Electric™ with quality control of acquisition.

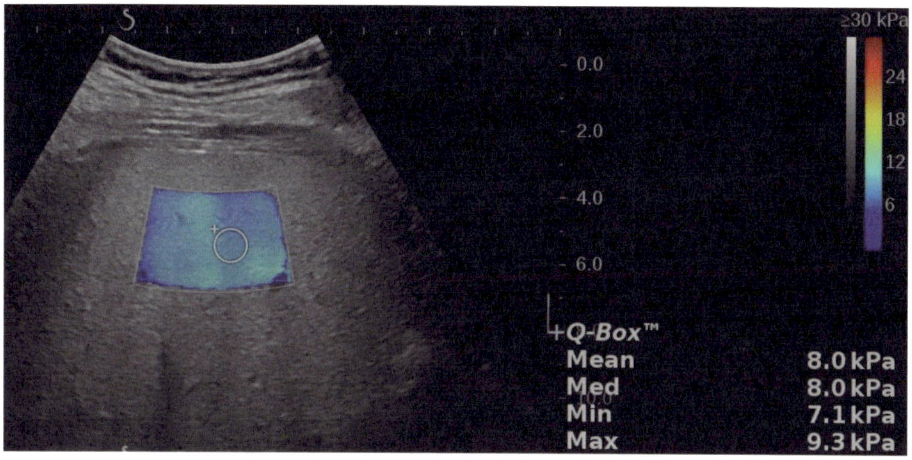

Figure 18.
2D-SWE from Aixplorer (Hologic™).

of which use liver biopsy as the gold standard—demonstrate the efficacy of SWE methods. These studies reveal that the AUROC curves for these methods tend to increase in parallel with the severity of fibrosis, frequently exceeding 90% for cases of liver cirrhosis [32–36].

Comparative studies between various SWE methods have demonstrated their equivalent practical value in assessing liver stiffness [37–42].

The latest EASL Guidelines regarding non-invasive tests for liver stiffness assessment highlight the pros and cons of various methods. These guidelines provide a comprehensive overview of several technologies, including serum markers, transient elastography (TE), point shear wave elastography (pSWE), 2D shear wave elastography (2D-SWE), and magnetic resonance elastography (MRE) (**Table 1**) [43].

The table compares the advantages and disadvantages of serum markers, transient elastography, pSWE, 2D-SWE, and MRE, providing insights into their efficacy, applicability, and potential limitations in the diagnosis and staging of liver fibrosis.

The use of SWE for evaluating portal hypertension (PH) has seen a notable increase in the recent years [30]. While VCTE was initially the primary method used for assessing PH noninvasively, there has been increasing literature supporting the use of ARFI techniques. ARFI has the distinct advantage of visualizing the spleen, thus allowing clinicians to optimally position the measurement box. For the assessment of PH, liver stiffness, spleen stiffness, or a combination of both, sometimes along with the platelet count, have been utilized. This multifaceted approach enables a more comprehensive evaluation of PH and reflects the evolving landscape of non-invasive liver diagnostics [44–46].

4. Liver inflammation

In patients with fatty liver disease, prognostic outcomes are determined not only by the presence of advanced fibrosis but also by the extent of inflammation and hepatocyte ballooning [47]. Although liver biopsy remains the gold standard for assessing these parameters, its practicality is limited considering the global prevalence of fatty liver, affecting over two billion people. In recent years, ultrasound manufacturers

Serum markers			Transient elastography	pSWE	2D-SWE	MRE
Advantages	Non-patented	Patented	• most widely used and validated technique • point-of-care(bedside, easy to learn, rapid) • quality criteria well defined • good reproducibility • high performance for cirrhosis • prognostic value in compensated cirrhosis well validated	• can be performed with regular ultrasound device • ROI smaller than TE and location chosen by the operator • higher applicability than TE • equivalent performance that of TE for advanced fibrosis and cirrhosis • prognostic value in cirrhosis • high applicability for spleen stiffness measurement	• can be performed with regular ultra-sound device • large ROI that can be adjusted in size and location chosen by the operator • measures liver stiff-ness in real time • good applicability • high performance for the diagnosis of advanced fibrosis and cirrhosis • prognostic value in cirrhosis	• can be implemented on a regular MRI machine • examination of the whole liver • higher applicability than TE(ascites and obesity) • -high performance for the earlier fibrosis stage and for diagnosis of cirrhosis
	• good reproducibility • high applicability • no cost and wide availability • well validated • can be performed in the outpatient clinic • validated prognos-tic value	• good reproducibility • high applicability • can be performed in the outpatient clinic • validated prognostic value				
Disadvantages	• non-liver specific • performance not as good as TE and patented serum markers • false-positive results with FIB4 and NFS in case of age > 65 yrs	• cost • non-liver specific • performance not as good as TE for cirrhosis • false-positive results in case of extrahepatic inflammatory condi-tions, profibrotic, extra-hepatic conditions and other (Gilbert syndrome, hemolysis)	• requires a dedicated device • ROI cannot be chosen • lower applicability than serum markers • false-positive in case of acute hepatitis, extrahepatic cholestasis, liver congestion, food intake, excessive alcohol intake.	• false positive in case of acute hepatitis, extrahepatic cholesta-sis, liver congestion, food intake, excessive alcohol intake.	• false positive in case of acute hepatitis, extrahepatic cholestasis, liver congestion, food intake, excessive alcohol intake.	• not applicable in case of iron overload • requires a MRI facility • time consuming • costly • not clear data on prognostic value

Table 1.
Overview of non-invasive tests for liver fibrosis (adapted after EASL guidelines).

have focused on developing techniques to measure the viscoelastic properties of liver tissue, which may serve as indicators of inflammation. By incorporating inflammation assessment, ultrasound technology evolves into a truly multiparametric approach for the comprehensive evaluation of patients with MASLD.

Clinically, patients with simple steatosis generally have a favorable prognosis when compared to those with steatohepatitis, now referred to as Metabolic Associated Steatohepatitis (MASH), which carries the risk of progression to advanced fibrosis and cirrhosis. Consequently, the ability to detect liver inflammation non-invasively, without the need for a liver biopsy, could significantly enhance the triaging process in clinical practice. Currently, only a select few publications and companies have incorporated a dedicated module for detecting inflammation within their devices.

Regarding the VCTE system using iLivTouch, a study by Gao et al. involving a cohort of 259 individuals with biopsy-proven non-alcoholic fatty liver disease explored the use of Radiofrequency (RF) and raw data. They identified two significant parameters that led to the development of a QUS score [48]. This score demonstrated a promising ability to discriminate NASH, with an AUROC of 0.798 (95% CI 0.731–0.865, $p = 0.755$) in the training set and 0.816 (95% CI 0.725–0.906; $p = 0.397$) in the validation set.

In another study using a system with integrated 2D-SWE, conducted by Sugimoto et al. on 120 patients undergoing liver biopsy for suspected fatty liver, biopsy specimens were scored by one expert pathologist according to the Nonalcoholic Steatohepatitis Clinical Research Network criteria. Sugimoto's study evaluated the effectiveness of 2D shear-wave elastography (SWE) parameters—dispersion slope, attenuation coefficient, and shear-wave speed—in diagnosing inflammation, steatosis, fibrosis, and nonalcoholic steatohepatitis (NASH) in NAFLD patients, finding that the dispersion slope was particularly effective in identifying various grades of lobular inflammation with AUCs of 0.95 for mild (A1), 0.81 for moderate (A2), and 0.85 for marked (A3) inflammation. The Attenuation Coefficient, which assesses steatosis, had an AUROC of 0.88 for S1, 0.86 for S2, and 0.79 for S3, while liver stiffness measurements had an AUROC of 0.88 for F2, 0.90 for F3, and 0.95 for F4 fibrosis. Ultimately, combining Dispersion Slope, Attenuation Coefficient, and SWE resulted in an AUC of 0.81 for the diagnosis of NASH [49].

In the study conducted by Lee et al., involving 102 patients with fatty liver who underwent liver biopsy, the effectiveness of Shear Wave Dispersion Slope (SWDS, measured in [m/s]/kHz) derived from 2D-SWE was assessed. The study discovered that lobular inflammatory activity corresponding to inflammation grades 1, 2, and 3 could be detected using this method. The AUROC values for these grades of inflammation were found to be 0.89, 0.85, and 0.78, respectively, with the highest values observed for mild inflammation. This suggests that SWDS from 2D-SWE could potentially be used as a non-invasive marker for detecting varying degrees of inflammation in patients with fatty liver disease [50].

In a recent prospective multicenter study that included a cohort of 132 patients with fatty liver diagnosed *via* liver biopsy, Jang et al. evaluated the diagnostic performance of multiparametric ultrasound. They focused on the Attenuation Coefficient (AC) from attenuation imaging (ATI), liver stiffness, and dispersion slope (DS) from 2D-SWE. The authors developed a risk score system by summing the unweighted scores of AC and DS. This system demonstrated high diagnostic performance for detecting NASH, with an AUROC of 0.94 (95% confidence interval: 0.89 to 0.98, $p < 0.05$) [51].

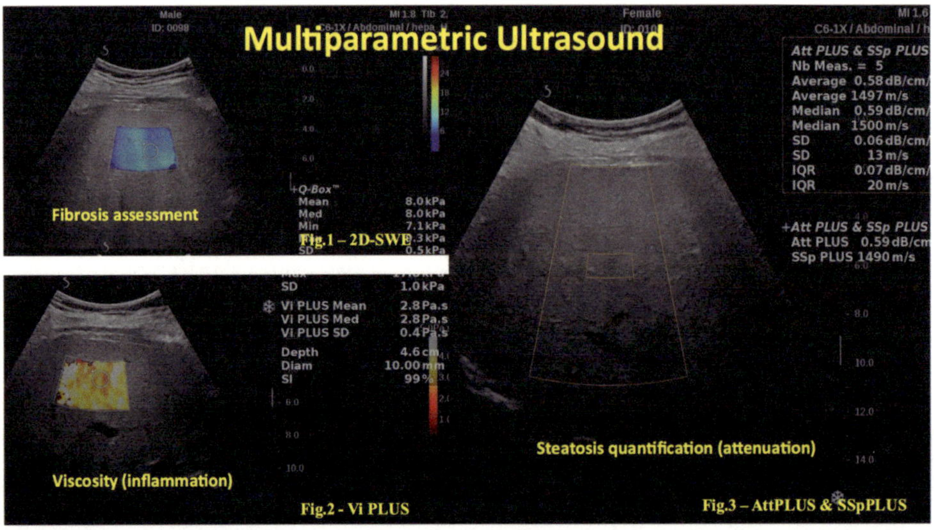

Figure 19.
MPUS evaluation process for patients with MASLD.

Another system was used to evaluate liver inflammation, employing Viscosity Plane-wave UltraSound (Vi.PLUS) technology. In a cohort of 204 subjects who did not undergo liver biopsy, multivariate regression analysis revealed that Vi.PLUS values were correlated with body mass index (BMI) and Liver Stiffness Measurements obtained using the Hologic ultrasound-system [52, 53].

Although only a few studies have demonstrated the capability of ultrasound to evaluate inflammation, the future advancement of this technique will be crucial in clinical practice. It will especially aid in differentiating between simple steatosis and steatohepatitis through non-invasive means. The integration of modules for assessing steatosis, stiffness, and inflammation within a single ultrasound device truly establishes a MPUS system for evaluating patients with MASLD (**Figure 19**).

5. Conclusion

The introduction of MPUS represents a major leap forward in the evaluation of fatty liver disease, combining key assessments—steatosis, fibrosis, and inflammation—into a single, rapid evaluation, often completed in less than 5 minutes. This positions MPUS as a leading tool for screening in high-risk groups. Its potential is particularly notable in screening individuals with T2DM, as well as those who are overweight, obese, or have metabolic disorders, offering a rapid and non-invasive means to stratify risk and guide clinical intervention [54].

As we conclude this review, it is evident that multiparametric ultrasound for patients with MASLD opens an exciting, non-invasive avenue for evaluating a large patient group. This innovative approach paves the way to detect the disease early, enhancing our ability to manage it more effectively. Looking ahead, integrating MPUS with artificial intelligence may well amplify the effectiveness of screening programs in the future. It is a development that promises to transform our approach to liver health, offering a beacon of hope for earlier, more accurate diagnoses and the promise of better outcomes for patients worldwide [55].

Conflict of interest

The authors declare no conflict of interest.

Author details

Ioan Sporea[1,2]*, Alexandru Popa[1,2] and Alina Popescu[1,2]

1 Department of Internal Medicine II, Division of Gastroenterology and Hepatology, "Victor Babeș" University of Medicine and Pharmacy, Timișoara, Romania

2 Advanced Regional Research Center in Gastroenterology and Hepatology, "Victor Babeș" University of Medicine and Pharmacy, Timișoara, Romania

*Address all correspondence to: isporea@umft.ro

References

[1] Younossi ZM, Golabi P, Paik JM, Henry A, Van Dongen C, Henry L. The global epidemiology of nonalcoholic fatty liver disease (NAFLD) and nonalcoholic steatohepatitis (NASH): A systematic review. Hepatology. 2023;**77**(4):1335-1347

[2] Younossi ZM, Koenig AB, Abdelatif D, Fazel Y, Henry L, Wymer M. Global epidemiology of nonalcoholic fatty liver disease—Meta-analytic assessment of prevalence, incidence, and outcomes. Hepatology. 2016;**64**(1):73-84

[3] Younossi ZM, Golabi P, de Avila L, Paik JM, Srishord M, Fukui N, et al. The global epidemiology of NAFLD and NASH in patients with type 2 diabetes: A systematic review and meta-analysis. Journal of Hepatology. 2019;**71**(4):793-801

[4] En Li Cho E, Ang CZ, Quek J, Fu CE, Lim LKE, Heng ZEQ, et al. Global prevalence of non-alcoholic fatty liver disease in type 2 diabetes mellitus: An updated systematic review and meta-analysis. Gut. 2023;**72**(11):2138-2148

[5] Eslam M, Sanyal AJ, George J. MAFLD: A consensus-driven proposed nomenclature for metabolic associated fatty liver disease. Gastroenterology. 2020;**158**(7):1999-2014.e1

[6] Rinella ME, Lazarus JV, Ratziu V, Francque SM, Sanyal AJ, Kanwal F, et al. A multisociety Delphi consensus statement on new fatty liver disease nomenclature. Hepatology. 2023;**78**(6):1966-1986

[7] Ferraioli G, Barr RG, Berzigotti A, Sporea I, Wong VW, Reiberger T, et al. WFUMB guidelines/guidance on liver multiparametric ultrasound. Part 2: Guidance on liver fat quantification. Ultrasound in Medicine & Biology [Internet]. 2024;**50**(8):1088-1098. Available from: https://www.sciencedirect.com/science/article/pii/S0301562924001431

[8] Hamaguchi M, Kojima T, Itoh Y, Harano Y, Fujii K, Nakajima T, et al. The severity of ultrasonographic findings in nonalcoholic fatty liver disease reflects the metabolic syndrome and visceral fat accumulation. The American Journal of Gastroenterology. 2007;**102**(12):2708-2715

[9] Hernaez R, Lazo M, Bonekamp S, Kamel I, Brancati FL, Guallar E, et al. Diagnostic accuracy and reliability of ultrasonography for the detection of fatty liver: A meta-analysis. Hepatology. 2011;**54**(3):1082-1090

[10] Ferraioli G. Quantitative assessment of liver steatosis using ultrasound controlled attenuation parameter (Echosens). Journal of Medical Ultrasonics. 2021;**48**(4):489-495

[11] Lupsor-Platon M, Feier D, Stefănescu H, Tamas A, Botan E, Sparchez Z, et al. Diagnostic accuracy of controlled attenuation parameter measured by transient elastography for the non-invasive assessment of liver steatosis: A prospective study. Journal of Gastrointestinal and Liver Diseases. 2015;**24**(1):35-42

[12] Karlas T, Petroff D, Sasso M, Fan JG, Mi YQ, de Lédinghen V, et al. Individual patient data meta-analysis of controlled attenuation parameter (CAP) technology for assessing steatosis. Journal of Hepatology. 2017;**66**(5):1022-1030

[13] Shi KQ, Tang JZ, Zhu XL, Ying L, Li DW, Gao J, et al. Controlled attenuation parameter for the detection of steatosis severity in chronic liver disease: A meta-analysis of diagnostic accuracy. Journal of Gastroenterology and Hepatology. 2014;**29**(6):1149-1158

[14] Eddowes PJ, Sasso M, Allison M, Tsochatzis E, Anstee QM, Sheridan D, et al. Accuracy of FibroScan controlled attenuation parameter and liver stiffness measurement in assessing steatosis and fibrosis in patients with nonalcoholic fatty liver disease. Gastroenterology. 2019;**156**(6):1717-1730

[15] Chan WK, Nik Mustapha NR, Mahadeva S, Wong VWS, Cheng JYK, Wong GLH. Can the same controlled attenuation parameter cut-offs be used for M and XL probes for diagnosing hepatic steatosis? Journal of Gastroenterology and Hepatology. 2018;**33**(10):1787-1794

[16] Qu Y, Song YY, Chen CW, Fu QC, Shi JP, Xu Y, et al. Diagnostic performance of FibroTouch ultrasound attenuation parameter and liver stiffness measurement in assessing hepatic steatosis and fibrosis in patients with nonalcoholic fatty liver disease. Clinical and Translational Gastroenterology. 2021;**12**(4):e00323

[17] Park J, Lee JM, Lee G, Jeon SK, Joo I. Quantitative evaluation of hepatic steatosis using advanced imaging techniques: Focusing on new quantitative ultrasound techniques. Korean Journal of Radiology. 2022;**23**(1):13-29

[18] Ferraioli G, Maiocchi L, Raciti MV, Tinelli C, De Silvestri A, Nichetti M, et al. Detection of liver steatosis with a novel ultrasound-based technique: A pilot study using MRI-derived proton density fat fraction as the gold standard. Clinical and Translational Gastroenterology. 2019;**10**(10):e00081

[19] Bae JS, Lee DH, Lee JY, Kim H, Yu SJ, Lee JH, et al. Assessment of hepatic steatosis by using attenuation imaging: A quantitative, easy-to-perform ultrasound technique. European Radiology. 2019;**29**(12):6499-6507

[20] Fujiwara Y, Kuroda H, Abe T, Ishida K, Oguri T, Noguchi S, et al. The B-mode image-guided ultrasound attenuation parameter accurately detects hepatic steatosis in chronic liver disease. Ultrasound in Medicine & Biology. 2018;**44**(11):2223-2232

[21] Imajo K, Toyoda H, Yasuda S, Suzuki Y, Sugimoto K, Kuroda H, et al. Utility of ultrasound-guided attenuation parameter for grading steatosis with reference to MRI-PDFF in a large cohort. Clinical Gastroenterology and Hepatology. 2022;**20**(11):2533-2541.e7

[22] Jeon SK, Lee JM, Joo I, Park SJ. Quantitative ultrasound radiofrequency data analysis for the assessment of hepatic steatosis in nonalcoholic fatty liver disease using magnetic resonance imaging proton density fat fraction as the reference standard. Korean Journal of Radiology. 2021;**22**(7):1077-1086

[23] Jung J, Han A, Madamba E, Bettencourt R, Loomba RR, Boehringer AS, et al. Direct comparison of quantitative US versus controlled attenuation parameter for liver fat assessment using MRI proton density fat fraction as the reference standard in patients suspected of having NAFLD. Radiology. 2022;**304**(1):75-82

[24] Ferraioli G, Kumar V, Ozturk A, Nam K, de Korte CL, Barr RG. US attenuation for liver fat quantification: An AIUM-RSNA QIBA pulse-Echo quantitative ultrasound initiative. Radiology. 2022;**302**(3):495-506

[25] Ferraioli G, Raimondi A, Maiocchi L, De Silvestri A, Poma G, Kumar V, et al. Liver fat quantification with ultrasound: Depth dependence of attenuation coefficient. Journal of Ultrasound in Medicine [Internet]. 2023;**42**(10):2247-2255. DOI: 10.1002/jum.16242

[26] de Franchis R. Expanding consensus in portal hypertension: Report of the Baveno VI consensus workshop: Stratifying risk and individualizing care for portal hypertension. Journal of Hepatology. 2015;**63**(3):743-752

[27] Dietrich CF, Bamber J, Berzigotti A, Bota S, Cantisani V, Castera L, et al. EFSUMBguidelinesandrecommendations on the clinical use of liver ultrasound elastography, update 2017 (long version). Ultraschall in der Medizin. 2017;**38**(4):e16-e47

[28] Cosgrove D, Piscaglia F, Bamber J, Bojunga J, Correas JM, Gilja OH, et al. EFSUMBguidelinesandrecommendations on the clinical use of ultrasound elastographypart 2: Clinical applications. Ultraschall in der Medizin. 2013;**34**(3):238-253

[29] Ferraioli G, Barr RG, Berzigotti A, Sporea I, Wong VW, Reiberger T, et al. WFUMB guideline/guidance on liver multiparametric ultrasound: Part 1. Update to 2018 guidelines on liver ultrasound elastography. Ultrasound in Medicine & Biology [Internet]. 2024;**34**(3):238-253. Available from: https://www.sciencedirect.com/science/article/pii/S030156292400142X

[30] de Franchis R, Bosch J, Garcia-Tsao G, Reiberger T, Ripoll C. Baveno VII - Renewing consensus in portal hypertension. Journal of Hepatology. 2022;**76**(4):959-974

[31] Barr RG, Wilson SR, Rubens D, Garcia-Tsao G, Ferraioli G. Update to the society of radiologists in ultrasound liver elastography consensus statement. Radiology. 2020;**296**(2):263-274

[32] Friedrich-Rust M, Ong MF, Martens S, Sarrazin C, Bojunga J, Zeuzem S, et al. Performance of transient elastography for the staging of liver fibrosis: A meta-analysis. Gastroenterology. 2008;**66**(5):1022-1030

[33] Tsochatzis EA, Gurusamy KS, Ntaoula S, Cholongitas E, Davidson BR, Burroughs AK. Elastography for the diagnosis of severity of fibrosis in chronic liver disease: A meta-analysis of diagnostic accuracy. Journal of Hepatology. 2011;**54**(4):650-659

[34] Herrmann E, de Lédinghen V, Cassinotto C, Chu WCW, Leung VYF, Ferraioli G, et al. Assessment of biopsy-proven liver fibrosis by two-dimensional shear wave elastography: An individual patient data-based meta-analysis. Hepatology. 2018;**67**(1):260-272

[35] Feng JC, Li J, Wu XW, Peng XY. Diagnostic accuracy of supersonic shear imaging for staging of liver fibrosis: A meta-analysis. Journal of Ultrasound in Medicine. 2016;**35**(2):329-339

[36] Jiang TNA, Tian G, Zhao Q, Kong D, Cheng C, Zhong L, et al. Diagnostic accuracy of 2D-shear wave elastography for liver fibrosis severity: A meta-analysis. PLoS One. 2016;**11**(6):e0157219

[37] Cassinotto C, Boursier J, de Lédinghen V, Lebigot J, Lapuyade B, Cales P, et al. Liver stiffness in nonalcoholic fatty liver disease: A comparison of supersonic shear imaging, FibroScan, and ARFI with liver biopsy. Hepatology. 2016;**63**(6):1817-1827

[38] Lefebvre T, Wartelle-Bladou C, Wong P, Sebastiani G, Giard JM, Castel H, et al. Prospective comparison of transient, point shear wave, and magnetic resonance elastography for staging liver fibrosis. European Radiology. 2019;**29**(12):6477-6488

[39] Xiao G, Zhu S, Xiao X, Yan L, Yang J, Wu G. Comparison of laboratory tests, ultrasound, or magnetic resonance elastography to detect fibrosis in patients with nonalcoholic fatty liver disease: A meta-analysis. Hepatology. 2017;**66**(5):1486-1501

[40] Furlan A, Tublin ME, Yu L, Chopra KB, Lippello A, Behari J. Comparison of 2D shear wave elastography, transient elastography, and MR elastography for the diagnosis of fibrosis in patients with nonalcoholic fatty liver disease. AJR. American Journal of Roentgenology. 2020;**214**(1):W20-W26

[41] Selvaraj EA, Mózes FE, Jayaswal ANA, Zafarmand MH, Vali Y, Lee JA, et al. Diagnostic accuracy of elastography and magnetic resonance imaging in patients with NAFLD: A systematic review and meta-analysis. Journal of Hepatology. 2021;**75**(4):770-785

[42] Imajo K, Honda Y, Kobayashi T, Nagai K, Ozaki A, Iwaki M, et al. Direct comparison of US and MR elastography for staging liver fibrosis in patients with nonalcoholic fatty liver disease. Clinical Gastroenterology and Hepatology. 2022;**20**(4):908-917.e11

[43] Berzigotti A, Tsochatzis E, Boursier J, Castera L, Cazzagon N, Friedrich-Rust M, et al. EASL clinical practice guidelines on non-invasive tests for evaluation of liver disease severity and prognosis – 2021 update. Journal of Hepatology. 2021;**75**(3):659-689

[44] Hu X, Huang X, Hou J, Ding L, Su C, Meng F. Diagnostic accuracy of spleen stiffness to evaluate portal hypertension and esophageal varices in chronic liver disease: A systematic review and meta-analysis. European Radiology. 2021;**31**(4):2392-2404

[45] Reiberger T. The value of liver and spleen stiffness for evaluation of portal hypertension in compensated cirrhosis. Hepatology Communications. 2022;**6**(5):950-964

[46] Segna D, Mendoza YP, Lange NF, Rodrigues SG, Berzigotti A. Non-invasive tools for compensated advanced chronic liver disease and portal hypertension after Baveno VII - An update. Digestive and Liver Disease : Official Journal of the Italian Society of Gastroenterology and the Italian Association for the Study of the Liver. 2023;**55**(3):326-335

[47] Raeman R. Inflammation: The straw that broke the NAFLD liver! Cellular and Molecular Gastroenterology and Hepatology. 2022;**13**(4):1273-1274

[48] Gao F, He Q, Li G, Huang OY, Tang LJ, Wang XD, et al. A novel quantitative ultrasound technique for identifying non-alcoholic steatohepatitis. Liver International. 2022;**42**(1):80-91

[49] Sugimoto K, Moriyasu F, Oshiro H, Takeuchi H, Abe M, Yoshimasu Y, et al. The role of multiparametric US of the liver for the evaluation of nonalcoholic steatohepatitis. Radiology. 2020;**296**(3):532-540

[50] Lee DH, Cho EJ, Bae JS, Lee JY, Yu SJ, Kim H, et al. Accuracy of two-dimensional shear wave elastography and attenuation imaging for evaluation of patients with nonalcoholic steatohepatitis. Clinical Gastroenterology and Hepatology. 2021;**19**(4):797-805.e7

[51] Jang JK, Lee ES, Seo JW, Kim YR, Kim SY, Cho YY, et al. Two-dimensional shear-wave elastography and US attenuation imaging for nonalcoholic steatohepatitis diagnosis: A cross-sectional, Multicenter study. Radiology. 2022;**305**(1):118-126

[52] Popa A, Sporea I, Bende F, Popescu A, Fofiu R, Borlea A, et al. The non-invasive ultrasound-based assessment of liver viscosity in a healthy cohort. Diagnostics. 2022;**12**(6):1451

[53] Popa A, Bende F, Șirli R, Popescu A, Bâldea V, Lupușoru R, et al. Quantification of liver fibrosis, steatosis, and viscosity using multiparametric ultrasound in patients with non-alcoholic liver disease: A "real-life" cohort study. Diagnostics. 2021;**11**(5):783

[54] Zhang E, Wartelle-Bladou C, Lepanto L, Lachaine J, Cloutier G, Tang A. Cost-utility analysis of nonalcoholic steatohepatitis screening. European Radiology. 2015;**25**(11):3282-3294

[55] Decharatanachart P, Chaiteerakij R, Tiyarattanachai T, Treeprasertsuk S. Application of artificial intelligence in non-alcoholic fatty liver disease and liver fibrosis: A systematic review and meta-analysis. Therapeutic Advances in Gastroenterology. 2021;**14**:17562848211062808

Chapter 13

Ultrasound-Based Methods for the Assessment of Advanced Liver Disease and Portal Hypertension

Rareș Crăciun, Tudor Mocan and Zeno Spârchez

Abstract

The current book chapter delves into the intricacies of ultrasonographic (US) assessment in patients with advanced liver disease and portal hypertension, offering a comprehensive, clinically oriented exploration of the most frequently employed tools in this domain. The chapter seeks to familiarize readers with a standardized US approach to advanced liver disease, encompassing standard B-mode imaging, Doppler US, elastography, and contrast-enhanced US (CEUS). Beyond the fundamental techniques, the chapter discusses specific clinical scenarios, providing valuable insights into transjugular intrahepatic portosystemic shunt (TIPS) assessment, post-transplantation follow-up protocols, the nuanced evaluation of vascular liver disease, and the management of incidental and treated liver nodules. This thorough exploration caters to the needs of clinicians and researchers and serves as a practical guide for medical practitioners involved in the day-to-day care of patients with complex liver conditions. The chapter aspires to be a useful resource in the field, offering an up-to-date and insightful overview that bridges the gap between theoretical knowledge and its practical application in the dynamic landscape of liver disease assessment using ultrasonography.

Keywords: cirrhosis, portal hypertension, ultrasonography, multiparametric ultrasonography, contrast-enhanced ultrasonography

1. Introduction

In the dynamic landscape of medical imaging, the integration of advanced technologies has revolutionized diagnostic approaches, and the field of ultrasonography (US) was no exception. With its non-invasive nature, real-time imaging capabilities, and absence of ionizing radiation, US has long been a cornerstone in diagnostic medicine as a natural extension to the physical examination. Lately, there has been a surge in US-based techniques that significantly enhance the value of US and overcome some of its traditional limits. The concept of multiparametric ultrasonography (MPUS), which incorporates multiple additional variables assessing vascularization, such as Doppler-based modules, contrast-enhanced ultrasonography (CEUS), elastography, and fat quantification, has emerged as a powerful tool in enhancing diagnostic accuracy and clinical decision-making [1–5].

MPUS represents a paradigm shift in ultrasonography by simultaneously assessing multiple parameters, including vascularity, tissue stiffness, and perfusion dynamics, thereby offering a comprehensive evaluation of tissue characteristics. This multifaceted approach holds immense promise across various medical specialties, ranging from hepatology and oncology to musculoskeletal and urology, among others.

Central to the arsenal of MPUS techniques is CEUS, which introduces microbubble-based contrast agents to visualize microvascular perfusion in real-time. By exploiting the unique acoustic properties of microbubbles, CEUS enables the assessment of tissue vascularity with unprecedented detail and sensitivity. Unlike traditional Doppler ultrasonography, CEUS provides exquisite delineation of microvascular architecture and perfusion dynamics, facilitating the characterization of focal lesions and monitoring of treatment response. Furthermore, CEUS offers distinct advantages over other imaging modalities, particularly in scenarios where iodinated contrast agents for computed tomography (CT) or gadolinium-based contrast agents for magnetic resonance imaging (MRI) are contraindicated, such as in patients with renal insufficiency or allergies. Its safety profile, portability, and cost-effectiveness make CEUS a valuable adjunct to conventional imaging techniques [6–8].

In addition to CEUS, elastography has emerged as a pivotal component of MPUS, providing valuable insights into tissue stiffness and elasticity. By quantifying the mechanical properties of tissues, elastography aids in the characterization of focal lesions, differentiation of benign and malignant masses, and guidance of interventional procedures. Various elastographic techniques, including strain elastography, shear wave elastography, and acoustic radiation force impulse imaging, offer complementary information about tissue elasticity, expanding the diagnostic repertoire of US [9–12].

The integration of CEUS and elastography into routine clinical practice has transformed diagnostic algorithms and therapeutic decision-making across a spectrum of medical disciplines. In the setting of advanced liver disease, CEUS plays a crucial role in the characterization of focal liver lesions in a standardized manner using the CEUS-Liver Imaging Reporting and Data System (LiRADS) system [13], assessing vascular liver disease [14, 15], guiding interventional procedures [16], post-procedural follow-up [17, 18] and liver transplantation [19]. On the other hand, elastography has revolutionized the assessment of liver fibrosis and cirrhosis in the past two decades, enabling non-invasive staging of liver disease and guiding therapeutic interventions. Elastography has virtually replaced liver biopsy for staging purposes in advanced liver disease and has largely limited the role of invasive hepatic venous pressure gradient (HVPG) measurements to select scenarios in expert facilities and research settings. The role of elastography has been recently reinforced by the Baveno VII consensus [20] and has become a *sine qua non* measurement in the diagnosis and follow-up of advanced liver disease [21–23].

In summary, the advent of multiparametric ultrasonography, encompassing all of its modes and features, represents a transformative leap in diagnostic imaging. By providing a holistic assessment of tissue vascularity, perfusion dynamics, and mechanical properties, MPUS enhances diagnostic accuracy, facilitates treatment planning, and improves patient outcomes across diverse clinical scenarios. This book chapter aims to elucidate the principles, applications, and clinical utility of MPUS. The following pages offer clinically driven insights into its evolving role in contemporary medical practice, starting from B-mode US to Doppler-based features, elastography, and CEUS.

2. B-mode and conventional Doppler ultrasonography

As stated above, recent advancements in digital imaging technology have introduced a diverse array of imaging modalities, encompassing color/power Doppler, harmonic imaging for contrast enhancement, three-dimensional visualization, and fusion imaging. These modalities have demonstrated enhanced diagnostic capabilities across various clinical contexts. Nevertheless, it is imperative to acknowledge that fundamental tissue imaging predominantly relies on B-mode sonography.

In the realm of portal hypertension, B-mode sonography assumes a pivotal role in the characterization of cirrhosis, assessment of vessel diameter and spleen dimensions, and detection of ascites and anomalous collateral pathways [24]. Despite its straightforward methodology, B-mode sonography furnishes invaluable insights for both diagnosing and monitoring portal hypertension-associated conditions [25, 26]. However, it is pertinent to recognize that while B-mode findings may infer the presence of portal hypertension, they serve as indirect indicators. Consequently, the applicability of B-mode ultrasound in predicting portal pressure and gauging the severity of portal hypertension is somewhat constrained.

From a clinical standpoint, discerning between the compensated and decompensated stages of cirrhosis holds paramount significance, given its pivotal role in prognostication [20, 27]. Abdominal ultrasound emerges as a valuable tool in this context, facilitating the diagnosis and quantification of decompensatory events such as ascites and hepatic hydrothorax and enabling the evaluation of cirrhosis-related complications and portal hypertension. These include the assessment of collateral circulation, portal axis status, splenomegaly, and hepatocellular carcinoma.

Liver cirrhosis epitomizes the terminal phase of an amalgamation of chronic liver pathologies, thereby elucidating the morphological heterogeneity observed in cirrhotic livers. Furthermore, the sonographic presentation of cirrhotic liver pathology spans a continuum, ranging from nearly normal morphology, encountered in chronic liver diseases exhibiting fibrosis at the border of the cirrhotic range and subclinical portal hypertension, to decompensated cirrhosis in its terminal phase [24, 28]. The principal alterations encountered with varying frequency within the context of cirrhosis and cirrhotic portal hypertension are systematized in **Table 1** and illustrated in **Figures 1–5**.

Liver Morphology	
Dimensions	Alterations in lobar size: • Right lobe atrophy (**Figure 1**) • Caudate lobe ± left-lobe hypertrophy
Echostructure	Inhomogeneous: • Micronodular (below 3 mm) • Macronodular (above 3 mm) • Mixed (**Figure 2**)

Liver Morphology	
Capsular contour	• Irregular, bosselated (**Figure 3**)
Margins	• Round
Vasculature	
Portal vein	• ± dilation ≥12 mm • Slow hepatopetal flow (Vmax ≤20 cm/s in the main portal vein, Vmax ≤15 cm/s in the right branch) • Hepatofugal flow • Complete/partial portal vein thrombosis
Hepatic artery	• Increase in the hepatic artery resistivity index (HARI) ≥0.8 (arterialization of the hepatic circulation)
Collateral circulation	• Recanalization of the round ligament (hepatofugal flow) • Perigastric • Perisplenic • Splenorenal shunt
Decompensating events	
Ascites [29]	• Grade I – perihepatic • Grade II – moderate amount (perisplenic, pelvis, latero-cholic, perimesenteric) • Grad III – entire abdominal cavity (**Figure 4**)
Hepatic Hydrothorax	• Pleural effusion, typically right-sided; can be bilateral
Liver nodules	• Regeneration nodules • Dysplastic nodules • Hepatocellular carcinoma • Other malignant nodules
Consequences of portal hypertension on other organs	
Spleen	• Splenomegaly (≥130 mm)
Gallbladder	• Thickening/doubling of the gallbladder walls (**Figure 5**)

Table 1.
The most frequent alterations encountered in cirrhosis and portal hypertension.

Doppler US is a readily available complement to B-mode in assessing the complications of advanced liver disease and can reliably detect signs of portal hypertension (PHT). While the correlation between the gold standard for PHT, namely HVPG measurement, and Doppler US findings is relatively low, Doppler US can provide a dichotomial yes/no answer for the presence of PHT due to numerous indirect findings.

Portal vein diameter fluctuates in liver disease, enlarging beyond 12 mm but not necessarily correlating with portal hypertension severity. As portal hypertension progresses, collateral circulation develops, causing the portal vein size to diminish. In advanced stages, with reversed portal vein flow (**Figure 6**), the diameter consistently measures <10 mm [28]. Portal vein velocity (PVV) significantly decreases in PHT

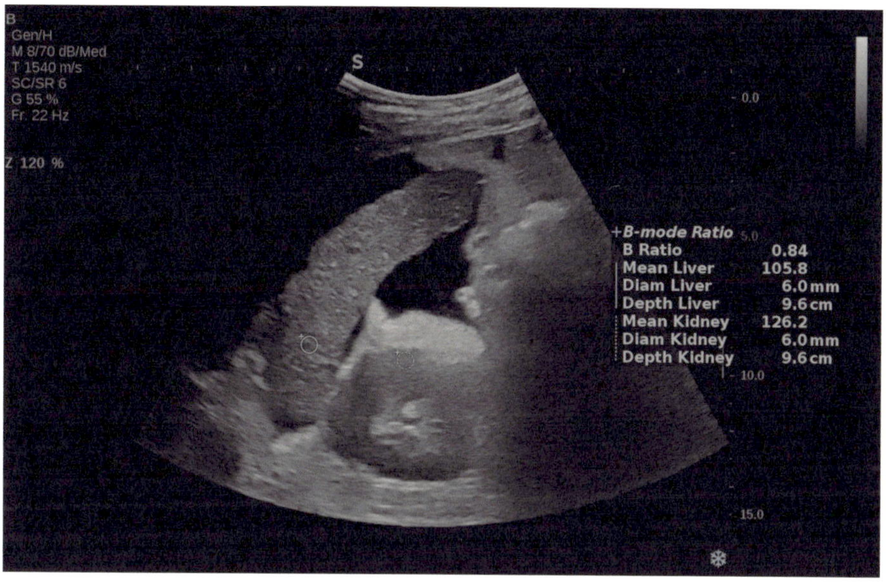

Figure 1.
Right liver lobe atrophy in a patient with alcohol-related decompensated cirrhosis.

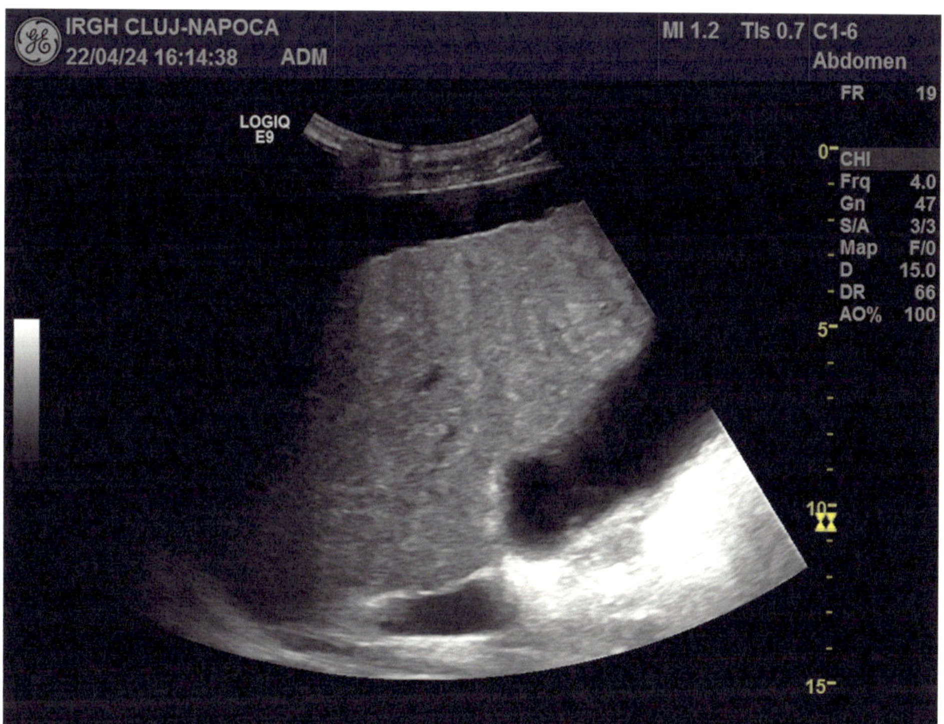

Figure 2.
Mixed-type macro- and micronodular inhomogeneous echostructure of the right liver lobe in a patient with decompensated cirrhosis and ascites.

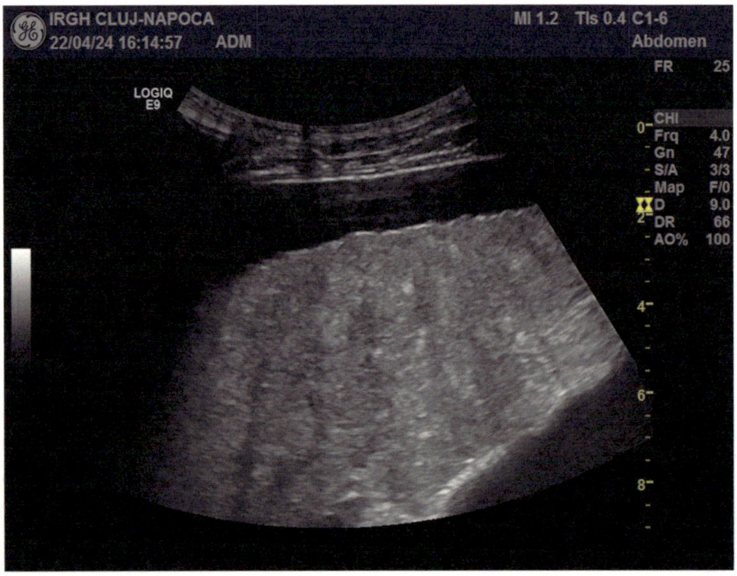

Figure 3.
Irregular capsular contour of the hepatic dome in a patient with decompensated cirrhosis and ascites.

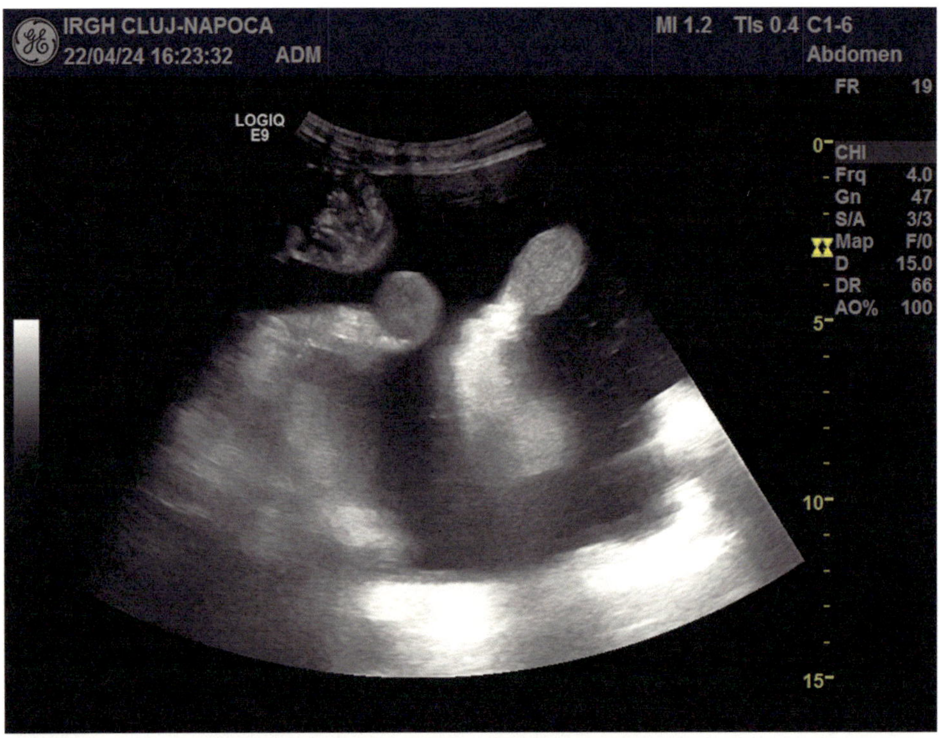

Figure 4.
Grade III ascites, with visible small bowel loops and corresponding mesentery in the periumbilical area.

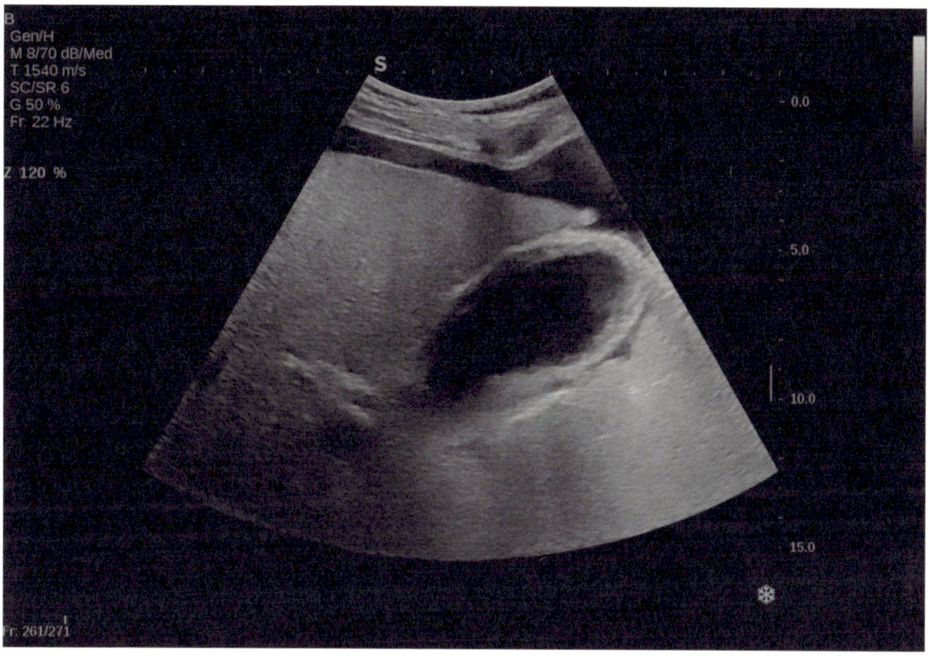

Figure 5.
Thickening of the gallbladder walls in a patient with MASLD cirrhosis and portal hypertension.

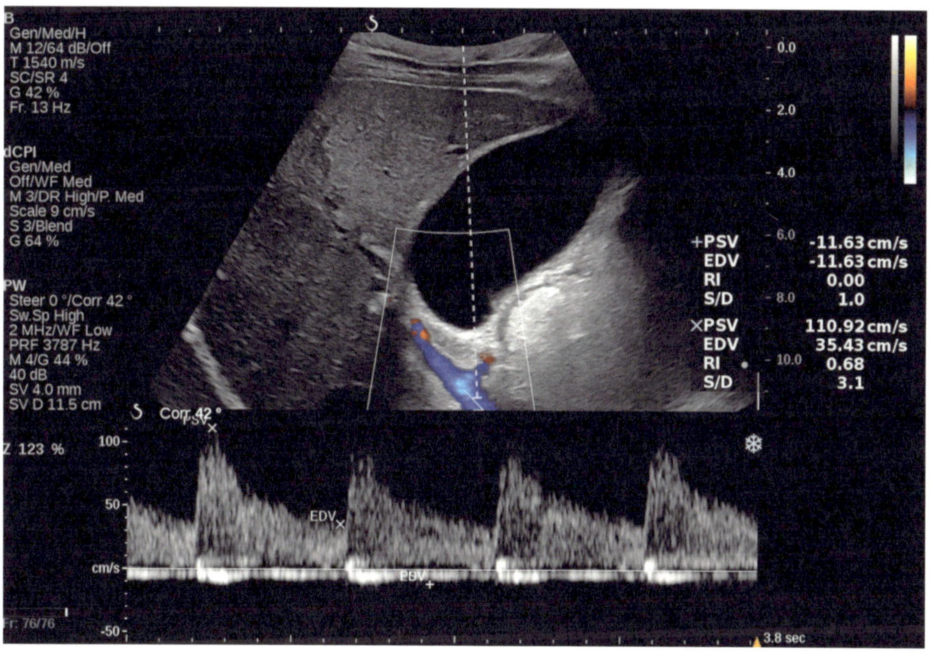

Figure 6.
Hepatofugal flow in the portal vein in a patient with severe alcoholic hepatitis.

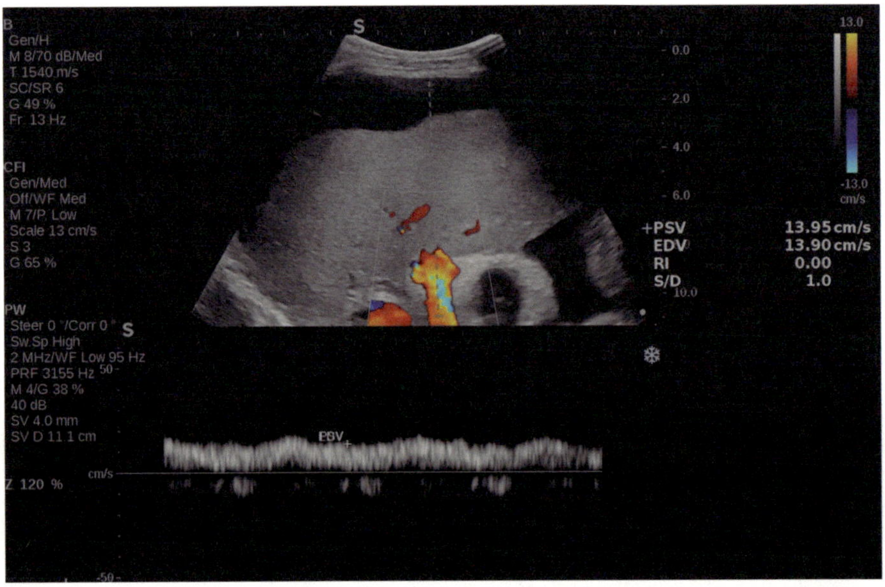

Figure 7.
Reduced portal vein velocity in a patient with decompensated cirrhosis and refractory ascites.

(**Figure 7**), as values of 18–20 cm/s are typically considered the threshold for normal portal flow. However, the relationship between PHT and PVV is non-linear, as numerous factors influence PVV, such as the presence of collateral circulation or thrombosis [30–32]. Moreover, portal vein flow can be reversed (hepatofugal), most often in severely decompensated patients, and can be highly suggestive of acute-on-chronic liver failure [33].

Evidence has shown that hepatic arterial vascular resistance or hepatic arterial resistivity index (HARI) increases proportionally to the severity of PHT [34]. The most validated threshold for HARI is 0.8, and an increase in HARI is correlated with a more advanced liver disease [34–37] and post-transplantation outcomes [38].

Beyond assessing the liver parenchyma and vasculature, conventional B-mode + Doppler US can provide additional hints about the severity of PHT. Therefore, splenomegaly, congestion of the gallbladder or colonic walls, and collateral circulation are all frequently encountered in patients with advanced liver disease and PHT [24, 28].

3. Ultrasound-based elastography techniques

Liver disease and its complications, including PHT, present significant challenges in clinical management and prognosis. Traditionally, liver biopsy and other invasive procedures (upper gastrointestinal endoscopy, HVPG measurement) have been the gold standard for assessing the degree of liver fibrosis and portal hypertension. However, their invasive nature, sampling variability, and potential complications have led to the development of non-invasive alternatives, of which ultrasound-based elastography techniques play a central role.

Ultrasound-based elastography utilizes the principle that the mechanical properties of liver tissue change with fibrosis and congestion, allowing for the estimation of liver stiffness. Transient elastography (TE), shear wave elastography (SWE), and acoustic radiation force impulse (ARFI) imaging are among the most widely studied techniques in this realm and are becoming increasingly available to clinicians across the world. These methods offer several advantages over biopsy, including non-invasiveness, repeatability, and real-time assessment. They provide quantitative measures of liver stiffness, which correlate well with histological fibrosis stages and portal pressure in liver disease [11, 20, 21, 39].

Chronic liver disease (CLD) encompasses a spectrum of pathological changes, ranging from mild fibrosis to advanced cirrhosis. The advent of elastography in clinical practice has revolutionized the early identification of patients with untreated or active CLD who are at risk of developing clinically significant portal hypertension (CSPH) and subsequent decompensation leading to liver-related mortality. To capture this continuum of disease severity, the term "compensated advanced chronic liver disease (cACLD)" has been introduced [40], aiming to stratify patients based on liver stiffness measurement (LSM), irrespective of histological staging. The following paragraphs summarize the most recent Baveno VII recommendations regarding the use of elastography in assessing fibrosis and the probability of CSPH in clinical practice [20]. While most of the recommendations rely on transient elastography (TE), as it is the older technique and has significantly more validation, all LSM methods have shown a high reliability [41–43] and have been incorporated, albeit cautiously, in the recent guidelines [20, 21].

Defining cACLD relies on LSM values conventionally obtained through TE. Values below 10 kPa, without other clinical or imaging signs, rule out cACLD, while values between 10 and 15 kPa suggest its presence, and values exceeding 15 kPa highly indicate cACLD. Notably, patients with an LSM <10 kPa have a minimal 3-year risk of decompensation and liver-related death [44]. Monitoring individuals with LSM values between 7 and 10 kPa, alongside ongoing liver injury, is crucial for detecting progression to cACLD. However, TE may yield false positives, necessitating repeat LSM under fasting conditions or supplementing with serum markers of fibrosis [45].

In cACLD, LSM serves as a prognostic indicator both at the index investigation and during follow-up. The "rule of 5" for LSM by TE (10–15–20-25 kPa) delineates escalating relative risks of decompensation and liver-related death across varying LSM thresholds, independent of the underlying etiology of CLD (**Table 2**) [20], and has been widely validate following the publication of the Baveno VII position paper [46, 47].

Regular LSM monitoring, ideally every 12 months, allows for early detection of significant changes in liver stiffness. A clinically significant decrease in LSM, defined as a reduction of ≥20% associated with LSM <20 kPa or any decrease to <10 kPa, signifies substantially reduced risks of decompensation and liver-related mortality, indicating a favorable response to therapy.

The diagnosis of CSPH, while traditionally HVPG-driven, has seen a shift toward non-invasive methods in clinical practice. In patients with cACLD, a combination of LSM by TE and platelet count offers a reliable means of CSPH exclusion when LSM ≤15 kPa and platelet count $\geq 150 \times 10^9$/L, with sensitivity and negative predictive value exceeding 90%. For patients with virus- and/or alcohol-related cACLD or non-obese (body mass index (BMI) <30 kg/m^2) non-alcoholic steatohepatitis (NASH)-related cACLD, an LSM value by TE of ≥25 kPa serves as a significant indicator of CSPH presence, with specificity and positive predictive value exceeding 90%. This delineates a subgroup at a higher risk of decompensation and necessitates closer monitoring [39, 48, 49].

Liver Stiffness (kPa)	Interpretation	Additional Notes	Clinical Action or Assumption
≤5	Normal		Exclude cACLD
>5 – <10	Borderline/Unclear		May consider further assessment
≥ 10	Possible cACLD		Begin considering cACLD
≥ 15	Likely clinically significant	Platelets ≥150 → Exclude CSPH	Consider avoiding endoscopy per Baveno VI
≥ 20	High suspicion of cACLD		Assume cACLD
≥ 25	Very high (suggests CSPH)	Common in HCV, HBV, ALD, non-obese MASLD	Assume CSPH

cACLD – compensated advanced chronic liver disease; CSPH – clinically significant portal hypertension; HCV – hepatitis C virus; HBV – hepatitis B virus; ALD – alcohol-related liver disease; MASLD – metabolic dysfunction-associated steatotic liver disease.

Table 2.
The "rule-of-five" criteria for predicting clinically significant portal hypertension according to the Baveno VII consensus [20].

In those with cACLD and LSM <25 kPa, the ANTICIPATE model offers a predictive tool for CSPH risk stratification. Notably, patients falling within LSM ranges of 20–25 kPa or 15–20 kPa, coupled with specific platelet count thresholds, exhibit a CSPH risk exceeding 60% [39]. Furthermore, in patients with NASH-related cACLD, the ANTICIPATE-NASH model integrating LSM, platelet count, and BMI holds promise for CSPH risk prediction, pending further validation [50].

Compensated cirrhotic patients ineligible for non-selective beta-blockers (NSBBs) due to contraindication or intolerance necessitate variceal screening *via* endoscopy if LSM by TE exceeds 20 kPa or platelet count falls below $150x10^9$/L. Alternatively, annual TE and platelet count monitoring can identify candidates warranting endoscopic evaluation based on LSM or platelet count changes [20].

Spleen stiffness measurement (SSM) by TE holds promise for CSPH assessment in cACLD stemming from viral hepatitis, with specific cut-offs indicating CSPH exclusion (<21 kPa) or inclusion (>50 kPa). However, validation using a 100 Hz specific TE probe, point-shear wave elastography, and 2D-shear wave elastography is warranted. Moreover, for non-NSBB candidates requiring endoscopic assessment based on Baveno VI criteria, SSM ≤40 kPa by TE can identify those at low risk of high-risk varices, obviating the need for endoscopy [51].

In contrast to TE, SWE poses additional standardization issues, primarily regarding the heterogeneity of the authorized devices and software. To this point, there have been multiple attempts to harmonize the data and provide cut-offs with similar reliability to TE, prompting their inclusion in the most recent Baveno recommendations [52–55]. A large-scale prospective study evaluated the diagnostic performance of three shear wave elastography (SWE) techniques—Philips ElastPQ, Siemens Virtual Touch Quantification (VTQ), and transient elastography (TE)—in 160 patients with chronic liver disease undergoing the same-day liver biopsy [55]. Each modality measured liver stiffness, and the results were compared with histological fibrosis staging. ElastPQ and TE demonstrated good diagnostic accuracy, while VTQ showed lower performance. The area under the receiver operating characteristic curve (AUROC) values for detecting significant fibrosis and cirrhosis were highest for TE, followed closely by ElastPQ. Left-lobe measurements were less reliable across techniques. Although the correlation between SWE results and fibrosis was significant, discrepancies persisted due to biopsy limitations, including sampling variability and anatomical mismatch. Despite these, SWE captured a broader tissue context than biopsy, explaining some discordances. The study advocates incorporating SWE into liver disease management and supports the recently proposed "rule of five" and "rule of four" stiffness thresholds for fibrosis staging. This research represents the first direct comparison of three SWE technologies with biopsy verification on the same day, providing critical insights into the real-world utility of these non-invasive tools. The proposed cut-off values are represented in **Table 3**.

While US-based elastography techniques have revolutionized non-invasive liver fibrosis assessment, they possess several limitations that might hinder their diagnostic utility in specific scenarios. A major challenge is the significant inter- and intra-operator variability, particularly in patients with high body mass index, ascites, or narrow intercostal spaces, which can impair acoustic penetration and reduce measurement reliability. Additionally, elastography measurements are susceptible to confounding factors such as hepatic inflammation, cholestasis, congestion, and food intake, all of

Fibrosis stage	Diagnostic performance	ELAST PQ	TE	VTQ
F0/1	Cut-off kPa	7.38	8.10	8.9
	AUC	0.828 (0.762–0.895)	0.810 (0.746–0.884)	0.741 (0.659–0.823)
	SE	0.79	0.75	0.80
	SP	0.79	0.75	0.64
	PPV	0.80	0.77	0.70
	NPV	0.79	0.73	0.75
F3/4	Cut-off kPa	8.32	9.70	10.88
	AUC	0.812 (0.734–0.889)	0.841 (0.771–0.910)	0.782 (0.702–0.861)
	SE	0.76	0.79	0.76
	SP	0.71	0.75	0.72
	PPV	0.97	0.91	0.89
	NPV	0.35	0.54	0.52
F4	Cut-off kPa	10.41	16.50	12.47
	AUC	0.856 (0.753–0.938)	0.939 (0.896–0.982)	0.826 (0.734–0.918)
	SE	0.83	0.91	0.69
	SP	0.73	0.88	0.78
	PPV	0.95	0.98	0.95
	NPV	0.40	0.57	0.57

AUC – area under the curve; SE – sensitivity; SP – specificity; PPV – positive predictive value; NPV – negative predictive value.

Table 3.
Diagnostic performance of ElastPQ, transient elastography and VTQ for hepatic fibrosis stage in different etiologies according to the dataset reported by Atzori et al. [55].

which can transiently increase liver stiffness independently of fibrosis. This can lead to false positives, particularly in acute hepatitis or heart failure. Moreover, discrepancies between different devices and lack of standardization across vendors result in poor cross-platform reproducibility, limiting longitudinal monitoring unless the same equipment is used. Sampling variability and heterogeneity in liver stiffness across different lobes further compound diagnostic uncertainty. Furthermore, elastography provides a global assessment of stiffness, which may not reflect localized fibrosis patterns captured by biopsy. While elastography is valuable for fibrosis staging and treatment monitoring, its results must be interpreted in conjunction with clinical context and biochemical data to avoid diagnostic pitfalls [56].

4. Contrast-enhanced ultrasonography

Cirrhosis and portal hypertension represent significant challenges in clinical practice, often necessitating accurate and timely diagnostic techniques for optimal management. Contrast-enhanced ultrasonography (CEUS) emerged as a promising modality in this landscape, offering distinct advantages over conventional ultrasound. By leveraging microbubble contrast agents, CEUS enhances vascular delineation, enabling real-time assessment of hepatic perfusion, portal hemodynamics, and liver nodule characterization with exceptional spatial and temporal resolution [14]. This capability holds particular relevance in cirrhosis, where traditional imaging modalities may encounter limitations due to parenchymal distortion and altered hepatic vasculature. In portal hypertension, CEUS facilitates the non-invasive evaluation of portosystemic collaterals, aiding in the stratification of bleeding risk and informing therapeutic decisions. Moreover, CEUS stands out for its safety profile, devoid of nephrotoxicity or ionizing radiation, making it well-suited for repeated examinations and vulnerable patient populations [57, 58]. Beyond diagnostic utility, CEUS demonstrates promise in prognostication, with emerging evidence correlating perfusion patterns obtained through CEUS with disease severity and clinical outcomes in cirrhotic patients [59, 60]. Furthermore, its versatility extends to therapeutic monitoring, enabling dynamic assessment of the treatment response [16] and early detection of complications such as portal vein thrombosis [15]. Despite these advancements, challenges remain, including standardization of imaging protocols and operator proficiency, necessitating ongoing research and collaborative efforts to fully realize the potential of CEUS in cirrhosis and portal hypertension. Nevertheless, the burgeoning body of evidence underscores the indispensable role of CEUS as a valuable adjunct to conventional imaging modalities, offering a non-invasive, safe, and clinically relevant approach to the comprehensive assessment of hepatic vascular dynamics in this complex patient population.

Portal vein thrombosis (PVT) poses a significant clinical challenge, complicating the management of cirrhosis, malignancy, and other hepatobiliary disorders. In this context, CEUS is a valuable tool for evaluating PVT, offering distinct advantages over traditional imaging modalities. By leveraging microbubble contrast agents, CEUS provides real-time assessment of vascular flow dynamics, allowing for the accurate detection and characterization of thrombotic occlusions within the portal vein system (**Figure 8**). Unlike conventional ultrasound, which may struggle to differentiate between bland thrombi and recanalized vessels, CEUS offers enhanced sensitivity and specificity, enabling precise delineation of thrombus extent and characterization of its composition, as well as an accurate distinction between benign and malignant

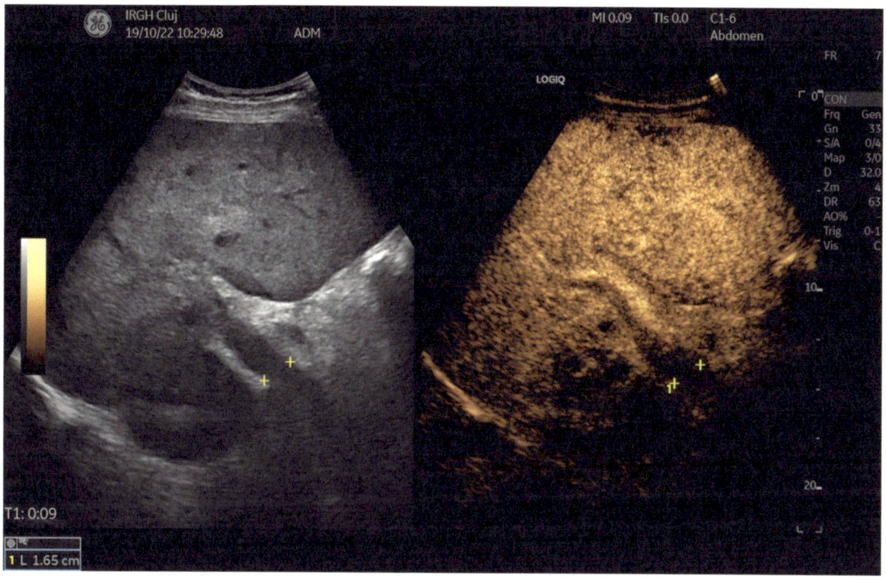

Figure 8.
Complete non-enhancement of the portal vein trunk (yellow markings) in a patient with non-cirrhotic portal vein thrombosis due to severe cholangitis.

PVT [61, 62]. Moreover, CEUS facilitates the assessment of collateral circulation and the identification of compensatory vascular pathways, which are crucial determinants of clinical management and prognostication in patients with PVT [63]. Through dynamic imaging, CEUS enables the visualization of portal blood flow patterns, including the presence of cavernous transformation (**Figure 9**) and portosystemic shunting, which carry important implications for therapeutic decision-making and risk stratification. Additionally, CEUS can aid in the differentiation between acute and chronic thrombotic events, guiding the timing and intensity of anticoagulation therapy in affected individuals. Furthermore, CEUS plays a pivotal role in the longitudinal monitoring of PVT, offering the ability to track thrombus resolution, assess treatment response, and detect potential complications such as portal hypertension and risk for variceal bleeding [64]. Its non-invasive nature and excellent safety profile make CEUS particularly well-suited for repeated examinations, facilitating close surveillance in high-risk patient populations.

In the context of cirrhosis, the presence of liver nodules poses a diagnostic dilemma, as distinguishing between benign regenerative nodules and hepatocellular carcinoma (HCC) is crucial for clinical management and prognosis. In this setting, CEUS is a useful adjunct to conventional imaging modalities, offering unique advantages in the characterization of liver nodules and potentalliy sparing further downstream costly investigations. Unlike conventional ultrasound, which may struggle to differentiate between nodular lesions due to inherent limitations in tissue contrast, CEUS leverages microbubble contrast agents to enhance vascular delineation and tissue perfusion, enabling real-time assessment of nodule vascularity and enhancement patterns. Through dynamic imaging, CEUS allows for the characterization of arterial-phase hyperenhancement, washout kinetics, and capsule appearance, which are key features in the diagnostic algorithm for HCC (**Figure 10**). Moreover, CEUS provides superior spatial and temporal resolution compared to computed tomography (CT) and magnetic resonance imaging (MRI), particularly in patients with compromised

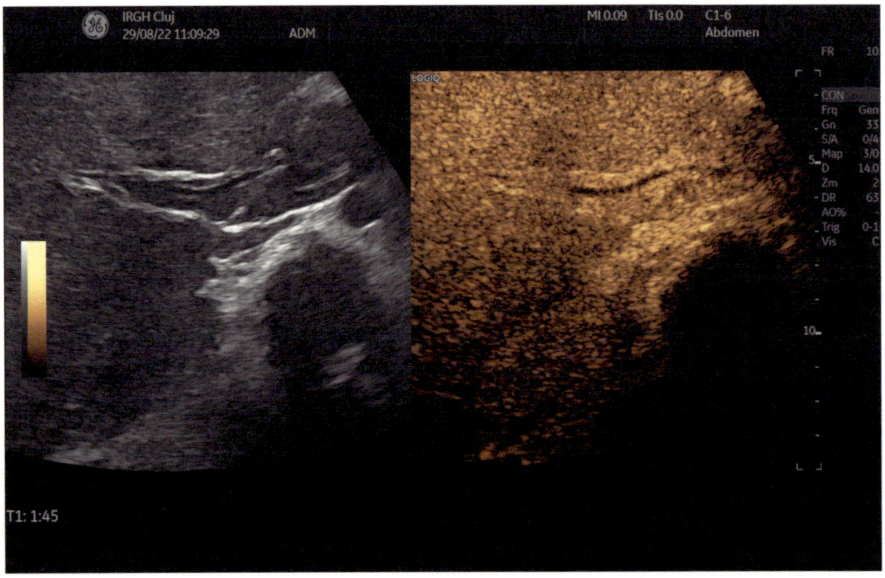

Figure 9.
Contrast-enhanced study of a patient with chronic portal vein thrombosis and cavernoma, revealing the central non-enhancing portal vein lumen and the peripheral hyperenhancement of the portal tract, corresponding to the cavernomatous venous transformation.

renal function or contraindications to iodinated contrast agents or gadolinium-based contrast agents [13].

Additionally, CEUS offers the advantage of real-time imaging, enabling immediate feedback during the procedure and facilitating targeted biopsy guidance, thus improving diagnostic accuracy and reducing the need for unnecessary invasive procedures. Its excellent safety profile, absence of ionizing radiation, and cost-effectiveness further contribute to its utility in the evaluation of liver nodules in cirrhosis. In the landscape of liver nodules within cirrhotic livers, the Liver Imaging Reporting and Data System (LiRADS) serves as a standardized framework for categorizing lesions, guiding clinical management decisions, and predicting malignancy risk [13, 65]. Within this framework, contrast-enhanced ultrasonography (CEUS) plays a pivotal role in the characterization and risk stratification of liver nodules, particularly in cases where other imaging modalities may yield equivocal results. Moreover, CEUS facilitates the visualization of ancillary features such as capsule appearance, rim enhancement, and threshold growth, which further inform lesion categorization within the LiRADS system (**Table 4**).

While CEUS LiRADS offers a structured approach to characterizing liver lesions in patients at risk of HCC, it carries notable limitations and potential biases. One primary limitation lies in its dependency on operator skill and image quality, which may lead to variability in lesion detection and interpretation [66]. Unlike CT or MRI, CEUS is more susceptible to suboptimal acoustic windows, particularly in obese patients or those with deeply located lesions. Furthermore, CEUS has limited ability to evaluate the entire liver comprehensively in a single examination, increasing the risk of missing multifocal or small lesions. Another challenge is the overlap in enhancement patterns between HCC and non-HCC malignancies, which can result in misclassification, particularly in the CEUS LR-M category. This is compounded by a lack of universally accepted thresholds for some imaging features, such as "mild" vs.

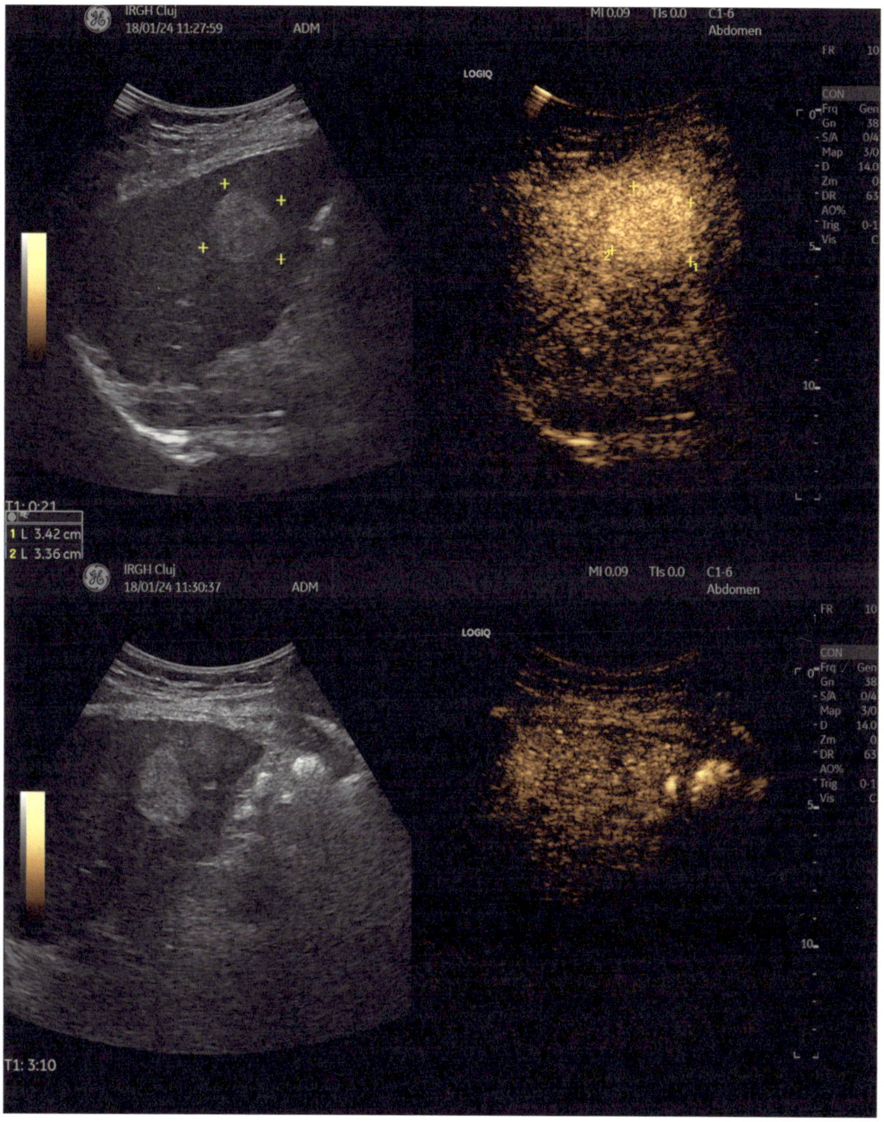

Figure 10.
Contrast-enhanced study of a hyperechoic liver nodule in a cirrhotic liver. The first image reveals an arterial-phase hyperenhancement of the nodule, while the image below reveals a late and mild washout 3 minutes after contrast injection. The perfusion of the nodule corresponds to LiRADS 5, suggesting a definite hepatocellular carcinoma diagnosis.

"marked" washout. Additionally, publication and selection biases may exist in validation studies, where high-quality CEUS exams in specialized centers may not reflect routine clinical practice. As such, while CEUS LiRADS provides valuable diagnostic guidance, it should be applied with an understanding of its inherent limitations and always interpreted in the context of clinical and laboratory findings [67].

Incorporating CEUS into the LiRADS algorithm enhances the accuracy and reliability of lesion characterization, ultimately improving patient outcomes through timely and appropriate management strategies. Despite ongoing challenges in standardizing imaging protocols and operator training, the integration of CEUS within

Category	Description	Criteria
CEUS LR-1	Definitely benign	Cyst; hemangioma; hepatic fat deposition/sparing
CEUS LR-2	Probably benign	Distinct isoenhancing solid nodule <10 mm; If isoenhancing nodule ≥10 mm, then apply CEUS LR-3; non-mass-like isoenhancing observation of any size not typical of hepatic fat deposition/sparing; CEUS LR-3 nodules with size stability for ≥2 years
CEUS LR-3	Intermediate malignancy probability	Nodule <20 mm with no APHE and no washout, or with late and mild washout; nodule ≥20 mm with no APHE and no washout; nodule <10 mm with APHE and no washout
CEUS LR-4	Probably HCC	Nodule ≥20 mm with no APHE and with late and mild washout; nodule <10 mm with APHE and with late and mild washout; nodule ≥10 mm with APHE and no washout
CEUS LR-5	Definitely HCC	Nodule ≥10 mm with APHE and with late and mild washout
CEUS LR-M	Probably or definitely malignant, not HCC specific	Rim (non-peripheral discontinuous globular) APHE; early (< 60 s) washout; marked washout
CEUS LR-TIV	Tumor in vein	Unequivocal enhancing soft tissue in vein, regardless of visualization of a parenchymal mass; Early visualization of intravenous contrast in the vein (approx. Same time as hepatic artery opacification) favors tumor in vein; Late visualization of intravenous contrast in the vein (approx. 10 seconds after hepatic artery opacification) favors portal flow in a patent non-occlusive or recanalized bland thrombus
CEUS LR-NC	Non-categorizable	Cannot be categorized due to image degradation or omission

APHE – arterial phase hyperenhancement; HCC – hepatocellular carcinoma.

Table 4.
The CEUS LiRADS classification system, adapted after [13].

the LiRADS framework represents a significant advancement in the comprehensive evaluation of liver nodules in cirrhotic patients, offering clinicians a valuable tool for optimizing diagnostic accuracy and therapeutic decision-making.

5. Multiparametric ultrasonography in specific scenarios

5.1 Transjugular intrahepatic portosystemic shunts

Multiparametric ultrasonography plays a crucial role in the surveillance of transjugular intrahepatic portosystemic shunts (TIPS), offering a non-invasive and comprehensive assessment of shunt patency and function. By integrating various ultrasound parameters from grayscale imaging to Doppler flow measurements and contrast-enhanced techniques, MPUS provides valuable information regarding intra-shunt velocity, direction, and morphology. Doppler ultrasound enables real-time evaluation of blood flow within the shunt and adjacent vessels, aiding in the detection of stenosis, thrombosis, or shunt dysfunction. Grayscale imaging allows for the visualization of shunt position and integrity, identifying any structural abnormalities or signs of shunt malfunction. Additionally, contrast-enhanced ultrasound enhances the assessment of shunt perfusion and identifies perfusion defects or areas of altered flow dynamics.

There have been multiple attempts to standardize the US evaluation of patients with TIPS, with the ultimate aim to reliably detect shunt dysfunction by circumventing the invasive hemodynamic assessment. While the diagnosis of stent thrombosis (**Figure 11**), occlusion, and stenosis are reliably identified, with a diagnostic accuracy exceeding 90% [68], the more subtle changes associated with an increase in portal pressure gradients (PPG) leading to TIPS dysfunction while the shunt is still fully permeable have yet to be adequately standardized [69]. In a seminal review written by Martin Rössle, one of the pioneers of TIPS, in 2013 [69] and recently updated [70], the author has proposed a

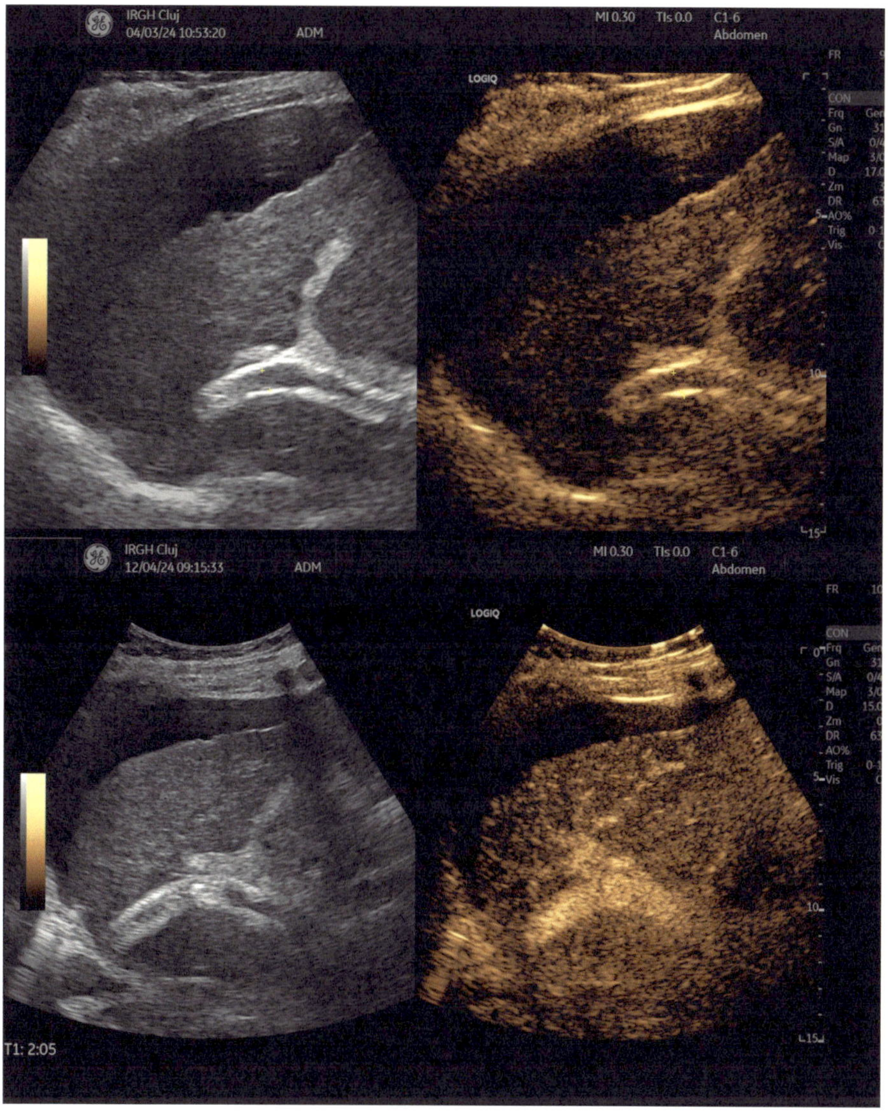

Figure 11.
Contrast-enhanced study of a patient with cirrhosis and inadequate control of ascites following transjugular intrahepatic portosystemic shunt (TIPS) placement. The first image reveals a complete filling defect within the stent, with no enhancement during the portal phase. The image below was acquired following TIPS revision and angioplasty, confirming shunt patency.

	Patent TIPS	TIPS dysfunction
Portal vein Velocity (cm/s) Intrahepatic flow	40 Hepatofugal	< 30 Hepatopetal
Stent Velocity (cm/s) Caliber (mm)	110 8–10	< 50 or > 180 < 8
Hepatic veins Velocity (cm/s)		> 180

Table 5.
Proposed criteria for transjugular intrahepatic portosystemic shunt dysfunction, adapted after Rössle [69].

multimodal approach for the detection of TIPS dysfunction, incorporating clinical elements (control of ascites, recurrence of PHT-related bleeding), grayscale US assessment and Doppler-based variables such as portal vein velocity (PVV), intrahepatic portal flow directionality, and peak in-stent velocity (**Table 5**).

Recent evidence has shown that CEUS can be used as a complementary method to Doppler US assessment of patients with TIPS, significantly increasing the diagnostic yield for TIPS dysfunction while sparing additional sectional imaging investigations [18, 71]. Thus, the patients can be referred to a hemodynamic revision quicker, without the additional (material and ionizing radiation) cost of a contrast-enhanced computed tomography, following a routine US follow-up.

Through its multifaceted approach, multiparametric ultrasonography facilitates early detection of complications, guides clinical decision-making, and optimizes patient management strategies in TIPS surveillance. Its non-invasive nature and ability to provide real-time, detailed information make it an invaluable tool in ensuring the long-term efficacy and safety of TIPS procedures.

However, US still poses some significant limitations. As shown in one of our recently published articles, Doppler parameters like PVV and its dynamics (ΔPVV) offer only moderate diagnostic accuracy (AUROC up to 0.78) for detecting hemodynamic dysfunction (PPG $\geq$12 mmHg). Many patients with normal ultrasound findings still had elevated PPG on invasive testing, highlighting ultrasound's limited sensitivity, especially for clinically silent dysfunction. Variability due to patient anatomy, ascites, and operator experience further restricts reliability. Therefore, ultrasound is useful for screening but insufficient to replace systematic hemodynamic evaluation post-TIPS placement [72]. **Table 6** summarizes the diagnostic performance of different cut-offs and variables for detecting TIPS dysfunction.

5.2 Liver transplantation

MPUS plays an essential role in post-liver transplantation (LT) follow-up as it can reliably detect most potential complications. Grayscale US can reveal perihepatic hematomas in the early post-LT period, reactive perihilar lymph nodes, and periportal edema. Depending on the type of biliary anastomosis, the common bile duct should not be dilated, or pneumobilia can be normal in hepato-jejunal anastomosis [73]. The Doppler US assessment of the transplanted liver should resemble the examination of a normal liver and should include measures of portal vein velocity, hepatic arterial resistivity index, and hepatic outflow evaluation.

Cut-off value	PVV - 40.5 cm/s	PVV - 39 cm/s + hepatopetal flow	PVV - 31 cm/s	PVV - 28 cm/s + hepatofugal flow	ΔPVV − 9.5 cm/s	PVV + ΔPVV*
Sensitivity (%, 95% C.I.)	83.8 (66.2–94.5)	67.7 (46.7–83.3)	48.3 (30.1–66.9)	32.3 (16.6–51.3)	96.7 (83.3–99.9)	87.1 (70.1–96.3)
Specificity (%, 95% C.I.)	50 (34.5–65.4)	61.3 (45.5–75.6)	79.5 (64.7–90.2)	93.1 (81.3–98.5)	35 (20.6–51.6)	60 (43.3–75.1)
Positive predictive value (%, 95% C.I.)	52.8% (44.5–60.9)	53.8 (42.8–64.5)	62.5 (45.6–76.8)	76.9 (49.9–91.7)	53.5 (47.6–59.3)	62.7 (53–71.6)
Negative Predictive Value (%, 95% C.I.)	82.3 (66.4–91.6)	74 (61.9–83.3)	68.6 (60.1–76)	66.1 (60.1–71.6)	93.3 (66–99)	85.7 (63.9–93.9)
Accuracy	63.5 (51.6–74.3)	63.9 (52–74.6)	66.6 (54.8–77.1)	68 (56.2–78.3)	61.9 (49.6–73.2)	71.8 (59.9–81.8)
p value (McNemar Test)	—	<0.01	<0.01	<0.01	0.02	<0.01

*PVV – portal vein velocity. *Using a cut-off value of 40.5 cm/s for PVV and 9.5 cm/s for ΔPVV; PVV – portal vein velocity; C.I. – confidence interval.*

Table 6.
Diagnostic test evaluation for portal vein velocity cut-off values, adapted with permission after Crăciun et al. [72].

Vascular complications	
Hepatic artery *60% of complications*	• Early hepatic artery thrombosis (high mortality) • Delayed thrombosis: stenosis, chronic rejection, sepsis • Stenosis • Pseudoaneurysms
Portal vein *1–2% of complications*	• Thrombosis: signs of portal hypertension
Hepatic outflow *<1% of complications*	• Budd-Chiari syndrome
Biliary complications 35% of complications	
Biliary leaks *Biliary strictures*	• Most common in end-to-end anastomosis, it leads to the formation of perihepatic bilomas • Non-anastomotic: ischemia, rejection, infection • Anastomotic
Gallstone disease	• Positive findings of choledocholithiasis
Other biliary complications	• Oddi dysfunction • Recurrence of primary sclerosing cholangitis
Focal liver lesions	
Hepatocellular carcinoma	• Recurrent or de novo, can be diagnosed using LiRADS criteria
Post-transplantation lymphoproliferative disorder	• Hypoechoic lesions or diffuse infiltrations due to unregulated lymphoid expansion secondary to immunosuppression
Benign focal lesions	• Infarction • Abcess • Biloma

Table 7.
The most frequent post-liver transplantation complications, adapted after O'Brien et al. [74].

The essential aspect of post-LT follow-up is, however, the prompt recognition of complications. In the setting of LT, complications can arise at any level, involving all vascular structures, the biliary tree, the occurrence of post-LT liver nodules or other parenchymal lesions or perihepatic anomalies [74]. The most common post-LT complications are summarized in **Table 7**.

6. Conclusion

In conclusion, multiparametric ultrasonography stands as a pivotal tool in the comprehensive assessment of patients with advanced liver disease and portal hypertension. Its non-invasive nature, versatility, and ability to provide a multifaceted evaluation make it indispensable in clinical practice. From assessing liver parenchyma to detecting complications like portal hypertension and its associated sequelae, multiparametric ultrasonography offers valuable insights guiding timely interventions and management strategies. As technology advances and techniques refine, its role is set to expand further, promising improved patient outcomes and enhanced diagnostic accuracy. Embracing multiparametric ultrasonography is pivotal in navigating the complexities of liver disease management in modern medicine.

Acknowledgements

We want to thank Dr. Horia Ștefănescu for providing images from his personal archives and valuable insights in writing this book chapter.

The authors also acknowledge the use of ChatGPT 4.5 (OpenAI, San Francisco, California, United States) and Grammarly Premium Editor (Grammarly Inc., San Francisco, California, United States) for phrasing, language polishing, and structural feedback. All of the primary data included in the manuscript has been written and verified by the authors. The responsibility for the content, including the parts produced by the AI tools, lies entirely with the authors, and the authors are liable for any breach of publication ethics.

Author details

Rareș Crăciun[1,2*], Tudor Mocan[1,3] and Zeno Spârchez[1,2]

1 Department of Internal Medicine, "Iuliu Hațieganu" University of Medicine and Pharmacy, Cluj-Napoca, Romania

2 Gastroenterology Clinic, "Prof. Dr. O. Fodor" Regional Institute of Gastroenterology and Hepatology, Cluj-Napoca, Romania

3 UBBMED Department, "Babeș-Bolyai" University, Cluj-Napoca, Romania

*Address all correspondence to: craciun.rares.calin@elearn.umfcluj.ro

References

[1] Sidhu PS. Multiparametric ultrasound (MPUS) imaging: Terminology describing the many aspects of ultrasonography. Ultraschall in der Medizin. 2015;**36**(4):315-317

[2] Peltec A, Sporea I. Multiparametric ultrasound as a new concept of assessment of liver tissue damage. World Journal of Gastroenterology. 2024;**30**(12):2219-2840

[3] Popescu A. Multiparametric ultrasound (MPUS) or "the many faces" of ultrasonography. Medical Ultrasonography. 2019;**21**(4):369-370

[4] Grgurevic I, Tjesic Drinkovic I, Pinzani M. Multiparametric ultrasound in liver diseases: An overview for the practising clinician. Postgraduate Medical Journal. 2019;**95**(1126):425-432

[5] Kloth C, Kratzer W, Schmidberger J, Beer M, Clevert DA, Graeter T. Ultrasound 2020 - Diagnostics & therapy: On the way to multimodal ultrasound: Contrast-enhanced ultrasound (CEUS), microvascular Doppler techniques, fusion imaging, sonoelastography, interventional sonography. RoFo Fortschritte auf dem Gebiet der Rontgenstrahlen und der Bildgebenden Verfahren. 2021;**193**(1):23-32

[6] Chernyak V, Fowler KJ, Kamaya A, Kielar AZ, Elsayes KM, Bashir MR, et al. Liver imaging reporting and data system (LI-RADS) version 2018: Imaging of hepatocellular carcinoma in at-risk patients. Radiology. 2018;**289**(3):816-830

[7] Maruyama H, Tobari M, Nagamatsu H, Shiina S, Yamaguchi T. Contrast-enhanced ultrasonography for the management of portal hypertension in cirrhosis. Frontiers in Medicine. 2022;**9**(6):1057045

[8] Sidhu PS, Cantisani V, Dietrich CF, Gilja OH, Saftoiu A, Bartels E, et al. The EFSUMB guidelines and recommendations for the clinical practice of contrast-enhanced ultrasound (CEUS) in non-hepatic applications: Update 2017 (long version). Ultraschall in der Medizin. 2018;**39**(2):e2-e44

[9] Minciuna I, Taru M, Fodor A, Nicoara Farcau O, Fischer P, Radu C, et al. Multiparametric ultrasound evaluation of liver fibrosis, steatosis, and viscosity in patients with chronic liver disease. Medical Ultrasonography. 2024;**26**(2):117-124

[10] Reiberger T. The value of liver and spleen stiffness for evaluation of portal hypertension in compensated cirrhosis. Hepatology Communications. 2022;**6**(5):950-964

[11] Mandorfer M, Hernández-Gea V, García-Pagán JC, Reiberger T. Noninvasive diagnostics for portal hypertension: A comprehensive review. Seminars in Liver Disease. 2020;**40**(3):240-255

[12] Buechter M, Manka P, Theysohn JM, Reinboldt M, Canbay A, Kahraman A. Spleen stiffness is positively correlated with HVPG and decreases significantly after TIPS implantation. Digestive and Liver Disease. 2018;**50**(1):54-60

[13] Van der Pol CB, McInnes MDF, Salameh JP, Levis B, Chernyak V, Sirlin CB, et al. CT/MRI and CEUS LI-RADS major features association with hepatocellular carcinoma: Individual patient data meta-analysis. Radiology. 2022;**302**(2):326-335

[14] Dietrich CF, Nolsøe CP, Barr RG, Berzigotti A, Burns PN, Cantisani V, et al. Guidelines and good clinical practice recommendations for contrast-enhanced

ultrasound (CEUS) in the liver–update 2020 WFUMB in cooperation with EFSUMB, AFSUMB, AIUM, and FLAUS: WFUMB in cooperation with EFSUMB, AFSUMB, AIUM and FLAUS. Ultrasound in Medicine and Biology. 2020;**46**(10):2579-2604

[15] Chen J, Zhu J, Zhang C, Song Y, Huang P. Contrast-enhanced ultrasound for the characterization of portal vein thrombosis vs tumor-in-vein in HCC patients: A systematic review and meta-analysis. European Radiology. 2020;**30**(5):2871-2880

[16] Sparchez Z, Mocan T, Craciun R, Sparchez M, Nolsøe C. Contrast enhancement for ultrasound-guided interventions: When to use it and what to expect? Ultrasonography. 2022;**41**(2):263-278

[17] Micol C, Marsot J, Boublay N, Pilleul F, Berthezene Y, Rode A. Contrast-enhanced ultrasound: A new method for TIPS follow-up. Abdominal Imaging. 2012;**37**(2):252-260

[18] Gao X, Wang HH, Zhang YZ, Liu XB, Qin XC. Contrast-enhanced ultrasound at high mechanical index: A new method for transjugular intrahepatic portosystemic shunt follow-up. Clinical Radiology. 2019;**75**(4):302-307

[19] Como G, Montaldo L, Baccarani U, Lorenzin D, Zuiani C, Girometti R. Contrast-enhanced ultrasound applications in liver transplant imaging. Abdominal Radiology. 2021;**46**(1):84-95

[20] de Franchis R, Bosch J, Garcia-Tsao G, Reiberger T, Ripoll C, Abraldes JG, et al. Baveno VII – Renewing consensus in portal hypertension. Journal of Hepatology. 2021;**76**(4):959-974

[21] Berzigotti A, Tsochatzis E, Boursier J, Castera L, Cazzagon N, Friedrich-Rust M, et al. EASL clinical practice guidelines on non-invasive tests for evaluation of liver disease severity and prognosis – 2021 update. Journal of Hepatology. 2021;**75**(3):659-689

[22] Sterling RK, Asrani SK, Levine D, Duarte-Rojo A, Patel K, Fiel MI, et al. AASLD practice guideline on non-invasive liver disease assessments of portal hypertension. Hepatology. 2024;**81**(3):1060-1085

[23] Sterling RK, Duarte-Rojo A, Patel K, Asrani SK, Alsawas M, Dranoff J, et al. AASLD practice guideline on imaging-based non-invasive liver disease assessments of hepatic fibrosis and steatosis. Hepatology. 2024;**81**(3):1060-1085

[24] Gerstenmaier JF, Gibson RN. Ultrasound in chronic liver disease. Insights into Imaging. 2014;**5**(4):441-455

[25] Maruyama H, Yokosuka O. Ultrasonography for noninvasive assessment of portal hypertension. Gut and Liver. 2017;**11**(4):464-473

[26] Vilgrain V, Lebrec D, Menu Y, Scherrer A, Nahum H. Comparison between ultrasonographic signs and the degree of portal hypertension in patients with cirrhosis. Gastrointestinal Radiology. 1990;**15**:218-222

[27] Angeli P, Bernardi M, Villanueva C, Francoz C, Mookerjee RP, Trebicka J, et al. EASL clinical practice guidelines for the management of patients with decompensated cirrhosis. Journal of Hepatology. 2018;**69**(2):406-460

[28] Aubé C, Bazeries P, Lebigot J, Cartier V, Boursier J. Liver fibrosis, cirrhosis, and cirrhosis-related nodules: Imaging diagnosis and surveillance. Diagnostic and Interventional Imaging. 2017;**98**(6):455-468

[29] Moore KP, Wong F, Gines P, Bernardi M, Ochs A, Salerno F, et al. The management of ascites in cirrhosis: Report on the consensus conference of the international ascites Club. Hepatology. 2003;**38**(1):258-266

[30] Robinson KA, Middleton WD, Al-Sukaiti R, Teefey SA, Dahiya N. Doppler sonography of portal hypertension. Ultrasound Quarterly. 2009;**25**(1):3-13

[31] Zironi G, Gaiani S, Fenyves D, Rigamonti A, Bolondi L, Barbara L. Value of measurement of mean portal flow velocity by Doppler flowmetry in the diagnosis of portal hypertension. Journal of Hepatology. 1992;**16**(3):298-303

[32] Liu C, Chen S, Yan X, Xiang Y, Hui J, Liu Z, et al. Diagnostic value of portal vein velocity for portal hypertension in patients with hepatitis B virus-related cirrhosis. Current Medical Imaging. 2021;**17**(11):1363-1368

[33] Bevilacqua M, De Marco L, Stupia R, Cattazzo F, Zonkape M, Paon V, et al. Hepatofugal portal flow is highly predictive of acute-on-chronic liver failure: A new hemodynamic patho-physiological hypothesis. Digestive and Liver Disease. 2024;**S1590-8658**(24):00208-00201

[34] Schneider AW, Kalk JF, Klein CP. Hepatic arterial pulsatility index in cirrhosis: Correlation with portal pressure. Journal of Hepatology. 1999;**30**(5):876-881

[35] Tana C, Tana M, Rossi S, Silingardi M, Schiavone C. Hepatic artery resistive index (HARI) and non-alcoholic fatty liver disease (NAFLD) fibrosis score in NAFLD patients: Cut-off suggestive of non-alcoholic steatohepatitis (NASH) evolution. Journal of Ultrasound. 2016;**19**(3):183-189

[36] Stulic M, Culafic D, Obrenovic R, Jankovic G, Alempijevic T, Lalosevic MS, et al. The clinical importance of cystatin C and hepatic artery resistive index in liver cirrhosis. Medicina (Lithuania). 2018;**54**(3):1-8

[37] Tana C, Schiavone C, Ticinesi A, Lauretani F, Nouvenne A, Dietrich CF, et al. Hepatic artery resistive index as surrogate marker for fibrosis progression in NAFLD patients: A clinical perspective. International Journal of Immunopathology and Pharmacology. 2018;**32**:2058738418781373

[38] Gaspari R, Teofili L, Mignani V, Franco A, Valentini CG, Cutuli SL, et al. Duplex Doppler evidence of high hepatic artery resistive index after liver transplantation: Role of portal hypertension and clinical impact. Digestive and Liver Disease. 2020;**52**(3):301-307

[39] Abraldes JG, Bureau C, Stefanescu H, Augustin S, Ney M, Blasco H, et al. Noninvasive tools and risk of clinically significant portal hypertension and varices in compensated cirrhosis: The "Anticipate" study. Hepatology. 2016;**64**(6):2173-2184

[40] De FR, Vi B. Position paper expanding consensus in portal hypertension report of the Baveno VI consensus workshop: Stratifying risk and individualizing care for portal hypertension. Journal of Hepatology. 2015;**63**(3):743-752

[41] Ferraioli G, De Silvestri A, Lissandrin R, Maiocchi L, Tinelli C, Filice C, et al. Evaluation of inter-system variability in liver stiffness measurements. Ultraschall in der Medizin. 2018;**40**(1):64-75

[42] Lin Y, Li H, Jin C, Wang H, Jiang B. The diagnostic accuracy of liver fibrosis

in non-viral liver diseases using acoustic radiation force impulse elastography: A systematic review and meta-analysis. PLoS One. 2020;**15**(1):1-20

[43] Herrmann E, de Lédinghen V, Cassinotto C, Chu WCW, Leung VYF, Ferraioli G, et al. Assessment of biopsy-proven liver fibrosis by two-dimensional shear wave elastography: An individual patient data-based meta-analysis. Hepatology. 2018;**67**(1):260-272

[44] Papatheodoridi M, Hiriart JB, Lupsor-Platon M, Bronte F, Boursier J, Elshaarawy O, et al. Refining the Baveno VI elastography criteria for the definition of compensated advanced chronic liver disease. Journal of Hepatology. 2021;**74**(5):1109-1116

[45] Piccinni R, Rodrigues SG, Montani M, Murgia G, Delgado MG, Casu S, et al. Controlled attenuation parameter reflects steatosis in compensated advanced chronic liver disease. Liver International. 2020;**40**(5):1151-1158

[46] Zhang X, Song J, Zhang Y, Wen B, Dai L, Xi R, et al. Baveno VII algorithm outperformed other models in ruling out high-risk varices in individuals with HBV-related cirrhosis. Journal of Hepatology. 2023;**78**(3):574-583

[47] Wong YJ, Zhaojin C, Tosetti G, Degasperi E, Sharma S, Agarwal S, et al. Baveno-VII criteria to predict decompensation and initiate non-selective beta-blocker in compensated advanced chronic liver disease patients. Clinical and Molecular Hepatology. 2023;**29**(1):135-145

[48] Szakács Z, Erőss B, Soós A, Mátrai P, Szabó I, Pétervári E, et al. Baveno criteria safely identify patients with compensated advanced chronic liver disease who can avoid variceal screening endoscopy: A diagnostic test accuracy meta-analysis. Frontiers in Physiology. 2019;**10**(AUG):1-14

[49] Marot A, Trépo E, Doerig C, Schoepfer A, Moreno C, Deltenre P. Liver stiffness and platelet count for identifying patients with compensated liver disease at low risk of variceal bleeding. Liver International. 2017;**37**(5):707-716

[50] Rabiee A, Deng Y, Ciarleglio M, Chan JL, Pons M, Genesca J, et al. Noninvasive predictors of clinically significant portal hypertension in NASH cirrhosis: Validation of ANTICIPATE models and development of a lab-based model. Hepatology Communications. 2022;**6**(12):3324-3334

[51] Dajti E, Ravaioli F, Zykus R, Rautou P, Elkrief L, Grgurevic I, et al. Accuracy of spleen stiffness measurement for the diagnosis of clinically significant portal hypertension in patients with compensated advanced chronic liver disease: A systematic review and individual patient data meta-analysis. The Lancet Gastroenterology and Hepatology. 2023;**8**(9):816-828

[52] Sporea I, Bota S, Gradinaru-Taşcău O, Şirli R, Popescu A, Jurchiş A. Which are the cut-off values of 2D-shear wave Elastography (2D-SWE) liver stiffness measurements predicting different stages of liver fibrosis, considering transient Elastography (TE) as the reference method? European Journal of Radiology. 2014;**83**(3):e118-22

[53] Zaki M, Hazem M, Elsamman M. Shear wave elastography in assessment of liver stiffness and prediction of gastro-esophageal varices in patients with liver cirrhosis. Egyptian Journal of Radiology and Nuclear Medicine. 2019;**50**(1):16

[54] Lee HA. Liver fibrosis assessment in chronic liver diseases using elastography:

A comprehensive review of vibration-controlled transient elastography and shear wave elastography. Clinical Ultrasound [Internet]. 2024;**9**(2):70-84. DOI: 10.18525/cu.2024.9.2.70

[55] Atzori SM, Pasha Y, Maurice JB, Taylor-Robinson SD, Campbell L, Lim AKP. Prospective evaluation of liver shearwave elastography measurements with 3 different technologies and same day liver biopsy in patients with chronic liver disease. Digestive and Liver Disease. 2024;**56**(3):484-494

[56] Tapper EB, Lok ASF. Use of liver imaging and biopsy in clinical practice. New England Journal of Medicine. 2017;**377**(8):756-768

[57] Piscaglia F, Bolondi L, Aiani L, Luigi Angeli M, Arienti V, Barozzi L, et al. The safety of Sonovue® in abdominal applications: Retrospective analysis of 23188 investigations. Ultrasound in Medicine and Biology. 2006;**32**(9):1369-1375

[58] Tang C, Fang K, Guo Y, Li R, Fan X, Chen P, et al. Safety of Sulfur hexafluoride microbubbles in sonography of abdominal and superficial organs: Retrospective analysis of 30,222 cases. Journal of Ultrasound in Medicine. 2017;**36**(3):531-538

[59] Liu D, Qian L, Wang J, Hu X, Qiu L. Hepatic perfusion parameters of contrast-enhanced ultrasonography correlate with the severity of chronic liver disease. Ultrasound in Medicine and Biology. 2014;**40**(11):2556-2563

[60] Haimerl M, Poelsterl S, Beyer LP, Wiesinger I, Nießen C, Stroszczynski C, et al. Chronic liver disease: Quantitative MRI vs CEUS-based microperfusion. Clinical Hemorheology and Microcirculation. 2016;**64**(3):435-446

[61] Danilă M, Sporea I, Popescu A, Şirli R. Portal vein thrombosis in liver cirrhosis - The added value of contrastenhanced ultrasonography. Medical Ultrasonography. 2016;**18**(2):218-223

[62] Tarantino L, Ambrosino P, Di Minno MND. Contrast-enhanced ultrasound in differentiating malignant from benign portal vein thrombosis in hepatocellular carcinoma. World Journal of Gastroenterology. 2015;**21**(32):9457-9460

[63] Rafailidis V, Fang C, Yusuf GT, Huang DY, Sidhu PS. Contrast-enhanced ultrasound (CEUS) of the abdominal vasculature. Abdominal Radiology. 2018;**43**(4):934-947

[64] Boccatonda A, Gentilini S, Zanata E, Simion C, Serra C, Simioni P, et al. Portal vein thrombosis: State-of-the-art. Review. 2024;**13**(5):1517

[65] Bartolotta TV, Terranova MC, Gagliardo C, Taibbi A. CEUS LI-RADS: A pictorial review. Insights into Imaging. 2020;**11**(1):9

[66] Dai T, Zhu H, Qiao M, Song Y, Sun Y, Meng X, et al. Training on contrast-enhanced ultrasound LI-RADS classification for resident radiologists: A retrospective comparison of performance after training. Insights Into Imaging. 2024;**15**(1):205

[67] Cheng MQ, Huang H, Ruan SM, Xu P, Tong WJ, He DN, et al. Complementary role of CEUS and CT/MR LI-RADS for diagnosis of recurrent HCC. Cancers (Basel). 2023;**15**(24):5743

[68] Manatsathit W, Samant H, Panjawatanan P, Braseth A, Suh J, Esmadi M, et al. Performance of ultrasound for detection of transjugular intrahepatic portosystemic shunt

dysfunction: A meta-analysis. Abdominal Radiology. 2019;**44**:2392-2402

[69] Rössle M. Review TIPS: 25 years later. Journal of Hepatology. 2013;**59**(June):1081-1093

[70] Schultheiβ M, Bettinger D, Thimme R, Rössle M. 30 years of transjugular intrahepatic portosystemic shunt (TIPS): Casting a retrospective glance and future perspectives. Zeitschrift fur Gastroenterologie. 2020;**58**(9):877-889

[71] Marschner CA, Geyer T, Froelich MF, Rübenthaler J, Schwarze V, Clevert DA. Diagnostic value of contrast-enhanced ultrasound for evaluation of transjugular intrahepatic portosystemic shunt perfusion. Diagnostics. 2021;**11**(9):1593

Crăciun R, Ștefănescu H, Nicoară-Farcău O, Fischer P, Fodor A, Tanțău M, et al. Portal vein velocity and its dynamics: A potentially useful tool for detecting clinically silent transjugular intrahepatic porto-systemic shunt dysfunction using Doppler ultrasonography. Ultrasound International Open. 17 Dec 2024;**10**:a24228339

[72] Maheshwari E, Tublin ME. Sonography of liver transplantation. Abdominal Radiology. 2021;**46**(1):68-83

[73] O'Brien J, Buckley AR, Browne R. Comprehensive ultrasound assessment of complications post-liver transplantation. European Journal of Radiology. 2010;**74**(1):206-213

Chapter 14

Perspective Chapter: AI in Computer Aided Diagnosis for Focal Liver Lesions Evaluated by Contrast-Enhanced Ultrasound

Georgiana Simion, Cristina-Laura Sîrbu, Cătălin-Daniel Căleanu, Ghiță-Adrian Burdan, Tudor Moga and Ioan Sporea

Abstract

The prevalence of liver diseases is increasing globally, positioning these conditions as having the third highest mortality rate. Contrast-enhanced ultrasound (CEUS) is an advanced medical imaging technique used to detect and characterize focal liver lesions. CEUS offers several advantages, including shorter investigation times, real-time results, cost-effectiveness, and high accuracy. This chapter aims to summarize and highlight key approaches in the latest computer-assisted diagnosis systems specifically focused on CEUS-based FLL diagnosis using AI principles. The discussion covers various image analysis tasks within the CEUS context, such as pre-processing, detection, segmentation, tracking, feature extraction, and classification. Additionally, this work outlines the existing challenges and potential trends in applying AI to medical CEUS image analysis.

Keywords: contrast-enhanced ultrasound, CEUS, focal liver lesions, machine learning, deep neural networks

1. Introduction

In our increasingly technological world, the medical field stands out as one with tremendous potential for advancement. The synergy between human expertise and artificial intelligence is driving innovation within healthcare.

Over the past few decades, various medical imaging techniques, including computed tomography (CT), magnetic resonance imaging (MRI), ultrasound, positron emission tomography (PET), mammography, and X-ray, have played pivotal roles in the early detection, diagnosis, and treatment of diseases. Although human experts have traditionally been responsible for interpreting and analyzing medical images in clinical situations, the emergence of computer-aided diagnosis (CAD) has started to change this paradigm.

The development of CAD tools, particularly those that aid in the evaluation of focal liver lesions (FLL), is of paramount importance, considering that liver cancer ranks as the fifth most common form of cancer worldwide and is second in mortality rate. In liver medical imaging, physicians typically rely on visual assessment to detect, characterize, and monitor diseases. However, such assessments, based on individual expertise and experience, can sometimes be subjective and prone to inaccuracies.

Artificial intelligence (AI) offers a promising alternative by enabling quantitative assessments through automated recognition of imaging information. By replacing qualitative reasoning with automated analysis, AI has the potential to help physicians make more precise imaging diagnoses, while significantly reducing their workload.

The CEUS investigation offers several advantages. Firstly, its short investigation time, typically only a few minutes, makes it a convenient option. Secondly, it provides real-time imaging, allowing for detailed visualization of lesion vascularity. Additionally, CEUS is less invasive and cost-effective compared to contrast-enhanced CT and MRI for diagnosing liver lesions. In addition, it has high specificity and accuracy to detect or exclude metastatic disease.

Due to its non-invasive nature, time efficiency, and affordability, CEUS investigation has become widely utilized across various pathologies. These include liver lesions [1], thyroid nodules [2, 3], prostate cancer [4, 5], rectal cancer [6, 7], breast cancer [8, 9], as well as kidney cystic lesions or tumors [10, 11]. While different methods can be employed to diagnose these pathologies from CEUS imaging, only a few approaches, particularly in some pathologies, take advantage of deep neural networks (DNN) and their associated learning paradigm, deep learning (DL).

The CEUS protocol commences with the intravenous administration of a specific contrast-enhancing agent, typically microbubbles of gas. This results in the creation of numerous small yet highly echogenic surfaces [12]. Illustrated in **Figure 1** are the dynamics of the investigative process, including some associated time intervals:

- The arterial phase initiates 10–20 seconds after the injection of the contrast agent and concludes approximately 25–35 seconds post-injection.

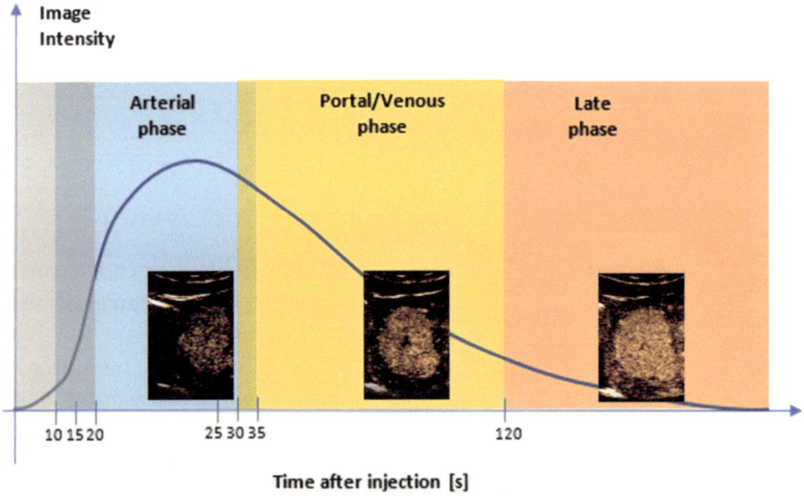

Figure 1.
CEUS investigation times according to the phase.

- The portal/venous phase spans from 30 to 120 seconds.
- Finally, the late phase encompasses times beyond 120 seconds.

To conclude the introduction, we may state that the aim in this context is to develop a computer-aided diagnosis system for FLL from CEUS data. Such systems could be of real help to practitioners and also fill an existing gap in commercially available medical investigation equipment. In the following, we will present state-of-the-art solutions which address every necessary step in the development of such a system.

2. Dataset

The collection of medical data represents one of the most problematic aspects in the effort to create a CAD system. This is due to the tedious acquisition process, data preprocessing, for example, ROI identification, difficulties in labelling/diagnosing large and heterogenous amount of medical data, and the lack of public datasets availability.

To our best knowledge, there is only one publicly available dataset with CEUS investigations, in which only three types of liver lesions are present: the SYSU-CEUS dataset [13, 14] comprises the next types of FLLs: 186 instances of hepatocellular carcinoma (HCC), 109 instances of hemangioma (HEM), and 58 instances of focal nodular hyperplasia (FNH), totaling 186 malignant instances and 167 benign instances. These data were collected from the First Affiliated Hospital, Sun Yat-sen University. The imaging equipment used for data acquisition was the Toshiba Medical System Aplio SSA-770A. All instances in the dataset have a resolution of 768 × 576 pixels and were obtained from different patients, resulting in substantial variations in the appearance and enhancement patterns of the FLLs, including differences in sizes, contrasts, shapes, and locations. Sample images from the SYSU-dataset are depicted in **Figure 2**.

Among some existing private datasets, we could mention UMFT acquired by the Department of Gastroenterology and Hepatology at the "Victor Babes" University of Medicine and Pharmacy in Timisoara, Romania. In this case, all examinations were performed using an Acuson S2000 ultrasound machine manufactured by Siemens (Berlin, Germany). A total of 91 patients were selected for this study. During the examination process, the ultrasound probe is intermittently lifted from contact with the patient to prevent the dissipation of echogenic gas bubbles injected for the procedure. The dataset consists of a total of 273 processed video files, covering five types of liver lesions. The distribution of patients in different categories of lesions is presented in **Table 1**.

For each video file, the ROIs were manually identified and labeled by experienced physicians, classified as Level II (advanced) and Level III (expert) operators according to the Romanian Society of Ultrasound in Medicine and Biology classification. All examinations adhered to the standard protocol outlined in the 2012 European Federation of Societies for Ultrasound in Medicine and Biology (EFSUMB) guidelines for contrast-enhanced ultrasound (CEUS). Additionally, contrast-enhanced CT, MRI, or histology data were available for each case to confirm the final diagnosis.

A total of 50 samples were selected from each phase of the investigation, resulting in approximately 150 ROI images per patient. Sampling during the arterial phase occurred when echogenicity began to increase. In total, 12,119 images were acquired, with varying sizes.

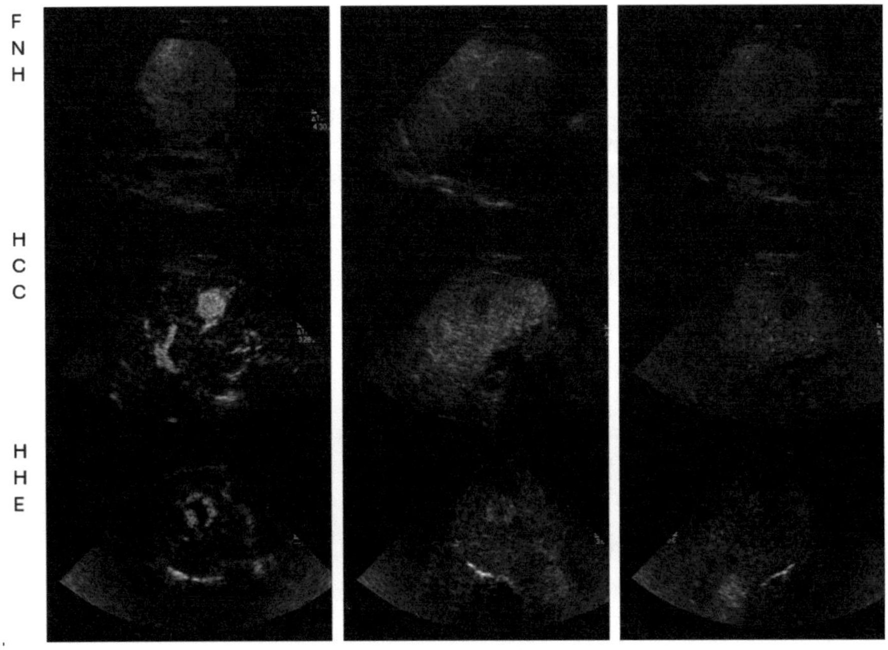

Figure 2.
Images from the SYSU-dataset showing different types of liver lesions.

FLL	No. of patients
FNH	16
HCC	30
HMG	23
HYPERM	11
HYPOM	11
Total:	**91**

Table 1.
The UMFT dataset: number of patients for each FLL type.

Samples from this dataset can be examined in **Figure 3**.

3. Detecting and tracking algorithms in CEUS videos

The detection step is crucial in the automated labelling of CEUS data. A possible approach to this field is described in [15], where the authors are using optical flow to detect areas of pixels with consistent illumination and coherent movement. Optical flow algorithms indeed assume that pixel color and intensity remain relatively constant between consecutive frames, allowing them to track motion accurately. To apply optical flow for lesion detection, the following steps should be taken into account:

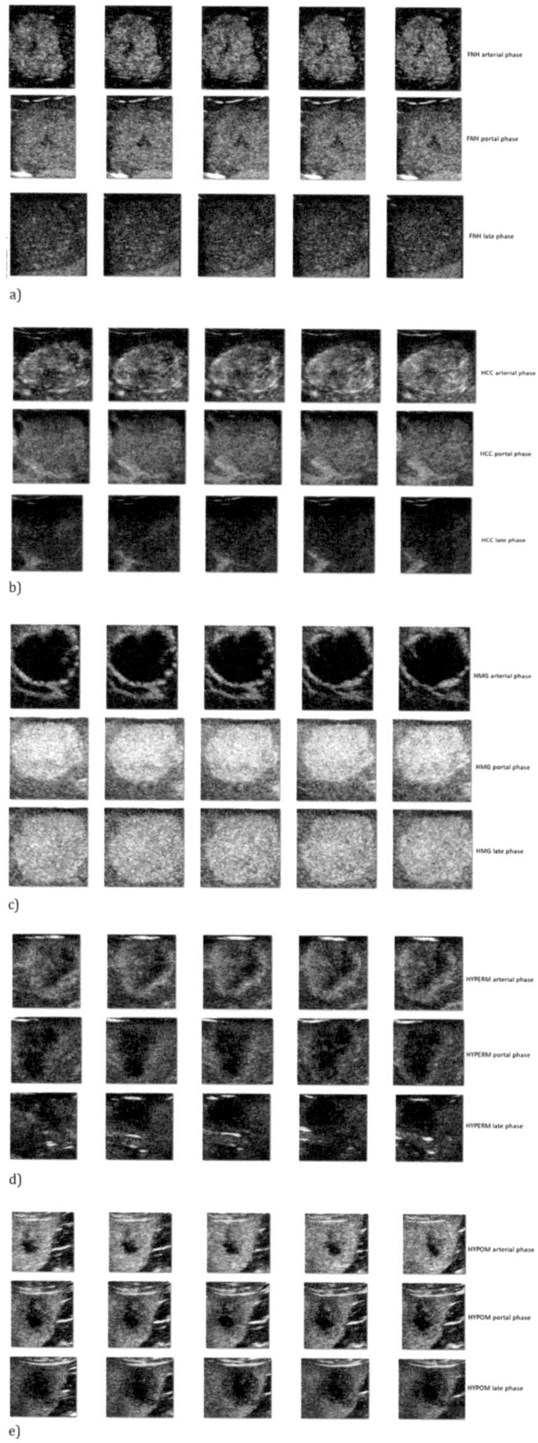

Figure 3.
CEUS representative ROIs from different phases—arterial, portal, late—sampled at 10 frame differences: (a) FNH; (b) HCC; (c) HMG; (d) HYPERM; (e) HYPOM.

- *Preprocessing*: preprocess image frames to enhance features relevant to lesion detection, such as contrast enhancement or noise reduction.

- *Optical flow computation*: apply an optical flow algorithm to calculate the motion vectors of pixels between consecutive frames. Common optical flow algorithms include Lucas-Kanade, Horn-Schunck, or more modern deep learning-based methods.

- *Motion analysis*: analyze the computed motion vectors to identify areas where pixels exhibit coherent movement in the same direction. This can be achieved by clustering or thresholding the motion vectors to group together pixels with similar motion.

- *Lesion detection*: define criteria for identifying lesions based on the results of the motion analysis. For example, you could look for regions with a high concentration of pixels exhibiting abnormal motion characteristics compared to the surrounding areas.

- *Validation and refinement*: validate the detected lesions and refine the detection algorithm as necessary. This may involve manual inspection of detected lesions to confirm their accuracy and adjusting parameters or algorithms to improve detection performance.

- *Integration with clinical workflow*: integrate the lesion detection algorithm into the clinical workflow, ensuring seamless integration with existing diagnostic processes and tools.

The effectiveness of lesion detection using optical flow depended on various factors such as image quality, motion characteristics, and the specific properties of the lesions was also estimated. Some intermediary steps of this process are presented in **Figure 4**.

Next to detection, comes the tracking phase. In [16], the authors use the optical flow algorithm to initialize the tracking phase. They investigate the performance of various tracking algorithms to efficiently generate training images, in the context of

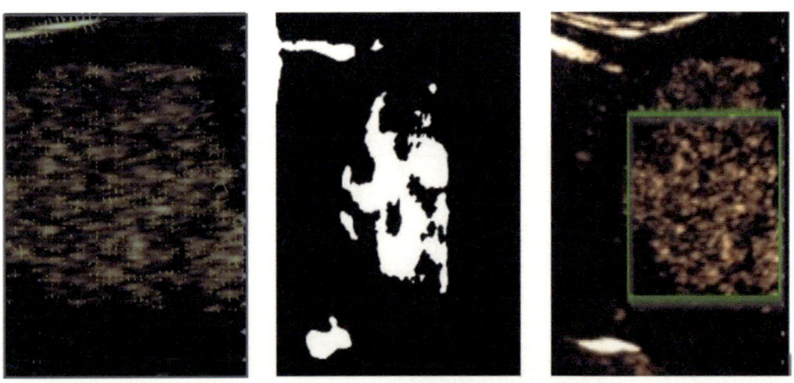

Figure 4.
Detection stages. (a) Velocity vectors. (b) Binarization. (c) ROI extraction.

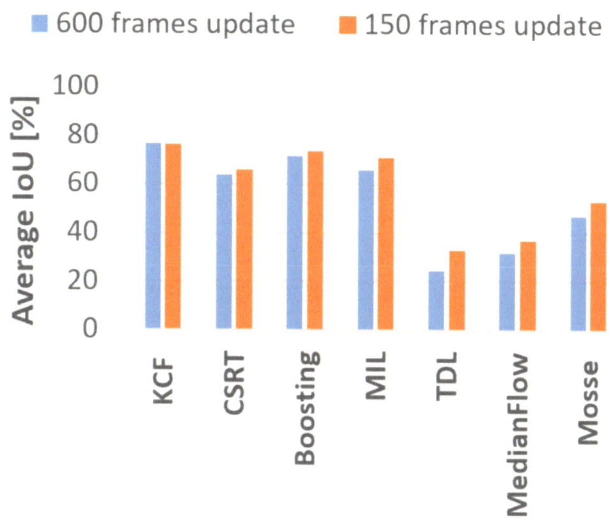

Figure 5.
Average IoU performance of the tracking algorithms.

contrast-enhanced ultrasound imaging. The aim is to automate the process of generating training datasets, which can then be used to train deep neural network (DNN) models for the classification of focal liver lesions in CEUS recordings. Investigating tracking algorithms to automate the labelling and extraction of Regions of Interest (ROIs) from video files is a crucial step in streamlining the process of developing computer-aided diagnosis systems. It is indeed labor-intensive to manually label entire video files, making automation highly desirable. Leveraging tracking algorithms can significantly alleviate this burden, particularly when dealing with CEUS images characterized by speckle noise and low contrast.

It has been concluded that the Kernelized Correlation Filter (KCF) tracking algorithm outperforms other solutions in terms of quality (76% intersection over union) while maintaining a short runtime (37.7 frames per second) [16]. This indicates its potential for effectively and efficiently tracking lesions in CEUS images. In **Figure 5**, one can see the results for the average IoU performance of the tracking algorithms that were tested.

4. The temporal approach

In an early work, the authors of [17] investigate temporal features extracted from contrast-enhanced ultrasound video frames to identify discriminative parameters to be used in developing a computer-aided diagnosis system for focal liver lesions. The aim of the system is to enable safe, inexpensive, early, and widely accessible detection of hepatic diseases. In this study, the improvement was achieved by introducing a robust fitting procedure and defining/selecting temporal descriptors. The focus was on the arterial phase (15–30 seconds post-injection) from CEUS investigation. The study characterizes the hemodynamic behavior for hepatocellular carcinoma, hemangioma, focal nodular hyperplasia, and hypervascular metastasis. In the proposed approach, CEUS video frames were evaluated by experienced physicians and categorized based on histology, biopsy, or contrast-enhanced CT/

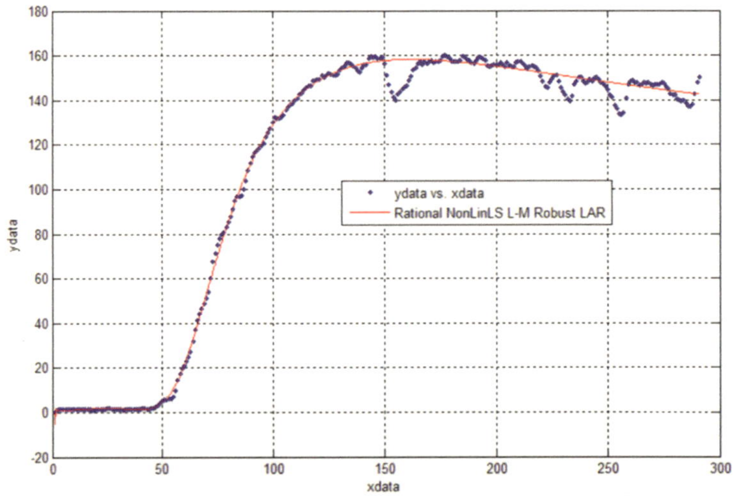

Figure 6.
Results of the intensity curve adjustment using the proposed model of [17].

MR imaging. A database comprising 37 cases of various FLL types was created. Subsequently, the arterial phase of the videos was analyzed, involving manual ROI localization and intensity calculation. Signal smoothing techniques were applied to minimize noise and motion effects, with alternative solutions proposed for robust fitting (the LAR LM parametric fitting rational regression model). The results can be seen in **Figure 6**.

Feature extraction was then performed, selecting significant temporal descriptors based on interclass and intraclass standard deviations. The top five descriptors (rise time, settling times, and peak time) were chosen for further analysis. Next, SVM was used to classify the feature vectors into one of the four predefined classes. The experimental outcomes showed the following classification accuracies: 37% for hepatocellular carcinoma, 82% for hemangioma, 65% for focal nodular hyperplasia, and 72% for hypervascular metastasis, with an overall classification rate of 64%.

5. The spatial approach

The CAD system proposed in one of our early works [18] adopts a different approach compared to existing methods by not relying on hand-crafted features; instead, it utilizes a variant of the Bag of Features (BoF) method. First, point selection is performed using a fixed 4 × 4 pixels grid, and multi-scale feature descriptors are extracted from square blocks of sizes 32, 64, 96, and 128 pixels. The number of clusters generated by K-means is set to k = 400. Next, the bag of visual words is used to encode images into histograms of visual words. These histograms serve as positive and negative samples to train a Support Vector Machine (SVM) multiclass classifier using the error-correcting output codes (ECOC) approach. The block diagram of the CAD system architecture is depicted in **Figure 7**, illustrating the flow of the processing steps.

Three BoF-based classifiers are trained, one for each phase of CEUS. Classifiers output prediction scores, which are converted to confidence scores. The fusion of

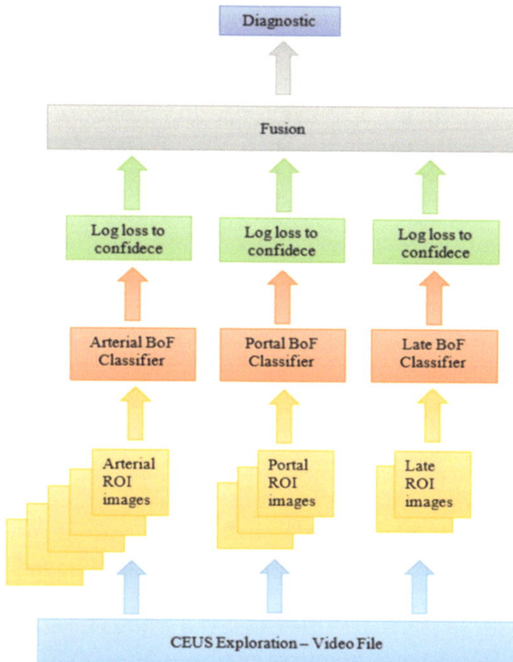

Figure 7.
CAD system architecture used in [18].

responses from the three classifiers can be done using either a soft-voting or a hard-voting strategy:

- Soft-voting: the CAD system predicts the class label based on the argmax of the sums of the predicted probabilities. This strategy is recommended for an ensemble of well-calibrated classifiers.

- Hard-voting: class labels are predicted using majority-rule voting. This strategy simplifies the decision-making process by selecting the class with the highest number of votes.

This approach aims to provide a robust and automated solution to FLL classification using CEUS images, leveraging the power of machine learning without relying on manually crafted features. The soft voting fusion scheme provided the best results, with an average accuracy of 64%.

Next, we seek to improve FLL diagnosis by harnessing the power of Deep Learning [19] to analyze CEUS images and classify lesions with high accuracy. Compared to existing approaches to that time, the novelty of this work was the use of 2D-DCNN to implement an automated diagnosis system that discriminates between a broader range of focal liver lesion types.

The dataset used contains 285 CEUS video sequences (from 95 patients) of five types of lesions, provided by the Department of Gastroenterology and Hepatology, 'Victor Babes' University of Medicine and Pharmacy, Timisoara. The dataset also includes Region of Interest (ROI) markings made by an expert radiologist, stored in associated text files. Uniform sampling was conducted on these ROIs, extracting 50 images per phase for each patient. To address noise and artifacts inherent in ultrasound images, the dataset underwent re-evaluation, resulting in a final set of 12,119 samples after removing inconsistent pictures.

The most successful model was a 12-layer 2D-DCNN trained with the ADAM optimiser over 50 epochs, employing a 32-batch size and input dimensions of 180 × 180 pixels. This model achieved an accuracy of 95.71% (averaged over 10 experiments) when tested with 2423 images.

In our following work [19], custom DNN designs are compared with state-of-the-art architectures, either pre-trained or trained from scratch. Our work improved and broadened previous works in the field in several aspects:

- New evaluation procedure: a leave-one-patient-out (LOPO) evaluation procedure is introduced, which is a more realistic evaluation method compared to the standard training/validation/testing split. This approach ensures that the evaluation is not biased by images from the same patient.

- Patient-orientated lesion diagnosis: different voting schemes are implemented for patient-oriented lesion diagnosis, such as hard voting and soft voting, which utilize predicted class labels or probabilities for decision-making.

- Utilization of modern DNN architectures: the study employs modern Deep Neural Network (DNN) architectures available through Keras Applications. These architectures come with pre-trained weights and are suitable for tasks such as transfer learning, fine-tuning, or training from scratch. Special emphasis is placed on TinyML/small-memory footprint models for potential deployment in medical embedded systems.

Transfer learning is a powerful technique in deep learning, where features learnt on one dataset, typically a large one like ImageNet, are applied to a new dataset with fewer data for training. Although the images in ImageNet may not be related to medical images, models trained on this dataset can capture general image features such as edges, textures, and shapes. This knowledge is then transferred to the new dataset, improving the performance of the model in tasks such as classification. In practice, transfer learning is implemented using pre-trained models, which are neural network architectures trained on large datasets like ImageNet. These pre-trained models are then fine-tuned on the new dataset to adapt their learnt features to the specific characteristics of the new data.

Data augmentation techniques, such as randomly flipping each image horizontally, rotating, and zooming by 10%, are applied to enhance the diversity of the training data and improve the robustness of the model. The results of applying transfer learning, as described, are presented in **Table 2**.

In contrast to transfer learning, in the train-from-scratch approach, the feature extraction layers' weights are trained; this means that the weights are initialized randomly and updated during training on the new dataset. The model learns the features directly from the new dataset without relying on pre-trained knowledge. This approach might be necessary when the new dataset significantly differs from the dataset the pre-trained weights were trained on, or when the available pre-trained models are not suitable for the task. The results for the modern DNNs trained from scratch can be seen in **Table 3**.

The results obtained through the pre-trained/transfer learning approach showed a top accuracy of 71%, as presented in **Table 2**. However, better results were achieved

Model/patients	11 FNH	11 HCC	11 HMG	11 MPER	11 MPO	55 patients
MobileNetV2	73	94	71	31	71	68
NASNetMobile	54	100	76	44	58	66
EfficientNetB0	85	94	70	33	54	68
DenseNet121	72	100	88	31	62	71
ResNet50	69	95	72	43	62	68

Table 2.
Average test accuracy [%]. Modern DNN, hard vote, 40 training epochs, and 20 early stopping patience, equal number of examples per class.

Model/patients	16 FNH	30 HCC	23 HMG	11 MPER	11 MPO	91 patients
MobileNetV2	100	100	93	36	72	80
NASNetMobile	100	88	82	68	83	84
EfficientNetB0	81	100	90	74	63	82
DenseNet121	92	100	94	78	70	87
ResNet50	100	100	100	72	67	88

Table 3.
Average test accuracy [%]. Modern DNN, hard vote, 40 training epochs, and 20 early stopping patience, unbalanced number of examples per class.

by training the model from scratch, albeit with longer training times (see **Table 3**). Specifically, employing the DenseNet121 architecture led to a significant improvement, achieving an average accuracy of 87%.

These results demonstrate that while transfer learning provides a good starting point by leveraging pre-trained weights, train from scratch allows for better adaptation to the specific characteristics of the new dataset, resulting in higher accuracy. It is noteworthy that despite DenseNet121 being a smaller architecture compared to others like ResNet or ResNetV2, it still achieved comparable results. For instance, both ResNet and ResNetV2 architectures achieved an average test accuracy of 88%, demonstrating the effectiveness of DenseNet121 in this context. Through a hard voting classification scheme, the study achieved a top accuracy of 88% in automatically diagnosing five types of FLLs, accounting for both intra- and inter-class imagistic differences that impact diagnostic accuracy. Compared to similar CAD systems, this deep learning-based method yields comparable or superior results for an increased number of FLL types. Furthermore, a state-of-the-art comparison [20–25] (see **Table 4**) showcases the performance of other CAD systems. For instance, Hassan et al. achieved a 97.2% accuracy in distinguishing cysts, hemangiomas (HEM), and hepatocellular carcinomas (HCC), while Pan et al. achieved a 93.1% accuracy in distinguishing focal nodular hyperplasia (FNH) and HCC.

One of our latest research papers [26] explores the potential of Transformer Neural Network (TNN) architectures in improving AI-based automated diagnosis, particularly in the field of medicine, focusing on the characterization of focal liver lesions (FLL) using contrast-enhanced ultrasound (CEUS). Traditionally, TNN architectures have excelled in various data processing applications, such as text, voice, image, and video, often outperforming conventional, convolutional, or recurrent deep neural network (DNN) models.

Reference	Lesions	General accuracy (%)
Hassan et al. [20]	Cyst, HEM, HCC	97.2
Pan et al. [21]	FNH, HCC	93.1
Guo et al. [22]	Malign, Benign	90.4
Vancea et al. [23]	HCC	80.3
Wu et al. [24]	HCC, CH, META, LFS	86.3
Streba et al. [25]	HCC, HYPERM, HYPOM, HEM, FFC	87.1
Ours	FNH, HCC, HMG, HYPERM, HYPOM	88

Table 4.
Comparison with state-of-the-art.

The study begins with a review of TNN architectures commonly used in image classification tasks, aiming to identify a suitable TNN variant for characterizing FLLs using CEUS. However, due to the limited availability of large datasets in the medical domain, including CEUS datasets, the effectiveness of TNNs in this context may be hindered, as these models typically require extensive data for training. Despite the challenges posed by limited data availability, the research compares the proposed TNN-based approach with other machine learning solutions reported in the literature. Remarkably, the proposed method demonstrates comparable accuracy to existing solutions while classifying a higher number of FLL types than most previous CEUS Computer-Aided Diagnosis systems. Vision Transformers (ViTs) have gained significant traction in the computer vision (CV) industry due to their exceptional performance and versatility. Originally introduced as a customized vanilla transformer architecture, ViTs have become one of the most popular and effective designs in the field [27, 28]. They excel in a wide range of machine vision tasks and have demonstrated outstanding performance on various benchmarks. At the core of ViTs lies a multi-head self-attention mechanism, which allows them to effectively capture contextual information from image patches. This adaptability enables ViTs to process images holistically, considering both local and global contexts. Over time, numerous variations of ViT architectures have been developed, each tailored to specific tasks and domains. One of the key advantages of ViTs is their ability to surpass traditional convolutional neural networks (CNNs) in image classification tasks, particularly when provided with sufficient training data [29]. This is attributed to their attention mechanism, which enables them to effectively capture long-range dependencies in images. We explored the performance of Vision Transformer (ViT) architectures in comparison to previously designed Convolutional Neural Network (CNN) architectures for characterizing focal liver lesions (FLLs) using contrast-enhanced ultrasound (CEUS) images. The ViT architecture that yielded the best results is illustrated in **Figure 8**.

In this case, the dataset comprised 12,119 images distributed across five subdirectories, each representing a different FLL type: focal nodular hyperplasia (FNH), hepatocellular carcinoma (HCC), hemangioma (HMG), hypervascular metastasis (METAHIPER), and hypovascular metastasis (METAHIPO). In our experiments, 90% (10,908 images) were used for training and 10% (1211 images) were used for validation. All images were resized to an input shape of (200, 200, 3) without augmentation. The accuracy obtained by the model was 86.5%.

This research underscores the potential of TNN architectures to advance automated diagnosis in the medical domain, particularly in characterizing FLLs using

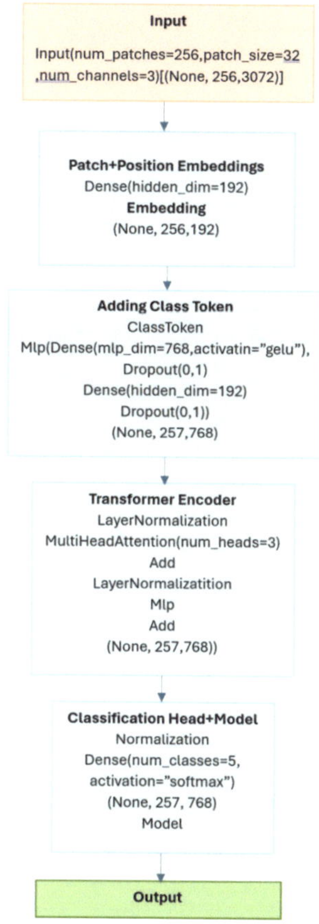

Figure 8.
ViT architecture that yielded the best results.

CEUS. Despite data limitations, the proposed approach offers promising results and expands the scope of FLL classification beyond what was previously achieved by CAD systems.

6. The spatio-temporal approach

The system architecture proposed in [30] for processing CEUS liver medical imaging videos is illustrated in **Figure 9**.

The process involves extracting a uniformly sampled preset number of frames from each CEUS video file. These frames serve as an input for a feature extractor layer, which utilizes a widely recognized deep convolutional neural network (DCNN) architecture, VGG16, available through the Keras Applications framework. Transfer learning (TL) is used, taking advantage of the knowledge gained by solving a problem (e.g., image classification on ImageNet) and applying it to another related problem (CEUS liver medical imaging). In this case, VGG16 is pre-trained on the ImageNet dataset, comprising approximately 1.2 million training images. To process the spatio-temporal inputs, the extracted feature vectors are fed into a Long Short-Term Memory (LSTM) network in a sequential manner. LSTM is a type of recurrent neural network (RNN) architecture that

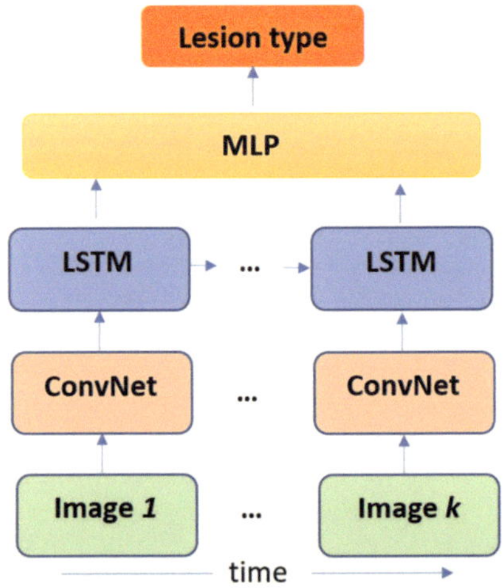

Figure 9.
The proposed system comprises (a) VGG16 ConvNet for spatial information feature extraction, (b) LSTM for temporal data processing, and (c) a fully connected layer multilayer perceptron (MLP) for the prediction task.

is well-suited for handling sequential data due to its ability to retain information over long periods. It consists of memory blocks with recurrent connections and three multiplicative units: input gate, forget gate, and output gate. The spatial features obtained from the DCNN and the temporal features obtained from the LSTM are combined and passed to a fully connected layer for classification of the entire input sequence. This integrated approach allows the model to effectively capture both spatial and temporal information from CEUS video sequences, enabling accurate classification of FLL types.

The detailed architecture of the resulting model is depicted in **Figure 10**, showing the interconnected components responsible for feature extraction, temporal processing, and classification.

The SYSU-CEUS dataset used for training and evaluation of our method contains three types of focal liver lesions (FLLs): hepatocellular carcinoma (HCC), hemangioma (HEM), and focal nodular hyperplasia (FNH). Specifically, the dataset comprises 186 cases of hepatocellular carcinoma (HCC), 112 cases of hemangioma (HEM), and 60 cases of focal nodular hyperplasia (FNH). The dataset includes 186 malignant instances (HCC) and 172 benign instances (HEM and FNH combined). This dataset provides a valuable resource for training and evaluating machine learning models for the automated diagnosis and classification of focal liver lesions using contrast-enhanced ultrasound (CEUS) imaging.

Our proof-of-concept study demonstrates the effectiveness of the proposed method by achieving an average classification accuracy of 86.67% for three types of focal liver lesions (FLLs) after conducting 10 sets of experiments. Although the results are slightly lower compared to similar approaches using CEUS video files as input, it is essential to note the following distinctions:

- Distinct train-test split: Pan et al. [21] used an 80–20% train validation split for the frames extracted from the videos, where images of the same patient could be present in both the train and the test data sets. In contrast, our implementation ensures a clear demarcation between the training and testing samples by using distinct patients for each of them.

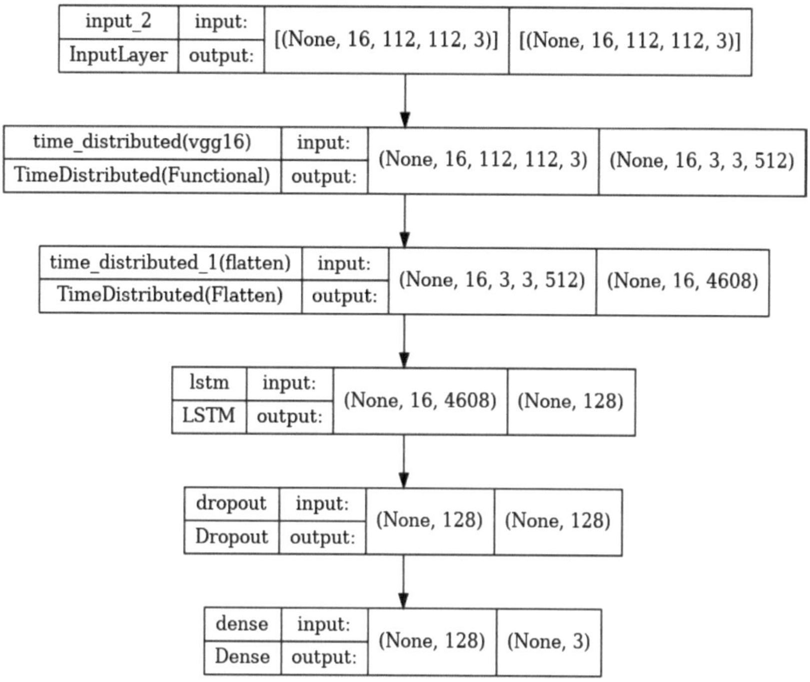

Figure 10.
Detailed architecture of the resulting model.

- ROI annotation process: unlike the approach in [21], where frames undergo a manual annotation procedure for Region of Interest (ROI) selection, our method does not rely on this selective process. This highlights the robustness of your approach, as it operates without the need for manual intervention.

- Lesion type discrimination: while the system proposed in [21] can classify only two types of lesions, our system demonstrates the ability to discriminate between three types of lesions. This expands the scope and applicability of our method, making it more versatile in clinical settings.

Overall, despite the slightly lower accuracy, our approach showcases its effectiveness in a more challenging scenario, offering distinct advantages such as patient-wise separation in the dataset, independence from manual annotation, and the ability to classify a broader range of lesion types. These factors contribute to the significance and validity of our proposed method in the domain of CEUS-based FLL diagnosis.

7. Conclusion and future directions

In this chapter, we investigated AI-based solutions used to implement a fully automated or an assisted/aided CEUS-based FLL diagnosis system. State-of-the-art methods for ultrasound data pre-processing, lesion detection, tracking, feature extraction, and classification are presented and compared. Special emphasis is given to the latter two tasks, as they play a crucial role within the diagnostic process.

From our analysis, one can conclude that there are two main categories of CAD for FLL designs: one based on features extracted from the time-intensity curve, for example, the work of [31, 32] and another in which the features describing normal parenchyma and various FLLs are extracted from images, for example, the work of [21, 25]. From the presented works, it is clear that deep learning based methods emerge as one of the most appealing technologies, although there is enough room for improvements.

Probably, better results could be obtained by using the combination of the first two approaches by blending the temporal information with spatial representation. To date, very few approaches have reported such results [21, 30]. One possible explanation for this fact is related to CAD input, typically represented in this case by video sequences, as they require substantial computing resources to be processed.

Although researchers are reporting encouraging results, actual CAD implementations still have many open issues. For example, automated identification of the reference/normal and FLL ROIs in the liver region remains a challenging task.

The future research directions should go toward employing SOTA DNN architectures, for example, transformers/ViTs or new learning paradigms, for example, federated learning.

Author details

Georgiana Simion[1*], Cristina-Laura Sîrbu[1], Cătălin-Daniel Căleanu[1], Ghiță-Adrian Burdan[2], Tudor Moga[2] and Ioan Sporea[2]

1 Politehnica University Timișoara, Romania

2 Victor Babeș University of Medicine and Pharmacy Timișoara, Romania

*Address all correspondence to: georgiana.simion@upt.ro

References

[1] Sporea I, Badea R, Martie A, Sirli R, Socaciu MPA, Dănilă M. Contrast enhanced ultrasound for the characterization of focal liver lesions. Medical Ultrasonography. 2011;**13**:38-44

[2] Liu Q, Cheng J, Li J, Gao X, Li H. The diagnostic accuracy of contrast-enhanced ultrasound for the differentiation of benign and malignant thyroid nodules: A PRISMA compliant meta-analysis. Medicine. 2018;**97**:e13325

[3] Wan P, Chen F, Liu C, Kong W, Zhang D. Hierarchical temporal attention network for thyroid dule recognition using dynamic CEUS imaging. IEEE Transactions on Medical Imaging. 2021;**40**:1646-1660

[4] Posteman AW, Scheltema MJ, Mannaerts CK, Van Sloun RJ, Idzenga T, Mischi M, et al. The prostate cancer detection rates of CEUStargeted versus MRI-targeted versus systematic TRUS-guided biopsies in biopsy-naïve men: A prospective, comparative clinical trial using the same patients. BMC Urology. 2017;**17**:27

[5] Feng Y, Yang F, Zhou X, Guo Y, Tang F, Ren F, et al. A deep learning approach for targeted contrast-enhanced ultrasound based prostate cancer detection. IEEE/ACM Transactions on Computational Biology and Bioinformatics. 2019;**16**:1794-1801

[6] Wang Y, Li L, Wang YXJ, Cui NY, Zou SM, Zhou CW, et al. Time-intensity curve parameters in rectal cancer measured using endorectal ultrasonography with sterile coupling gels filling the rectum: Correlations with tumor angiogenesis and clinicopathological features. BioMed Research International. 2014;**2014**:587806

[7] Qin L, Yin H, Zhuang H. Classification for rectal CEUS images based on combining features by transfer learning. In: Proceedings of the Third International Symposium on Image Computing and Digital Medicine—ISICDM, Xi'an, China. NY: ACM; 24-26 August. 2019. pp. 187-191

[8] Yang Z, Gong X, Guo Y, Liu W. A temporal sequence dual-branch network for classifying hybrid ultrasound data of breast cancer. IEEE Access. 2020;**8**:82688-82699

[9] Zhang F, Jin L, Li G, Jia C, Shi Q, Du L, et al. The role of contrast-enhanced ultrasound in the diagnosis of malignant non-mass breast lesions and exploration of diagnostic criteria. The British Journal of Radiology. 2021;**94**:20200880

[10] Erlichman DB, Weiss A, Koenigsberg M, Stein MW. Contrast enhanced ultrasound: A review of radiology applications. Clinical Imaging. 2020;**60**:209-215

[11] Gasnier A, Ardon R, Ciofolo-Veit C, Leen E, Correas JM. Assessing tumor vascularity with 3D contrast-enhanced ultrasound: A new semi-automated segmentation framework. In: Proceedings of the 2010 IEEE International Symposium on Biomedical Imaging: From Nano to Macro. Rotterdam, The Netherlands: IEEE; 14-17 April 2010. pp. 300-303

[12] Dancygier H. Clinical Hepatology: Principles and Practice of Hepatobiliary Diseases. Vol. 1. Berlin, Heidelberg: Springer; 2010

[13] Liang X, Cao Q, Huang R, Liang L. Recognizing focal liver lesions in contrast-enhanced ultrasound with discriminatively trained spatio-temporal model. In: 2014 IEEE 11th International Symposium on Biomedical Imaging (ISBI). Beijing, China. 2014. pp. 1184-1187. DOI: 10.1109/ISBI.2014.6868087

[14] Liang X, Liang L, Cao Q, Huang R, Wang Y. Recognizing focal liver lesions in CEUS with dynamically trained latent structured models. IEEE Transactions on Medical Imaging (T-MI). Mar 2016;**35**(3):713-727

[15] Sîrbu CL, Simion G, Căleanu C-D. Improving the diagnostic of contrast enhanced ultrasound imaging using optical flow for focal liver lesion detection. In: 2022 24th International Symposium on Symbolic and Numeric Algorithms for Scientific Computing (SYNASC), Hagenberg/Linz, Austria. 2022. pp. 258-263. DOI: 10.1109/SYNASC57785.2022.00048

[16] Sirbu CL, Seiculescu C, Burdan GA, Moga T, Caleanu CD. Evaluation of tracking algorithms for contrast enhanced ultrasound imaging exploration. In: Proceedings of the 2022 Australasian Computer Science Week (ACSW '22). 2022. pp. 161-167. DOI: 10.1145/3511616.3513111

[17] Căleanu C-D et al. A study over the importance of arterial phase temporal parameters in focal liver lesions CEUS based diagnosis. In: 2014 11th International Symposium on Electronics and Telecommunications (ISETC), Timisoara, Romania. 2014. pp. 1-4. DOI: 10.1109/ISETC.2014.7010799

[18] Căleanu C-D, Simion G. A bag of features approach for CEUS liver lesions investigation. In: Telecommunications and Signal Processing (TSP), Budapest, Hungary. IEEE; 1-3 July 2019. DOI: 10.1109/TSP.2019.8768851

[19] Caleanu CD, Sirbu CL, Simion G. Deep neural architectures for contrast enhanced ultrasound (CEUS) focal liver lesions automated diagnosis. Sensors. 2021;**21**(12). DOI: 10.3390/s21124126. WOS:000666412700001

[20] Hassan TM, Elmogy M, Sallam E-S. Diagnosis of focal liver diseases based on deep learning technique for ultrasound images. Arabian Journal for Science and Engineering. 2017;**42**:3127-3140

[21] Pan F, Huanq Q, Li X. Classification of liver tumors with CEUS based on 3D-CNN. In: 2019 IEEE 4th International Conference on Advanced Robotics and Mechatronics (ICARM), Toyonaka, Japan. 2019. pp. 845-849. DOI: 10.1109/ICARM.2019.8834190

[22] Guo L, Wang D, Xu H, Qian Y, Wang C, Zheng X, et al. CEUS-based classification of liver tumors with deep canonical correlation analysis and multi-kernel learning. In: Proceedings of the Annual International Conference IEEE Engineering Medicine and Biology Society, Jeju Island, Korea; 11-15 July 2017. pp. 1748-1751

[23] Vancea F, Mitrea D, Nedevschi S, Rotaru M, Stefanescu H, Badea R. Hepatocellular carcinoma segmentation within ultrasound images using convolutional neural networks. In: 2019 IEEE 15th International Conference on Intelligent Computer Communication and Processing (ICCP), Cluj-Napoca, Romania. 2019. pp. 483-490. DOI: 10.1109/ICCP48234.2019.8959687

[24] Wu K, Chenb X, Ding M. Deep learning-based classification of focal liver lesions with contrast-enhanced ultrasound. Optik. 2014;**125**:4057-4063

[25] Streba CT, Ionescu M, Gheonea DI, Sandulescu L, Ciurea T, Saftoiu A, et al. Contrast-enhanced ultrasonography parameters in neural network diagnosis of liver tumors. World Journal of Gastroenterology. 2012;**18**:4427-4434

[26] Mercioni M, Căleanu CD, Sîrbu CL. Computer aided diagnosis for contrast-enhanced ultrasound using transformer neural network. In: 2023 25th International Symposium on Symbolic and Numeric Algorithms for Scientific Computing (SYNASC), Nancy, France. 2023. pp. 256-259. DOI: 10.1109/SYNASC61333.2023.00044

[27] Parvaiz A, Khalid MA, Zafar R, Ameer H, Ali M, Fraz MM. Vision transformers in medical computer vision—A contemplative retrospection. Engineering Applications of Artificial Intelligence. 2023;**122**:106126

[28] Naseer MM, Ranasinghe K, Khan SH, Hayat M, Shahbaz Khan F, Yang M-H. Intriguing properties of vision transformers. Advances in Neural Information Processing Systems. 2021;**34**:23296-23308

[29] Cao YH, Yu H, Wu J. Training Vision Transformers with only 2040 Images. In: Avidan S, Brostow G, Cissé M, Farinella GM, Hassner T, editors. Computer Vision – ECCV. Lecture Notes in Computer Science. Vol. 13685. Cham: Springer; 2022. DOI: 10.1007/978-3-031-19806-9_13

[30] Schmiedt K, Simion G, Căleanu C-D. Preliminary results on contrast enhanced ultrasound video stream diagnosis using deep neural architectures. In: 2022 International Symposium on Electronics and Telecommunications (ISETC), Timisoara, Romania. 2022. pp. 1-4. DOI: 10.1109/ISETC56213.2022.10010032

[31] Ganeshan B, Miles KA, Young RCD, Chatwin CR. Texture analysis in non-contrast enhanced CT: Impact of malignancy on texture in apparently disease-free areas of the liver. European Journal of Radiology. 2009;**70**:101-110

[32] Rognin NG, Arditi M, Mercier L, Frinking PJA, Schneider M, Perrenoud G, et al. Parametric imaging for characterizing focal liver lesions in contrast-enhanced ultrasound. IEEE Transactions on Ultrasonics, Ferroelectrics, and Frequency Control. 2010;**57**:2503-2511

Section 6

Vascular

Chapter 15

Arteriovenous Fistula Ultrasound Assessment

Iulia Dana Grosu and Flaviu Bob

Abstract

Arteriovenous fistula (AVF) ultrasound (US) assessment is the first-line tool in addition to the physical examination to surveil, screen, and diagnose complications of the vascular access (VA) of chronic hemodialysis (HD) patients. The VA currently recommended by all guidelines as the "gold standard" for chronic HD patients is the AVF; therefore, creating long-lasting, complication-free fistulas is one of the targets considered by all nephrologists. US assessment is a noninvasive technique that offers detail regarding vascular morphology and hemodynamics, and may be performed at the patient's bedside. The clinical settings in which US assessment is currently performed are the presurgical screening of veins and arteries (presurgical mapping) or the diagnosis of AVF complications, usually when there are relevant clinical signs and symptoms. Moreover, AVF point-of-care US examination (POCUS) is used to assist and aid nurses in the cannulation procedure, with the scope of minimizing accidents. The current chapter aims to provide a guidebook regarding the multiple situations in which AVF US may be performed and to highlight the importance of this tool for the purpose of maintaining the long-term functionality of the VA of HD patients.

Keywords: hemodialysis, arteriovenous fistula, vascular access, end-stage renal disease, presurgical mapping

1. Introduction

End-stage renal disease (ESRD) is a rising global healthcare burden leading to an increasing need for renal replacement therapies (RRT). Currently, ESRD prevalence has surged by 43% from 2003 to 2016 [1], while chronic kidney disease (CKD) is expected to be the world's fifth leading cause of mortality by 2040 [2]. Even though renal transplantation is the most desirable therapeutic option for the patient with ESRD, kidney donation availability varies greatly among countries and cultures. The most used RRT modality worldwide nowadays is in-center HD. Survival rates on maintenance HD therapy are poor when compared to the age-matched general population, but they have increased steadily recently, reaching a 5-year survival of 42% [3]. However, the life span of HD patients may vary largely, depending on age, comorbidities, dialysis adequacy, vascular access, and treatment compliance.

Performing HD therapy requires a functional VA, accomplished either through central venous catheters (CVCs), AVFs, or arteriovenous grafts (AVGs). Initiating

IntechOpen

HD sessions on CVCs has been reported to carry a larger mortality risk, HR 1.55 (95%CI: 1.09, 2.21) [4, 5], with AVFs remaining the gold standard for vascular access in hemodialysis nowadays.

Referral to AVF formation should start when the estimated glomerular filtration rate (eGFR) drops below 15–20 ml/min/1.73 m^2, which, in general, is within at least 6 months of the estimated dialysis initiation [6]. Moreover, timely preservation of the vascular structures of the arm (no venipuncture or intravenous cannulation procedures) has proven of benefit in accomplishing a better primary AVF patency.

There are several types of autogenous AVFs, usually performed upon the upper limbs, such as radio-cephalic, brachio-cephalic, and brachio-basilic. The types of AVGs usually performed include the antecubital forearm loop graft, the upper-arm AVG, and only in rare cases lower extremity AVG or HeRO grafts. The choice of VA site should be based not only according to the current KDOQI vascular access guidelines [7] regarding the patient's end stage kidney disease (ESKD) life plan but also on presurgical ultrasound mapping criteria [8]. The current consensus is that, if permitted, the AVF site should be performed on the nondominant arm, starting distally, at the wrist. The anastomosis preferred is end-to-side (vein to artery) due to a lower incidence of distal venous hypertension, as compared to side-to-side anastomosis [9].

After maturation, AVFs should be able to withstand repeated cannulations, roughly 24 cannulations/week and should ensure proper blood flow (Qb) toward the HD machine to ensure adequacy. Cannulation techniques are very important to preserve complication-free VA. Typically, needle sizes start from 17G, increasing up to 15G, depending on AVF/AVG characteristics. The preferred cannulation techniques are rope ladder (which implies the use of the entire VA, by alternating needling sites) or the buttonhole technique (only for AVFs), while the area technique leads to multiple complications (aneurysms, long bleeding time) and is not recommended anymore.

2. Presurgical clinical examination and ultrasound mapping

2.1 Presurgical clinical examination

Clinical examination of both the arterial and venous systems prior to surgery is mandatory, and several studies have shown that a correct preoperative evaluation may have an approximately 70% success rate in predicting fistula maturation [10]. The patient's history of diabetes mellitus, presence of peripheral artery disease, and ipsilateral previous catheter placement may be useful in placing the patient in a high risk of VA failure category.

2.1.1 Arterial clinical examination

The preoperative arterial clinical examination should assess the patency of the arterial tree and potential detections of steno-occlusive disease. Therefore, the following should be performed:

- Assessment of the presence and quality of arterial pulses in the arterial, ulnar, and brachial arteries, with attention to potential asymmetries.

- Allen's Test: To confirm the patency of the palmar arch, the Allen test involves the following steps:
- Manual compression of the arteries at the wrist until distal pallor and lack of capillary refill occur.
- Decompression of the radial artery and assessment of the speed in which revascularization occurs. A normal arm flush occurs in 5–15 seconds.
- Repetition of the maneuver for the ulnar artery.

2.1.2 Venous clinical examination

The clinical examination of the veins implies following the cephalic and basilic veins at the forearm and antecubital fossa with and without a proximal tourniquet. The evaluation includes trajectory, tortuosity, and increase in diameter after tourniquet placement.

2.2 Ultrasound mapping

The latest clinical VA Society guidelines recommend that preoperative ultrasound examination should succeed in every clinical assessment. The patient should be placed lying supine, with their arms relaxed, in a warm room. The ultrasound scanning probe used is a high-frequency US probe, 7–12 MHz (5Mhz or higher for Doppler), and the modes involved in the examination are B-mode (for morphological information), spectral Doppler (for flow assessment), color Doppler (for flow detection and direction assessment). Grayscale (B-mode) is used to characterize anatomical features such as blood vessel diameters, depth from the skin surface, collateral veins, and blood vessel trajectories. The spectral Doppler technique allows the analysis of the blood flow velocity changes over time (regarded as cardiac cycles) in a small volume sample, therefore generating a spectrum with positive or negative curves. To achieve an accurate result, the technique requires consideration of the following aspects:

- Placing the transducer longitudinally, set the sample volume ("gate" size) for interrogation. The size should be 2/3 of the width of the vessel.
- Set the insonation angle lower than 60 degrees; usually, this means aligning it parallel to the long axis of the vessel.
- Adjust the gain setting to allow a clearly visible Doppler flow in the region of interest.
- Adjust the PRF (pulse repetition frequency, which changes the number of pulses transmitted by the transducer in 1 second) according to the velocity ranges. Higher PRF levels will allow the detection of higher velocities.
- Set the wall filter (if available) to eliminate any low-velocity frequency shifts.

The following parameters should be recorded after color and spectral Doppler analysis:

- Direction of flow.
- Type of curve (high resistance in the presurgical setting and low resistance in the functioning AVF).
- Peak systolic velocity (PSV), end-diastolic velocity (EDV), and resistive index (RI).
- Time average mean velocity (TA mean)—only for the AVF/AVG.
- Blood flow (Qb-ml/min) in the feeding artery.

The pressure placed on the ultrasound transducer should be minimal, and there should be plenty of ultrasound conduction gel to avoid the underestimation of the superficial venous calibers, which may be easily compressed. The insonation angle of the spectral Doppler scan should be lower than 60 degrees.

2.2.1 Presurgical mapping of the arterial system

The examination of the arterial system should start distally and should continue proximally. The following steps should be employed:

- B-mode examination in the transverse section at the wrist—note the internal diameter of the radial artery and the depth. Current guidelines (7) recommend a diameter of >2 mm for the radial artery (**Figure 1**)
- B-mode examination in longitudinal section—note calcifications, intimal irregularities, and wall thickening.

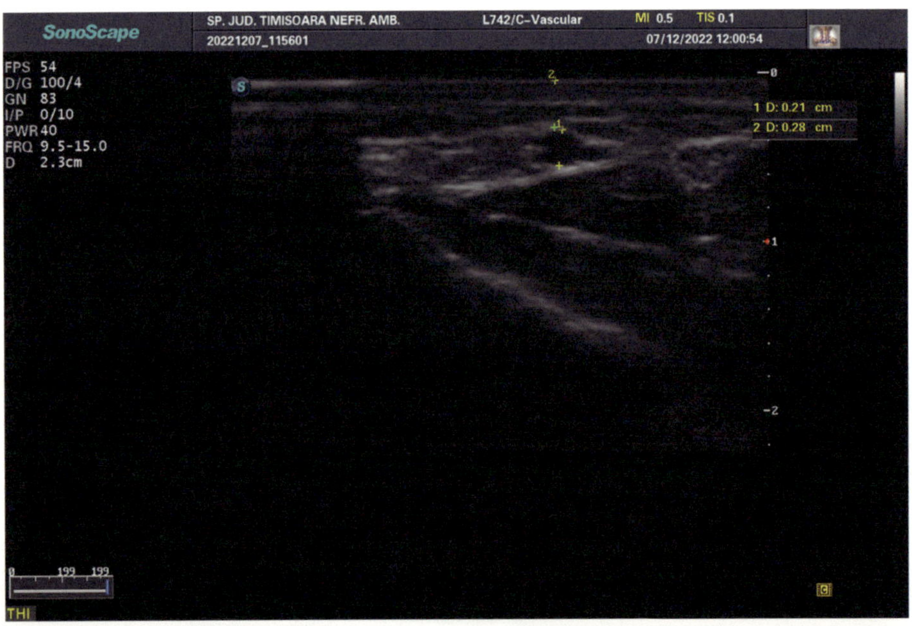

Figure 1.
B-mode transverse section of the radial artery (noted caliber and depth).

- Color and spectral Doppler examination in longitudinal scan—note peak systolic velocity (PSV) in the radial artery (which should be >50 cm/s) [11]. Perform hyperemic response (with PSV, end diastolic velocity (EDV), and resistive index (RI) quantifications) in the radial artery, which implies assessing the change in the spectral waveform after inducing distal ischemia by clenching the fist of the patient for 2 minutes. The waveform should be high resistance during ischemia and afterward should change into a moderate-resistance waveform during unclenching the fist (**Figures 2** and **3**). A study has found that a RI > 0,7 during reactive hyperemia predicted the failure of a future AVF [12]. The RI is an indirect indicator that the radial artery can provide an increased blood flow, as a response to a future anastomosis.

The RI may be calculated using the formula: RI = PSV-EDV/PSV.

- B-mode examination of the brachial artery in transverse and longitudinal sections assess wall morphology, diameter, and presence of calcifications.

- Color and spectral Doppler examination of the brachial artery include PSV and EDV measurements.

There is no current consensus on brachial artery measurement thresholds that predict the patency of a brachio-cephalic or brachio-basilic AVF.

2.2.2 Presurgical mapping of the venous system

The examination of the venous system should start distally and should continue proximally. All measurements should be performed before and after proximal tourniquet placement with sufficient gel use and without significant compression of the transducer. The increase in size of the vein after 2 min tourniquet placement reveals

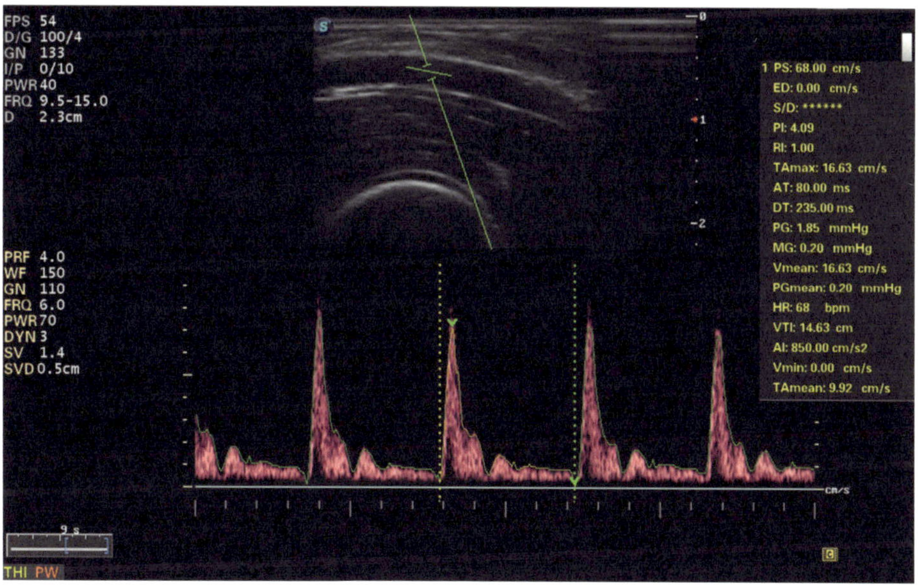

Figure 2.
Radial artery spectral Doppler scan with a clenched fist.

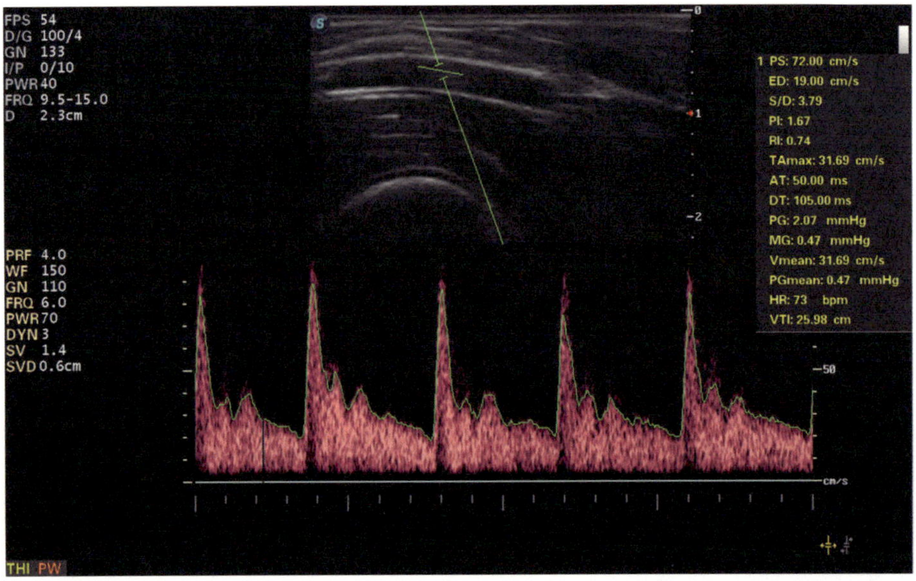

Figure 3.
Radial artery spectral Doppler scan after releasing the fist.

the venous capacity of distension, which should be at least 40%. The following steps should be employed:

- B-mode examination in transverse and longitudinal sections of the cephalic vein at the wrist—assess compressibility by pressing on the vein until it fully collapses. A minimum diameter of 2 mm is considered adequate for a future radio-cephalic AVF. Assess continuity, collaterals, depth, and caliber variations in its course toward the antecubital fossa.

- B-mode examination in transverse and longitudinal sections of the cephalic (**Figure 4**) and basilic veins of the arm—assess compressibility, depth, and

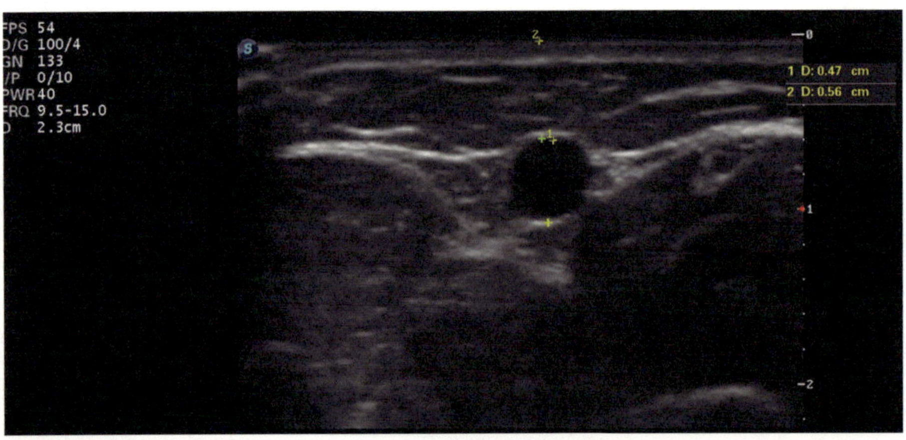

Figure 4.
B-mode transverse scan of a cephalic vein in the arm (noted caliber and depth).

diameters. A minimum venous diameter of 3 mm is considered sufficient for a brachio-cephalic or brachio-basilic vein. Follow the venous trajectories proximally. For the basilic vein, the depth is of relevance, because of its profound situation. At a depth of over 8 mm, a second surgical intervention is needed to raise the vein at a more superficial level.

- Color and spectral Doppler examination of the proximal veins shows respiratory phasicity. The lack of increase in flow during inspiration may be an indirect sign of stenosis or occlusion in the subclavian vein, brachio-cephalic trunk, or superior vena cava.

3. Arteriovenous fistula ultrasound assessment

The surveillance of AVFs through ultrasound assessment in the postoperative setting is not routinely performed. Usually, the first ultrasound scan occurs at 4–6 weeks after creation, to assess the level of maturation it has reached. Cannulations of immature AVFs may lead to premature AVF failure or thrombosis. The ideal AVF should fulfill the rule of 6 s: minimum 600 ml/min flow, minimum 6 mm diameter, and maximum 6 mm depth. There is no recommendation regarding routine, scheduled US surveillance; however, the current VA guidelines suggest AVF ultrasound be performed as a first-line investigation if there are suspected complications. The clinical examination that may indicate the need for US evaluation includes the following signs:

- Distal edema, cyanosis and multiple collateral veins may suggest central vein stenosis, thrombosis, or occlusion.
- Hand pain, cold fingers, steal syndrome, or distal ischemia.
- Low blood flow on dialysis, inflow artery stenosis, anastomotic stenosis
- Indurated AVF—hematoma, collections, thrombosis
- Lack of thrill and bruit complete thrombosis
- AVF with high pulsatility, low perceptible thrill, AVF stenosis
- Aneurysms and dilatations may suggest high-flow AVFs.
- Blood clots removed upon cannulation, segmental, or total AVF thrombosis.

The examination should be performed with a relaxed and supported extended arm, using a 7–12 MHz linear transducer. A widely recognized, systematic protocol has not been agreed on by the current VA or Nephrology guidelines; however, the available literature proposes the following methodological approach for the VA Duplex US examination [13, 14].

3.1 Inflow arterial examination

- B-mode, transverse section follows the feeding artery in a proximal direction toward the clavicle. Any variations in caliber should be noted. The brachial artery bifurcation should be identified because blood flow should be measured proximal to the bifurcation (regardless of the type of AVF).

- B-mode longitudinal section applies color and spectral Doppler on brachial artery and proceed to measure blood flow. The typical spectral curve involves high flow and low resistance. It is important to maintain an insonation angle of 60 degrees and a sample volume of minimum of 2/3 of the vessel parallel to the vessel walls. If the sample volume is too small, the flows tend to be overestimated. Once a stable curve is obtained, freeze the image and measure the diameter of the artery (the brachial artery radius is the diameter divided by 2). The US machine software will calculate the time averaged mean velocity (TA mean) and the resistive index (RI), and in some cases, the AVF flow as well (**Figure 5**). The AVF flow may be calculated using the following formula, as well:

AVF flow (ml/min) = 3,14 × brachial artery radius 2 × TA mean × 60.

Due to the variability of the AVF flow measurement, it is best to assess it three times, to ensure that the calculation is accurate and reproducible. The normal blood flow values for native AVFs are >500 ml/min and for AV grafts >600 ml/min.

The resistivity index is usually calculated by the US machine but has the following formula:

IR = PSV-EDV/PSV. If it is increased over 0,6, the AVF should be scanned thoroughly for the presence of stenosis.

3.2 Anastomosis examination

- B-mode transverse and longitudinal sections—measurement of the largest diameter of the anastomosis (**Figure 6**), to exclude an anastomotic stenosis.

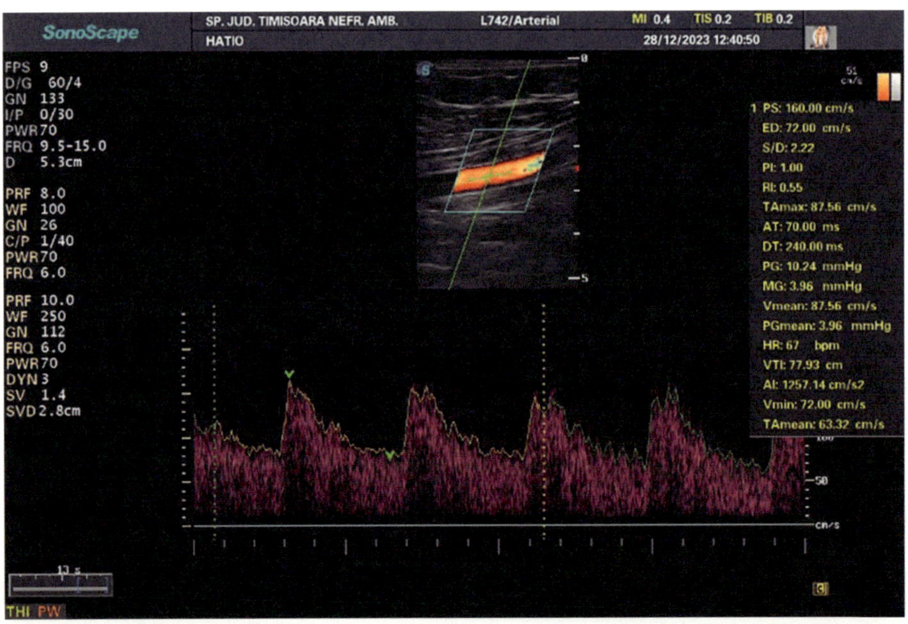

Figure 5.
Measuring the TA mean, RI in the brachial artery using color and Doppler scans.

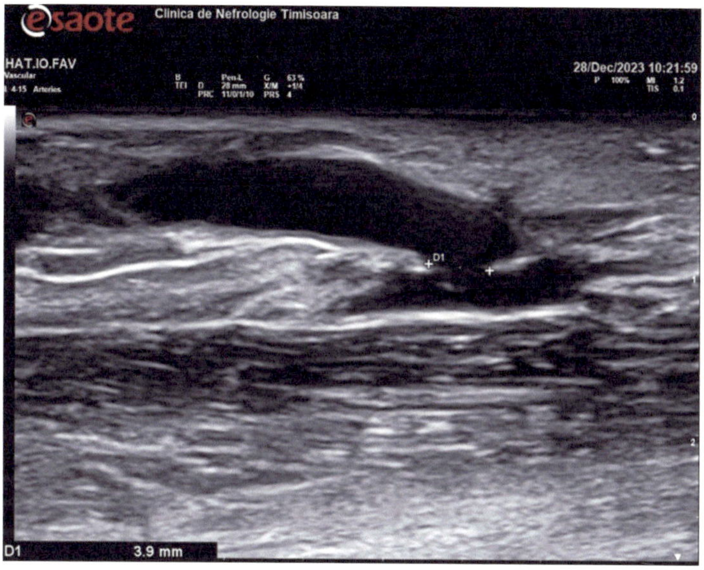

Figure 6.
End-to-side anastomosis in a B-mode transverse scan.

3.3 Venous examination

- B-mode transverse section—follow the course of the vein from the anastomosis proximally, until its drainage in the subclavian system. The following should be noted: vein caliber and caliber variation, depth, and possible sites for cannulation.

- B-mode longitudinal section—identify any anomalies or complications inside and outside the vessels such as stenosis (vessel caliber appears reduced), aneurysms/pseudoaneurysms, thrombi, hematomas, and edema. Describe them in relation to the surrounding anatomical structures. If luminal caliber differences are noted, they should be recorded before the stenosis and inside the stenosis. Using color and Doppler scans, the PSVs should be measured in the same places as the calibers.

4. Arteriovenous fistula complications

US is the first-line imagistic method to use when suspecting a malfunction or complicated AVF in a patient, as per current VA Society guidelines [7, 8]. The most frequent complications include stenosis, thrombosis (partial or occlusive), calcifications, steal syndrome, aneurysms or pseudoaneurysms, and high-flow AVF.

4.1 Stenosis

Stenoses are defined as vascular intraluminal narrowing that leads to hemodynamic and functional consequences. The hemodynamic modifications induced by a stenosis in the vascular wall are turbulences at the site of the stenosis and decreased flow in the post-stenotic segment. The causes of AVF stenoses are atherosclerotic calcified plaques (usually occurring in longstanding AVFs), partial thrombosis, outer compression due to hematomas or edema, and lastly intimal hyperplasia. The latter situation occurs when the walls of the vein cannot withstand the shear wall stress due to the increased blood flow. That is why, in most cases, AVF stenoses occur in the juxta-anastomotic segment (first 5 cm), but may occur in the middle segment as well, or in the central veins. For AVGs, stenoses may occur at the distal (venous) anastomosis usually. For brachio-basilic AVFs, a typical site for stenosis is the proximal swing segment, due to kinking of the vessel [15]. According to a study [16], the most frequent sites for native AVF stenosis are brachio-basilic proximal swing segment stenoses, juxta-anastomotic stenoses, and puncture site stenoses.

The clinical examination that supports the suspicion of a stenotic lesion in the AVF includes abnormal thrill (weak) in the stenotic area, abnormal high-pitched bruit in the stenotic area, reduction/failure of the AVF collapse during arm elevation, lack of pulse augmentation during arm elevation, ipsilateral extremity edema, prolonged bleeding (central stenosis), not achieving dialysis efficiency (eKt/v), and cannulation difficulty and low Qb delivered at the HD machine.

Ultrasound has an over 50% sensitivity for stenosis diagnosis, with respect to angiography which has a sensitivity of 76–95%. The advantages of the US are that it allows the visualization of the surrounding structures as well as the calculation of blood flow. Current literature is quite heterogeneous in defining clear criteria for AVF stenosis, due to small-scale studies, retrospective studies, lack of control groups, etc. Even so, there are several aspects to assess when an AVF stenosis is suspected.

The following steps should be employed when assessing a suspected AVF stenosis:

- B-mode transverse scan—visualize whether the caliber of the AVF is decreasing abruptly. Rotate the transducer in a longitudinal section and measure the intraluminal diameters in the pre-stenotic and stenotic regions.

% stenosis = (original lumen- residual lumen)/original residual lumen × 100.

This measurement is useful in AVGs; however, in a native AVF lumen reduction alone must be interpreted with caution due to possible wall caliber changes.

- Color and spectral Doppler longitudinal section scan—determine the peak systolic velocities in the pre-stenotic segment and in the stenotic segment. A PSV ratio between 2 and 3 (pre-stenosis/stenosis) indicates a hemodynamically significant stenosis (50–75%), while a ratio > 3 reflects a stenosis of >75%.

The Prague group has defined the following criteria for stenosis diagnosis, including both hemodynamic and morphological changes on which the examinator may rely when judging if a stenosis needs immediate action or just watchful waiting. The Prague group criteria are presented in **Table 1** [17].

In order to diagnose a significant stenosis, two main criteria and at least one additional criterion are needed; if less than two criteria are present, the patient needs to be reevaluated in 6–8 weeks. If only one main criterion is present, the stenosis is not considered significant.

Indirect arterial measurements in the brachial artery, highly suggestive of AVF stenosis, are high resistance Doppler wave, RI >0,6, and reduced flow.

4.2 Thrombosis

Ultrasonography is the first-line imaging technique employed when an AVF thrombosis is suspected. The clinical signs and symptoms that may lead to the

Significant	**Borderline**
Main Criteria Diameter reduction by >50% Peak systolic velocity increase >2–3 ×	
+ Additional criteria (≥ 1)	
Residual diameter < 1.9–2 mm	No additional criterion
Flow volume decreases by >25% (if previously >1000 ml/min)	
Flow volume < 600 ml/min for AVGs, < 500 ml/min for AVFs	

Table 1.
Prague group criteria for stenosis.

suspicion of AVF thrombosis are AVF with no thrill or bruit but with high pulsatility, AVF pain, redness, cannulation difficulties, drawing clots from the AVF after cannulation, and high HD machine arterial or venous pressures. AVF thrombosis may occur as a postoperative complication (usually during the first week after surgery) or after prolonged AVF use. The current existing data is conflicting regarding certain risk factors (demographics and comorbidities) that would absolutely contraindicate performing AVF. The risk factors associated with AVF thrombosis are:

- For early AVF thrombosis: hypotension, hypovolemia, and vascular trauma due to prior needling.

- For late AVF thrombosis: persistent hypotension, AVF stenosis, AVF vicinity compressions (seromas, hematomas, lymphatic collections, and compressive wound dressings), and hypercoagulability states.

A study by Yii et al. [18] assessed 511 AVFs and analyzed the ROC curves for TA mean, PSV, and EDV as predictive for thrombotic flow-related AVF dysfunction. They concluded that TA mean cutoffs of 45 cm/s for forearm AVFs and 49 cm/s for arm AVFs yielded the best AUC values (0.95).

When performing AVF ultrasound, the following findings suggest thrombosis:

- B-mode examination: The vein is not fully compressible, and intraluminal echogenic material can be noticed. The thrombus increases in echogenicity as it becomes older.

- Color and spectral Doppler examination—based on how occlusive the thrombus is, the flow will be reduced accordingly. In complete thrombosis, no AVF flows will be determined at the site of thrombosis (**Figure** 7).

Indirect signs or complete AVF occlusion due to thrombosis are similar to those of critical stenosis, that is, the high resistance triphasic Doppler wave in the feeding artery and a high resistive index.

4.3 Aneurysms and pseudoaneurysms

Diagnosing AVF aneurysms is typically clinical. An AVF aneurysm is a fusiform or saccular dilatation of the AVF, with a diameter exceeding two times the diameter of the undilated vessel. It usually occurs in longstanding fistulas, due to the reactivity of

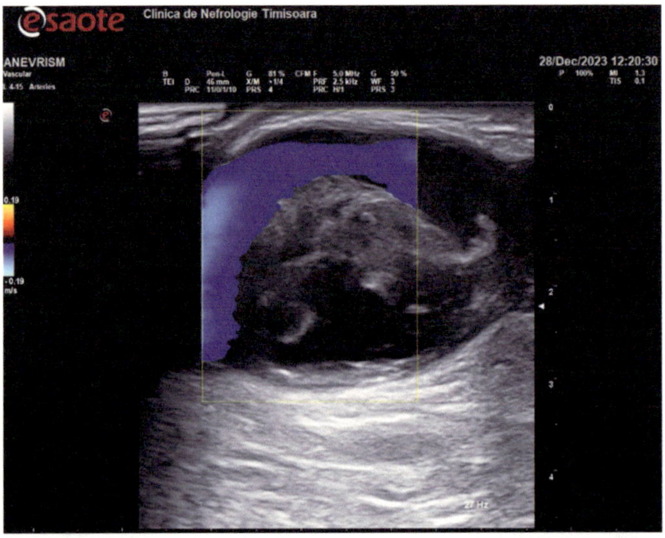

Figure 7.
Color Doppler transverse scan incomplete thrombosis of an aneurysmal brachio-cephalic AVF.

the endothelium to repeated cannulations, and usually grows gradually over time. The aneurysmal dilatation comprises all three layers of the wall, which makes it less prone to ruptures (**Figure 8**). Even if most aneurysms are stable lesions, other complications may occur inside the aneurysms, such as calcifications or segmental thrombosis (due to nonlinear local blood flow circulation).

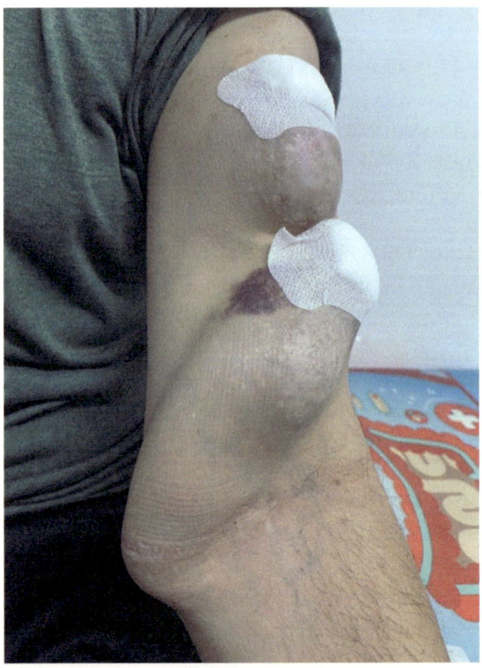

Figure 8.
Aneurysmal dilation of a brachio-cephalic AVF.

The pseudoaneurysm is a false vessel dilatation, which is not delimitated by the AVF walls, but by surrounding structures. It usually occurs abruptly, due to cannulation accidents, and implies blood flow from the AVF to a false saccular structure, adjacent to the AVF. It may occur next to the posterior or anterior walls and generally requires treatment as the risk of rupture is much higher than with true aneurysms. Anterior wall pseudoaneurysms are clinically present as a subcutaneous pulsating collection; the skin is lucent and thin, while posterior wall pseudoaneurysms may be asymptomatic.

From the US evaluation point of view, the aneurysm reveals only a dilated AVF. In the B-mode, the blood flow may describe a cigarette smoke-like pattern due to low blood flow velocities. In color Doppler, a red-blue vortex may appear (Korean flag appearance). Sometimes, local, punctiform calcifications may be visualized, appearing as hyperechogenic wall deposits.

In contrast, pseudoaneurysms require identifying an additional cavity or communication of the AVF with the adjacent structures. In B-mode, the communicating structure may be identified, while color and spectral Doppler show flows in a "to and fro" pattern [19]. When the sample volume of the spectral Doppler is placed at the collar region of the pseudoaneurysm, the flow curve shows both positive and negative waveforms, corresponding to the recirculation of the blood in the lesion. Angiography is the gold standard method for pseudoaneurysm diagnosis; however, it does entail more periprocedural complications. CT angiography also demonstrates a high sensitivity (95%) and specificity rate (99%) regarding diagnosis [20]. However, because the US is easy and quick to perform, it is noninvasive and has no contraindications as well as high (94%) sensitivity and high (97%) specificity rates; it is regarded as an essential tool for pseudoaneurysm diagnosis.

When identifying pseudoaneurysms, the treatment is either surgical repair, endovascular covered stenting, or percutaneous thrombin injections, which induce local thrombosis.

4.4 Hematomas

Hematomas typically occur in tissues surrounding the AVF due to improper cannulation or improper hemostasis. From a clinical point of view, the appearance is that of a localized subcutaneous blood suffusion. Its color varies according to the timing of the vessel injury, varying from red-bluish to green and ultimately yellowish. Typically, AVF hematomas do not require US confirmation; however, if additional, more severe complications (stenosis due to compression, AVF dysfunction) are suspected, it is reasonable to perform AVF US.

In the B-mode US evaluation, hematomas appear as local collections, not communicating with the AVF vessel walls. The margins of the hematomas are vaguely delimitated, many times accompanied by local edema in the surrounding tissue. If the color or spectral Doppler is implied, even when adjusting PRF for low velocities, no active blood flow should be detected in the hematoma. Most often, hematomas have a favorable evolution; however, some of them may become infected. US surveillance of AVF combined with US-guided cannulations reduced the occurrence of AVF hematomas from 2.63 to 1.71 episodes/patient/year in a prospective study [21]. The differential diagnosis between a local purulent collection and an uninfected hematoma is mainly clinical and does not have clear US criteria (**Figures 9** and **10**).

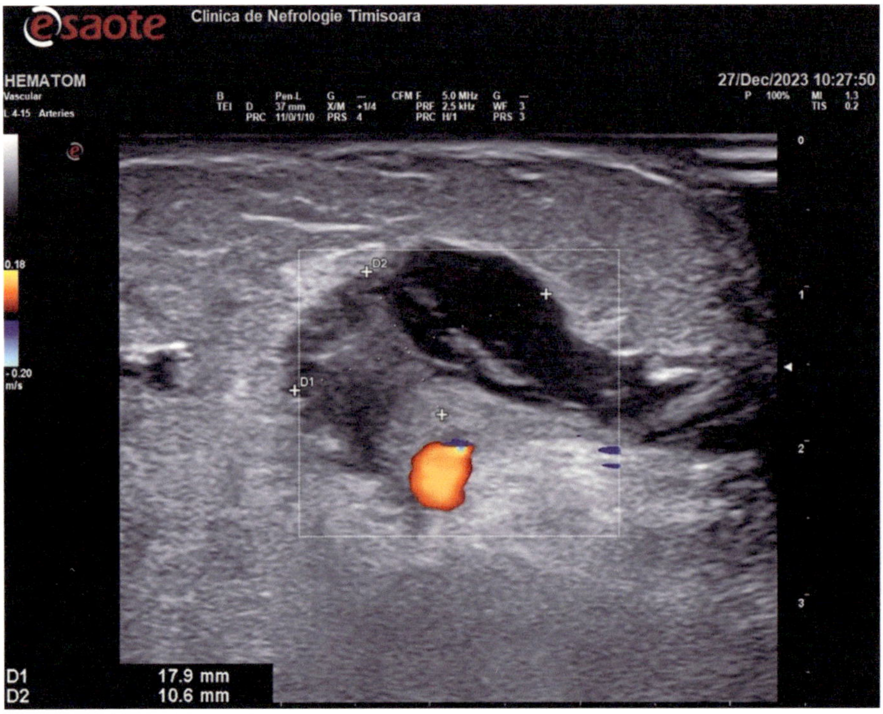

Figure 9.
Color Doppler transverse scan—Large hematoma surrounding the anastomotic site and the inflow artery (hematoma dimensions noted D1, D2). Note no color Doppler flow inside the hematoma.

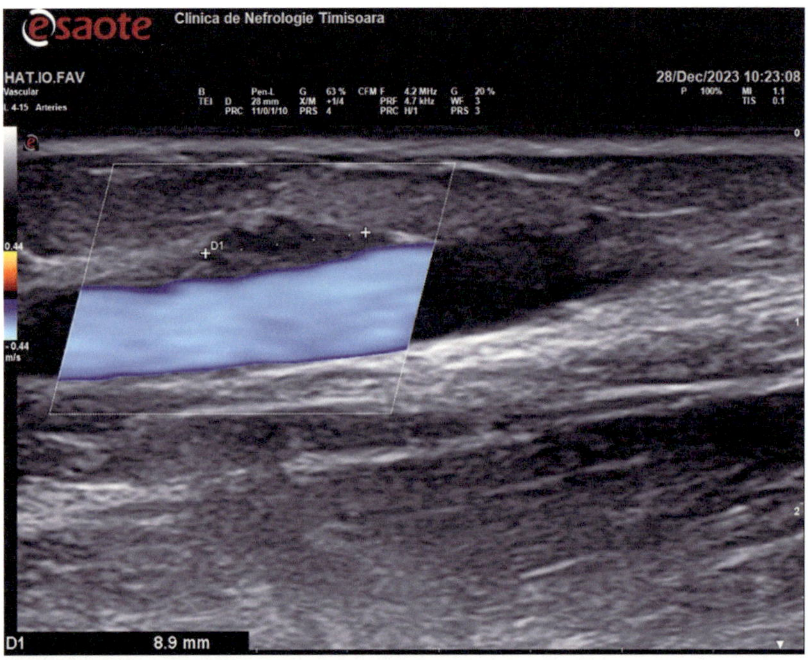

Figure 10.
Color Doppler longitudinal scan—Small hematoma over the anterior AVF wall (hematoma dimension noted D1). Note no color Doppler flow inside the hematoma.

4.5 Maturation deficit

The maturation period (meaning the time from ABF/AVG creation to its first cannulation) differs significantly worldwide [22]. Higher rates of AVF maturation occur in patients with lower body mass index, no peripheral vascular disease, and lack of smoking or diabetes. Diseases associated with hypercoagulation are at higher risk of maturation failure, and so are patients with high inflammatory status or hypo-albuminemia. The ideal and mature AVF according to the NKF-KDOQI guidelines presents the outflow vein diameter ⩾of 6 mm and blood flow ⩾of 600 mL/min.

In a study by Caputo et al. [23], the addition of Doppler US evaluation at 4–6 weeks after surgical creation had a better sensitivity of detecting AVF failure than physical examination alone. The detection of poor AVF flow (<500 ml/min) had a 67% sensitivity of predicting AVF maturation deficit, in comparison with only 42% sensitivity of the physical examination ($p < 0.001$).

According to Wilson [24], the US evaluation at 4 weeks after surgical creation divides AVFs into the following categories (**Table 2**):

4.6 Steal syndrome

Steal syndrome occurs when the structures situated distally from the AVF are poorly vascularized, and thus symptoms of ischemia occur. The risk factors associated with steal syndrome are: brachio-basilic or brachio-cephalic fistulas, diabetes mellitus, and coronary and peripheral artery disease. The hemodynamics governing AVF steal syndrome are complex and may include inflow arterial pathology, outflow vein low resistance, or the collateral arteries [25]. Therefore, the following situations should be considered:

- Proximal artery stenosis in the subclavian, axillary, or brachial arteries, leading to low inflow.
- Distal artery pathology: peripheral artery disease and vasculitis, leading to high distal arterial resistance in the ulnar and radial territory.
- Enlargement of the arteriovenous anastomosis or of the outflow vein—leading to low venous resistance.

The signs and symptoms associated with AVF steal syndrome include imperceptible radial and ulnar pulses, a digital brachial index lower than 0.6, and digital pressures

Type of AVF	AVF blood flow	Cannulation segment length	Other	Observations
Mature	>600 ml/min	At least 10 cm	>6 mm in diameter, < 6 mm in depth	May be cannulated
Still maturing	400–600 ml/min	<10 cm	Depth < 6 mm	Needs follow-up in max. 4 weeks
Unusable	>600 ml/min	>10 cm	Too deep to cannulate	Require s surgical superficialization
Requiring intervention	>400 ml/min	—	Stenosis detected	Requires percutaneous transluminal angioplasty

Table 2.
Types of AVFs at the 4-week US evaluation.

under 50 mmHg. If steal syndrome occurs in the acute setting the hand is cold and painful, the patient experiences tingling or numbness. In a chronic setting, the symptoms include muscular atrophy, nail changes, cutaneous ulcers, and gangrene.

The ultrasound examination of steal syndrome may include the following findings:

- Color and spectral Doppler scan: Abnormal waveforms in the radial or ulnar arteries, showing decreased PSV.
- Inverse flow in the distal artery, usually with an antegrade flow during systole and a retrograde flow during diastole.
- High flow in the brachial artery feeding the AVF (usually over 2–3 l/min).

4.7 High-flow AVF

High-flow AVFs are rarely diagnosed vascular access complications because the symptoms are unspecific and are usually related to right heart decompensation. High-flow AVFs are defined by an AVF blood flow of over 1500 ml/min [26]. The symptoms of this VA complication are shortness of breath, palpitations, orthopnea, and dyspnea upon exertion. Patients undergoing chronic HD treatment have a high rate of cardiovascular comorbidities, and high-flow AVFs add to this cardiovascular burden. A study by Saleh et al. [27] showed that high-flow AVFs lead to an increase in ventricular mass by 12,7% and a reduction in the ejection fraction.

The ultrasound examination of high-flow AVFs reveals spectral Doppler brachial flows over 1500 ml/24 h. Most authors recommend evaluating this blood flow in conjunction with the cardiac output. Thus, if the AVF blood flow/cardiac output ratio exceeds 40%, the patient may present symptoms of heart failure [28]. The procedures that may be implied to reduce AVF flows are either surgical or endovascular, venous banding, Miller banding technique using a PTA balloon, anastoplasty (reducing the size of the anastomosis), graft interposition, and graft inclusion.

4.8 Calcifications

Usually, calcifications occur in the inflow arteries and may be observed when performing presurgical mapping US. Even though arterial calcifications may reflect a poor vascular bed, two studies have shown that the presence of arterial wall calcifications determined on preoperative mapping was not associated with poor AVF maturation [29, 30].

Studies involving AVF calcifications are scarcer, even though the prevalence is high. The diagnosis of calcifications is mainly based on ultrasound examinations as they are asymptomatic in clinical practice. Upon B-mode ultrasound examination, these complications occur as intensely hyperechogenic areas, either punctiform or gross, usually at the cannulation sites. There is no current consensus regarding calcification quantification in terms of dimensions or position and the prospective impact on AVF functionality.

Most of the calcifications present with posterior wall shadowing (**Figures 11** and **12**). One study [31] showed that AVFs presenting calcifications had a higher 1-year chance of complete thrombosis and are associated with other VA complications as well, such as stenosis.

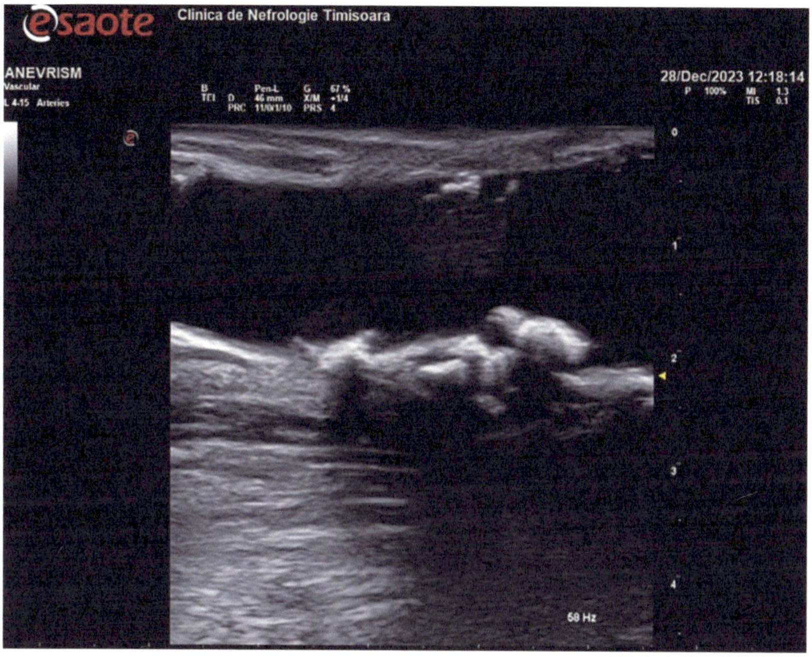

Figure 11.
B-mode longitudinal scan- hyperechogenic areas with posterior wall shadowing on the posterior AVF wall.

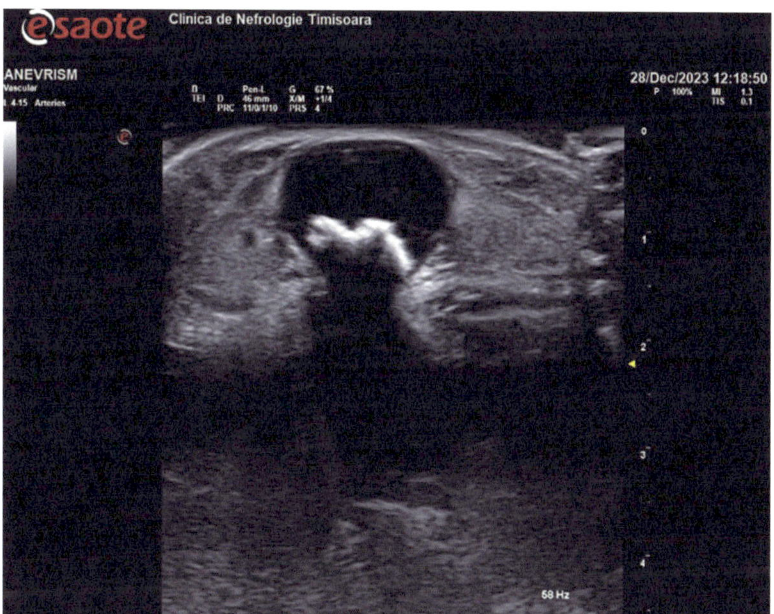

Figure 12.
B-mode transverse scan- hyperechogenic area with posterior wall shadowing on the posterior AVF wall.

5. Point-of-care ultrasound use (POCUS) for AVF evaluation

The aim of POCUS for AVF evaluation is to provide an additional tool in extension to the physical examination. Taking into account that in almost all centers, the cannulations are performed by the HD nurses, having expertise in POCUS may be regarded as a supporting technique for difficult cannulations or new AVFs. Therefore, the scope of POCUS is to answer quick questions regarding the morphology of the AVF (where to cannulate, at what depth, whether there are side branches, and whether there are acute ongoing complications). It is not meant for in-depth analysis, such as stenosis quantification or detailed flow measurements.

AVF POCUS is implied in the following situations, and in current practice, there are portable devices or wireless transducers that make the technique easy to perform at the patient's bedside:

5.1 First cannulation

The POCUS examination steps will include B-mode examination of the AVF morphology—depth, caliber, presence of site branches, and best site of cannulation (to avoid puncturing side branches) (**Figure 13**). Most centers use the "Rule of 6s" for the ideal AVF. It may also help draw a map of the AVF/AVG for the "rope ladder" cannulation technique.

5.2 Difficulty in cannulation

Most often, cannulation difficulties are encountered when the AVF is too deep and the needle does not reach it properly. In these situations, besides statically

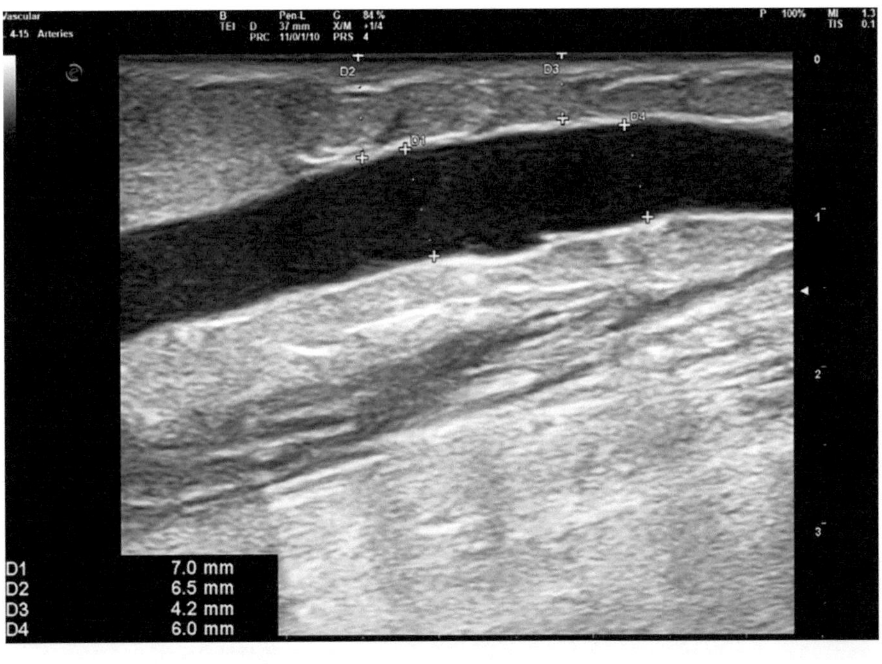

Figure 13.
B-mode longitudinal scan of the AVF noted various depths and calibers.

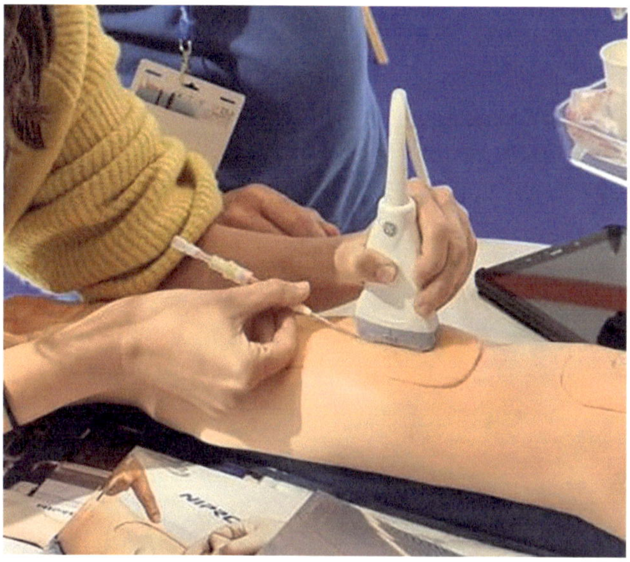

Figure 14.
Transverse probe and needle positioning on a mannequin model.

assessing AVF depth, an US-guided cannulation may be performed. US-guided cannulation requires the use of sterile gloves, sterile transducer gel, and a sterile sheath, to not risk contaminating the needling sites. Using a B-mode longitudinal scan, the long axis of the probe faces parallel to the vessel. The needle will be inserted below the ultrasound probe (example of cannulation position in **Figure 14**, using a mannequin).

The needle trajectory can be noticed on the screen as it progresses toward the middle of the vessel.

- Screening for hematomas or pseudoaneurysms—when clinically, there is swelling or blood infiltration around the AVF/AVG and may help avoid cannulation in a traumatized site.

6. Conclusions

To conclude, AVF US is an invaluable tool in daily clinical practice when managing chronic HD patients. It is an inexpensive and noninvasive technique that provides a quick diagnosis and assists in therapeutic management. Moreover, AVF US has the important advantage that it may be performed at the patient's bedside, helping to reduce AVF complications due to miscannulations. More programs should include VA US training for nephrologists so that HD patients will benefit from the advantages of this technique.

Author details

Iulia Dana Grosu[1,2,3]* and Flaviu Bob[1,2,3]

1 Department of Internal Medicine II, Division of Nephrology, "Victor Babeș" University of Medicine, and Pharmacy, Timisoara, Romania

2 University Clinic of Nephrology, "Pius Branzeu" County Emergency Hospital Timisoara, Romania

3 Faculty of Medicine, Centre for Molecular Research in Nephrology and Vascular Disease, "Victor Babeș" University of Medicine, and Pharmacy, Timisoara, Romania

*Address all correspondence to: grosu.iulia@umft.ro

References

[1] Thurlow JS, Joshi M, Yan G, Norris KC, Agodoa LY, Yuan CM, et al. Global epidemiology of end-stage kidney disease and disparities in kidney replacement therapy. American Journal of Nephrology. 2021;**52**(2):98-107. DOI: 10.1159/000514550. Epub 2021 Mar 22

[2] Foreman KJ, Marquez N, Dolgert A, Fukutaki K, Fullman N, McGaughey M, et al. Forecasting life expectancy, years of life lost, and all-cause and cause-specific mortality for 250 causes of death: Reference and alternative scenarios for 2016-40 for 195 countries and territories. Lancet. 2018;**392**(10159):2052-2090. DOI: 10.1016/S0140-6736(18)31694-5. Epub 2018 Oct 16

[3] Kramer A, Pippias M, Noordzij M, et al. The European renal association - European dialysis and transplant association (ERA-EDTA) registry annual report 2016: A summary. Clinical Kidney Journal. 2019;**12**(5):702-720

[4] Ravani P, Palmer SC, Oliver MJ, Quinn RR, MacRae JM, Tai DJ, et al. Associations between hemodialysis access type and clinical outcomes: A systematic review. Journal of the American Society of Nephrology. 2013;**24**(3):465-473. DOI: 10.1681/ASN.2012070643. Epub 2013 Feb 21

[5] Yeh LM, Chiu SH, Lai PC. The impact of vascular access types on hemodialysis patient long-term survival. Scientific Reports. 2019;**9**:10708. DOI: 10.1038/s41598-019-47065-z

[6] Shechter SM, Skandari MR, Zalunardo N. Timing of arteriovenous fistula creation in patients with CKD: A decision analysis. American Journal of Kidney Diseases. 2014;**63**(1):95-103. DOI: 10.1053/j.ajkd.2013.06.021. Epub 2013 Aug 24

[7] Lok CE, Huber TS, Lee T, Shenoy S, Yevzlin AS, Abreo K, et al. KDOQI clinical practice guideline for vascular access: 2019 update. American Journal of Kidney Diseases. 2020;**75**(4 Suppl. 2):S1-S164. DOI: 10.1053/j.ajkd.2019.12.001. Epub 2020 Mar 12. Erratum in: Am J Kidney Dis. 2021;77(4):551

[8] Schmidli J, Widmer MK, Basile C, de Donato G, Gallieni M, Gibbons CP, et al. Esvs Guidelines Reviewers, Mohaupt M, Ricco JB, Roca-Tey R, ESVS Guidelines Committee. Editor's Choice - Vascular Access: 2018 clinical practice guidelines of the European Society for Vascular Surgery (ESVS). European Journal of Vascular and Endovascular Surgery 2018;**55**(6):757-818. DOI: 10.1016/j.ejvs.2018.02.001. Epub 2018 May 2

[9] Wedgwood KR, Wiggins PA, Guillou PJ. A prospective study of end-to-side vs. side-to-side arteriovenous fistulas for haemodialysis. The British Journal of Surgery. 1984;**71**(8):640-642. DOI: 10.1002/bjs.1800710831

[10] Fullerton JK, McLafferty RB, Ramsey DE, et al. Pitfalls in achieving the dialysis outcome quality initiative (DOQI) guidelines for hemodialysis access? Annals of Vascular Surgery. 2002;**16**:613-617

[11] Sedlacek M, Teodorescu V, Falk A, Vassalotti JA, Uribarri J. Hemodialysis access placement with preoperative noninvasive vascular mapping: Comparison between patients with and without diabetes. American Journal of Kidney Diseases. 2001;**38**(3):560-564

[12] Malovrh M. Native arteriovenous fistula: Preoperative evaluation. American Journal of Kidney Diseases. 2002;**39**(6):1218-1225. DOI: 10.1053/ajkd.2002.33394

[13] Nalesso F, Garzotto F, Petrucci I, Samoni S, Virzì GM, Gregori D, et al. Standardized protocol for hemodialysis vascular access assessment: The role of ultrasound and color Doppler. Blood Purification. 2018;**45**(1-3):260-269. DOI: 10.1159/000485590

[14] Pichot O, Diard A, Bosc J-Y, Abbadie F, Franco G, Mahé G, et al. Standardized methodology for duplex ultrasound examination of arteriovenous access for hemodialysis: A proposal of the French Society of Vascular Medicine and the French-Speaking Society of Vascular Access. Ultrasound in Medicine & Biology. 2023;**49**(10):2213-2220. DOI: 10.1016/j.ultrasmedbio.2023.07.007, ISSN 0301-5629

[15] Quencer KB, Arici M. Arteriovenous fistulas and their characteristic sites of stenosis. AJR. American Journal of Roentgenology. 2015;**205**(4):726-734. DOI: 10.2214/AJR.15.14650

[16] Badero OJ, Salifu MO, Wasse H, Work J. Frequency of swing-segment stenosis in referred dialysis patients with angiographically documented lesions. American Journal of Kidney Diseases. 2008;**51**:93-98

[17] Malik J, de Bont C, Valerianova A, Krupickova Z, Novakova L. Arteriovenous hemodialysis access stenosis diagnosed by duplex Doppler ultrasonography: A review. Diagnostics. 1979;**2022**:12. DOI: 10.3390/diagnostics12081979

[18] Yii E, Yii MK, Thwaites S, Zhu J, Chong T, Tong L, et al. Receiver operating characteristic curve analysis of arteriovenous dialysis access flow using ultrasound. ANZ Journal of Surgery. 2022;**92**(3):461-465. DOI: 10.1111/ans.17378. Epub 2021 Nov 21

[19] Meola M, Marciello A, Di Salle G, Petrucci I. Ultrasound evaluation of access complications: Thrombosis, aneurysms, pseudoaneurysms and infections. The Journal of Vascular Access. 2021;**22**(1_suppl):71-83. DOI: 10.1177/11297298211018062. Epub 2021 Jul 27

[20] Saad NE, Saad WE, Davies MG, Waldman DL, Fultz PJ, Rubens DJ. Pseudoaneurysms and the role of minimally invasive techniques in their management. Radiographics. 2005;**25**(Suppl. 1):S173-S189. DOI: 10.1148/rg.25si055503

[21] Carneiro F. SP597, reducing adverse effects of arteriovenous fistula cannulation with Doppler ultrasound. Nephrology Dialysis Transplantation. 2018;**33**(suppl_1):i548-i549. DOI: 10.1093/ndt/gfy104.SP597

[22] Chytilova E, Jemcov T, Malik J, Pajek J, Fila B, Kavan J. Role of Doppler ultrasonography in the evaluation of hemodialysis arteriovenous access maturation and influencing factors. The Journal of Vascular Access. 2021;**22**(1_suppl):42-55. DOI: 10.1177/1129729820965064

[23] Caputo BC, Leong B, Sibona A, Jhajj S, Kohne C, Gabel J, et al. Arteriovenous fistula maturation: Physical exam versus flow study. Annals of Vascular Surgery. 2021;**77**:16-24. DOI: 10.1016/j.avsg.2021.05.022. Epub 2021 Aug 17

[24] Wilson SE. Vascular Access, principle and practice. Philadelphia: Lippincott Williams & Wilkins; 2010

[25] Bucktowarsing B. Available from: https://www.renalfellow.org/2019/06/30/an-overview-of-dialysis-access-associated-steal-syndrome/

[26] Basile C, Lomonte C, Vernaglione L, Casucci F, Antonelli M, Losurdo N. The relationship between the flow of arteriovenous fistula and cardiac output in haemodialysis patients. Nephrology, Dialysis, Transplantation. 2008;**23**(1):282-287. DOI: 10.1093/ndt/gfm549. Epub 2007 Oct 17

[27] Saleh MA, El Kilany WM, Keddis VW, El Said TW. Effect of high flow arteriovenous fistula on cardiac function in hemodialysis patients. The Egyptian Heart Journal. 2018;**70**(4):337-341. DOI: 10.1016/j.ehj.2018.10.007. Epub 2018 Nov 16

[28] MacRae JM, Pandeya S, Humen DP, Krivitski N, Lindsay RM. Arteriovenous fistula-associated high-output cardiac failure: A review of mechanisms. American Journal of Kidney Diseases. 2004;**43**:e17-e22

[29] Tang WJ, Adnan AS, Md Salleh MS, Mat Saad AZ. Microcalcification in the arterial wall and its relationship to the ultrasound criteria of maturation of the arteriovenous fistula. The Journal of Vascular Access. 2019;**20**(1):46-51. DOI: 10.1177/1129729818775359

[30] Gubensek J. Doppler ultrasound assessment of calcified radial arteries prior to radio-cephalic arterio-venous fistula placement: An observational study. The Journal of Vascular Access. 2022;**25**(3):897-903. DOI: 10.1177/11297298221143598

[31] Grosu ID, Stirbu O, Gadalean F, Bob F, Mihaescu A, Marc L, et al. MO790: Arteriovenous fistula calcifications—Risk factors and impact on arteriovenous fistula functionality. Nephrology Dialysis Transplantation. 2022;**37**(Supplement_3):gfac080.027. DOI: 10.1093/ndt/gfac080.027

Chapter 16

Childhood Obesity: Systemic Complications, Early Atherosclerosis and the Value of Carotid Intima-Media Thickness

Monica Simina Mihuta, Corina Paul, Andreea Borlea, Cristina Mihaela Roi, Denisa Pescari and Dana Liana Stoian

Abstract

Childhood obesity is a growing public health concern with long-term metabolic and cardiovascular consequences. It results from a complex interplay of genetic, environmental, and behavioral factors, leading to systemic inflammation, insulin resistance, dyslipidemia, and endothelial dysfunction—key contributors to early-onset atherosclerosis. Beyond excess adiposity, multiple risk factors influence vascular health, including maternal obesity, gestational diabetes, birth weight abnormalities, family history of cardiometabolic disease, smoking exposure, hypertension, physical inactivity, and sleep deprivation. Maternal health during pregnancy can impact fetal cardiovascular programming, while postnatal influences such as sedentary lifestyles and poor sleep further exacerbate metabolic dysfunction and vascular alterations. Carotid intima-media thickness (CIMT) is a well-established, non-invasive marker for subclinical atherosclerosis, offering valuable insights into early vascular changes in obese children. Studies demonstrate significant correlations between CIMT and metabolic parameters, making it a promising tool for cardiovascular risk stratification. However, its interpretation should consider the broader spectrum of obesity-related risk factors. A comprehensive approach to childhood obesity management must address metabolic dysfunction, vascular health, and early intervention strategies. Public health initiatives, maternal health optimization, and lifestyle modifications play a critical role in preventing long-term complications. Integrating CIMT assessment with clinical and biochemical evaluations enhances early risk detection, ultimately improving long-term cardiovascular outcomes in obese children.

Keywords: atherosclerosis, carotid intima-media thickness, obesity, insulin-resistance, serum TMAO

1. Introduction

Childhood obesity presents a significant global health challenge, with particular concern for the enduring cardiovascular implications that can affect the well-being of young adults in the long term. One key aspect of assessing cardiovascular health is the use of carotid intima-media thickness (CIMT), a non-invasive imaging marker. This marker is obtained through ultrasonographic (US) measurements of the thickness between the inner layers of the carotid artery. The CIMT serves as an important indicator for detecting early stages of atherosclerosis, and its correlation with changes in lipid and glucose metabolism enhances its value in identifying cardiovascular risk factors.

This chapter delves into the impact of childhood obesity on the early manifestations of cardiovascular changes, shedding light on various facets of the subject. It encompasses comprehensive background information on childhood obesity, exploring its complications, the underlying pathophysiology of vascular disruptions, and the heightened cardiovascular risk faced by obese children. By examining these aspects, we aim to gain a deeper understanding of the intricate interplay between childhood obesity and cardiovascular health, ultimately contributing to the broader discourse on pediatric cardiovascular risk assessment and management.

2. Defining childhood obesity

The excess of adipose tissue in an individual as a result of the imbalance between energy intake and energy expenditure defines primary obesity [1]. In pediatrics, obesity is defined using charts developed for age and sex for the value of the Body Mass Index (BMI) [2]. The globally acknowledged definitions of childhood obesity are those proposed by the Centers for Disease Control and Prevention (CDC) and the World Health Organization (WHO) [2–4].

According to CDC guidelines, a child ≥2 years old presenting:

- a BMI ≥ 85th percentile for age and sex is characterized as overweight,
- a BMI ≥ 95th percentile is characterized as obese (class 1 obesity);
- a BMI ≥ 120th percentile is characterized as severely obese (class 2 and 3 obesity) [2, 3].

The WHO recommends utilizing BMI Z-score thresholds:

- Z-score > 1 for identifying overweight;
- Z-score > 2 for diagnosing obesity;
- Z-score > 3 for diagnosing severe obesity.

The Z-score is calculated based on the number of standard deviations away from the average value [4].

3. Epidemiology of childhood obesity

In the European Region, recent epidemiological data spanning from 2018 to 2020 indicate that almost 60% of adults and 29% of school-aged children are grappling with issues related to weight excess [5]. Meanwhile, the United States, as per CDC reports from 2017 to 2020, has seen a prevalence of 19.7% for obesity in children aged two and older [6]. BMI statistics reveal a noteworthy trend during the SARS-CoV-2 pandemic, with reported rates nearly doubling [7]. Globally, the prevalence of childhood weight excess, be it overweight or obesity, is significantly higher in developed countries. Rates of obesity as high as 30% are reported in most countries in North and South America, as well as in the United Kingdom, Greece, Italy, Malta, Portugal, and Spain [8]. Lower rates are observed in Scandinavian countries, France, and Central Europe [9]. Eastern European countries and Russia report lower rates of overweight, at about 15%. China reports significantly higher rates of overweight in young children compared to adolescents [10].

4. Etiology of childhood obesity

The core concept behind weight gain centers on the idea of ingesting more calories than the body expends, resulting in an energy imbalance that leads to the storage of excess energy in the form of fat, ultimately causing an increase in body weight. However, a more profound understanding of the complex nature of the issue reveals a nuanced and intricate scenario.

Various factors, such as dietary patterns, social dynamics, economic factors, and environmental influences, play a role in the individuals' ability to maintain a balance [11]. Increased consumption of fast food is associated with weight gain, larger waist size, and an elevated risk of health issues [12]. Genetic predisposition and the intricate interplay between homeostatic circuits and brain reward systems can further amplify these effects. The accumulation of lipid metabolites and inflammatory signaling also substantially contribute to the development of obesity [13].

Family genetics and unhealthy lifestyles contribute to obesity susceptibility, especially for children with obese parents [14, 15]. Primary obesity is thus characterized by a polygenic nature, driven by genetic variations and environmental influences. This interplay results in decreased physical activity, increased food intake, and heightened fat storage. The early-life environment, including maternal nutrition, can induce epigenetic changes contributing to obesity [16].

The connections between neural, hormonal, and gut-brain axes influence hunger and satiety. Hormones like ghrelin stimulate hunger, while leptin suppresses appetite. Stress, disrupted sleep patterns [17–20], and psychiatric disorders elevate ghrelin levels, increasing appetite [21].

The gut microbiome regulates weight and links to conditions like obesity, diabetes, and mental health issues. Alterations result from factors like gestational age, delivery method, feeding practices [22–24], anxiety, depression [23, 24], and use of pro and antibiotics [24].

A considerably smaller proportion of childhood obesity cases, approximately up to 10%, can be linked to secondary causes. Endocrinological disorders involving thyroid and adrenal function (hypothyroidism and cortisol excess), growth hormone deficiency, and pseudohypoparathyroidism are recognized contributors to obesity. Conditions such as hypothalamic injury/disorders, ghrelin-leptin dysfunction, and genetic syndromes (Prader–Willi, Alstrom, Bardet-Biedl, Beckwith-Wiedeman, or Cohen syndrome) may also lead to excessive weight. Patients using medications such as glucocorticoids, sulphonylureas, tricyclic antidepressants, and antipsychotics, or being exposed to endocrine-disrupting chemicals like bisphenol A and dichlorodiphenyltrichloroethane, are also at risk of weight gain [17–20].

5. Pathogeny of childhood obesity

Adipogenesis involves precursor cells transforming into mature adipocytes, synthesizing adipokines [25]. Children's adaptable white adipose tissue plays a crucial role in obesity-related metabolic complications. It undergoes histological, metabolic, and endocrine changes due to factors like adipocyte metabolic capacity, chemokine production, recruitment of new adipocytes, and altered adipokine secretion [26, 27].

Children experience increased adipocyte numbers, especially in obesity, due to higher proliferation rates (hyperplastic model). This limits immediate impacts on adipokine secretion but raises the risk of severe obesity and metabolic comorbidities later in life [28]. In contrast, adults exhibit a hypertrophic model with expanded existing adipocytes, potentially affecting adipokine secretion profiles differently [29].

Leptin and adiponectin, crucial in energy homeostasis and insulin sensitivity, are influenced by factors such as body fat mass, adipocyte size, and pubertal development [30]. Leptin, signaling energy sufficiency, regulates food intake and can cause severe obesity at low levels [31]. Leptin levels relate to body fat mass, triglyceride content, and are influenced by gestational age and birth weight. Adiponectin, enhancing insulin sensitivity, shows varying levels in newborns, prepubertal children, and adults, inversely related to body fat in the latter [32, 33].

Metabolomic studies also reveal complex metabolite profiles associated with childhood obesity and insulin resistance, linking perturbations in amino acids, nucleotide metabolism, and lipids to the severity of obesity [34]. Notably, uric acid and serum lipids exhibit strong positive correlations with obesity severity [34, 35]. These metabolic disruptions are consequences of obesity, correctable through weight loss [36].

6. Obesity-driven vascular damage: The pathogeny of atherosclerosis

The metabolic changes in obesity lead to vascular disruptions affecting the structure and function of arterial walls, serving as drivers for the ongoing process of atherosclerosis. Atherogenesis initiates at damaged endothelial sites, influenced by factors like hypertension, elevated LDL-c levels, exposure to toxins from cigarette smoke, low serum HDL-C, insulin resistance, and metabolic alterations [37]. These drivers of vascular dysfunction and atherosclerosis commence in early childhood, with obesity exacerbating and accelerating potential complications [38].

The initial alteration in this process is the modification of flow-mediated dilatation, also known as nitric oxide-mediated dilation, assessing the earliest changes in endothelial dilation function [39]. Nitric oxide plays a crucial role in vasodilation, but various vasoactive substances are released from endothelial cells to regulate blood flow. Reduced nitric oxide activity represents endothelial dysfunction, the primary etiological cause of atherosclerosis, measured by Doppler ultrasound [40].

Intermediate alterations involve arterial stiffness, which affects both vessel function and structure [41]. The stiffening of arterial walls is influenced by shared mechanisms, including a reduced elastin/collagen ratio, elastin cross-linking generation, inflammation induced by reactive oxygen species, calcification, vascular smooth muscle cell stiffness, and endothelial dysfunction [41]. Various cardiovascular risk factors associated with obesity affect arterial vessel elasticity. High blood pressure induces stiffness in large vessels, while the renin-angiotensin system activation promotes inflammation, vascular smooth muscle cell proliferation, and glycation end product formation [42]. Hyperglycemia and insulin resistance impact the structure and function of large artery walls, promoting smooth muscle cell proliferation, glycation end product formation, and collagen cross-linking, resulting in early loss of arterial elasticity [43]. These factors represent the primary causes of obesity-related arterial stiffness. Underlying inflammation from visceral adiposity exacerbates dyslipidemia, hyperglycemia, and arterial hypertension [44], contributing to increased arterial stiffness, a reliable indicator of wall damage. While vessel elasticity is mainly influenced by the aging process [45], in the context of obesity, arterial stiffness is also affected by disruptions in nitric oxide and oxygenase balance due to inflammation [46], elevated blood pressure impacting hemodynamic forces [47], and insulin resistance along with high levels of LDL-c, irrespective of age [48].

The stage of subclinical atherosclerosis signifies advanced structural wall changes and can be US assessed through carotid intima-media thickness (CIMT) [49]. The progression of atherosclerosis is initiated by LDL-c particles infiltrating the subendothelial space, undergoing oxidative modifications [50]. In this dysfunctional state, endothelial cells express specific adhesion molecules and selectins, promoting the binding of circulating monocytes to the vascular endothelium [50]. Within the inflamed intima, monocytes differentiate into macrophages. Exposed to modified LDL-c, these macrophages internalize oxidized LDL-c and other particles, forming cytosolic lipid droplets and resembling lipid-laden foam cells over time [50]. Type T lymphocytes and other inflammatory and immune mediators invade the lesion site, releasing cytokines and growth factors. Smooth muscle cells migrate, proliferate, and secrete extracellular matrix components, contributing to fibrous cap formation over the lesion [50]. The ongoing inflammatory response in the vascular wall, mediated by cytokines like interleukin-6, triggers further uptake of LDL-c and leukocytes, promoting atherosclerotic lesion growth [37]. The atherosclerotic lesion expands at its base through mechanisms leading to the initial fatty streak formation, progressing throughout adulthood and causing chronic and acute complications [49].

In children with atherosclerotic risk factors such as obesity and metabolic syndrome, arterial wall changes are subtle but progressive. Obese children are more likely to exhibit subclinical atherosclerosis compared to their normal-weight peers [51, 52]. A substantial abdominal panniculus, indicative of visceral adiposity, has been linked to atherosclerotic lesions in young adults [53] and subclinical atherosclerosis in children [54, 55].

7. Risk factors for atherosclerosis progression in children

Apart from excess adiposity, various factors, both modifiable and non-modifiable, contribute to vascular health issues to varying degrees. Advancing age and male sex are direct influencers of increased CIMT values in adults [56]. Arterial stiffness is impacted by aging, with alterations in collagen and a reduction in elastin content being primary factors [57]. In children and young adults, age appears less significant in vascular damage development compared to pathologies like obesity and exposure to cardiometabolic risks.

Other risks include aspects related to pregnancy, maternal health, perinatal conditions concerning weight or nutrition, family history of cardiometabolic disease, exposure to smoking, elevated blood pressure, a lack of daily physical activity, and sleep disruptions [56].

A mother's health during pregnancy significantly influences fetal development and the child's future well-being [58]. Maternal obesity can lead to placental insufficiency, resulting in intrauterine growth delay and cardiovascular changes predisposing to high blood pressure, arterial stiffness, and atherosclerosis [59]. Maternal health during pregnancy can indirectly affect CIMT values by influencing the newborn's vulnerability to atherosclerosis. Childhood obesity correlates with maternal obesity and gestational diabetes [60]. High blood pressure in a pregnant woman can impact her child's blood pressure, especially in adulthood. A mother's cardiovascular profile is linked to her offspring's health [61]. In utero exposure to chronic autoimmune thyroiditis increases the risk of the offspring developing a thyroid disorder during childhood or adolescence [62]. Moreover, autoimmune thyroiditis in children contributes to atherosclerosis due to chronic inflammation affecting endothelial integrity [63]. Smoking during pregnancy leads to low birth weight and higher CIMT values in the child's young adulthood [64].

Regarding birth weight, low birth weight for gestational age is a significant risk for atherosclerosis, with a more severe deficit linked to a higher risk. Higher-than-normal birth weight is also a risk factor for elevated CIMT in young adulthood [64].

Postnatal nutrition, particularly breastfeeding, has universal protective characteristics, while artificial alimentation is associated with obesity, atherosclerosis, arterial hypertension, and insulin resistance [65].

Family medical history reflects genetic predispositions and behavioral components, associated with higher CIMT values and linked to factors like oxidant status, insulin resistance, and dyslipidemia [66].

Smoking impacts vascular wall integrity, triggers early atherosclerosis, and hastens arterial stiffness. Cigarette smoking increases CIMT values, making the vascular age of a regular smoker about 6–7 years older than that of non-smokers. Smoking exacerbates the effects of metabolic syndrome and aging on CIMT, impacting genders differently. Passive smoking in children has detrimental effects on vascular health, increasing the risk of atherosclerosis, and adolescents with smoking parents have a higher risk of becoming smokers themselves [67].

Sedentary behavior contributes to weight gain and influences glucose and lipid metabolism, reducing cardiovascular adaptability to physical exertion. Leading a sedentary lifestyle during childhood increases the risk of cardiometabolic issues and carotid plaque development in young adulthood [68].

Sleep deprivation in children, associated with behavioral and emotional problems, increases cardiovascular risk. Adequate sleep is crucial for cardiovascular health, with studies showing connections between sleep deprivation and high blood pressure in children, making it a valid cardiovascular risk factor [69].

8. Screening and evaluation of atherosclerosis in children

The standard method for assessing atherosclerosis in both children and adults is the measurement of carotid intima-media thickness. CIMT gauges the space between the intimal and medial layers of the common carotid artery, approximately 1–2 cm caudally from the carotid bulb, serving as an established indicator of generalized atherosclerosis [70]. An increase in CIMT is an initial observable sign of subclinical atherosclerosis, making it the most precise non-invasive method for early detection through US techniques. While clinical parameters and blood markers are commonly used in clinical settings to estimate early stages, recent advances in imaging technologies have shown that cardiovascular risk can be reliably assessed in pediatric patients as well [71].

CIMT, a non-invasive, painless, radiation-free, cost-effective, and easily reproducible method, is considered a potential cornerstone for risk evaluation in at-risk pediatric patients. Ongoing research is focusing on the predictive value of CIMT in children as a risk indicator, with substantial evidence indicating higher values in children with obesity. Farello et al. reported elevated CIMT values in both metabolically healthy and obese children, with early detection predicting cardiovascular disease in young adults [55].

While not the most accurate method for analyzing arterial walls, sonography-measured CIMT is the most suitable screening tool for children. Although MRI wall-thickness measurements may have superior prognostic value, its limitations, such as cost and reduced accessibility, make it more suitable for research than routine clinical practice. CT angiography, despite potential benefits in detecting vasa vasorum neovascularization, is unsuitable as a screening tool for children due to radiation exposure and poor contrast [72]. Fluorodeoxyglucose-PET, valuable in assessing plaque vulnerability, is unlikely to be useful in screening at-risk children [73]. Therefore, for everyday clinical risk assessment in pediatric patients, CIMT ultrasonography remains the only suitable imaging tool for evaluating subclinical atherosclerosis, despite its limitations, making it a practical and valuable option.

8.1 US technique

Ultrasonography of the carotid arteries, the standard method for obtaining reliable CIMT measurements, has a relatively short learning curve, of only 4 weeks. This is especially true in the case of using automated echography devices [74]. The operator sets up the ultrasound settings (B-mode) and selects a suitable linear ultrasound probe, taking into account variations in neck structure due to adipose tissue, particularly in obese children. Subjects are positioned to lie down and extend their necks backward to achieve a clearer view of both common carotid arteries.

Transversal scanning begins from the clavicle and moves upwards on each side, identifying the carotid bulb and the sequential bifurcation into internal and external carotids. Once located, the probe orientation shifts to longitudinal scanning, presenting the carotid in a longitudinal section with the bulb on the left side and a clear intima-media image. For CIMT measurement, the recommended region is the posterior carotid wall, approximately 1–2 cm caudally from the bulb [75]. In children, image acquisition is performed during end-diastole [76].

Automated echography devices streamline the process by automatically measuring CIMT after obtaining a clear intima-media image (refer to **Figure 1**) [77]. To ensure accuracy, it is recommended to take at least three measurements for each carotid artery. This meticulous approach enhances the precision of CIMT assessments in pediatric populations undergoing ultrasonography.

The latest technological advances have allowed the development of echography devices in which CIMT is measured in real-time, without freezing the image of interest. The device acquires multiple real-time measurements and provides the mean value. Utilizing real-time radio frequency data, the device provides enhanced accuracy compared to conventional 2D-based IMT methods that rely solely on grayscale image quality. This minimizes inter-operator variability and boosts confidence in the measurements [78].

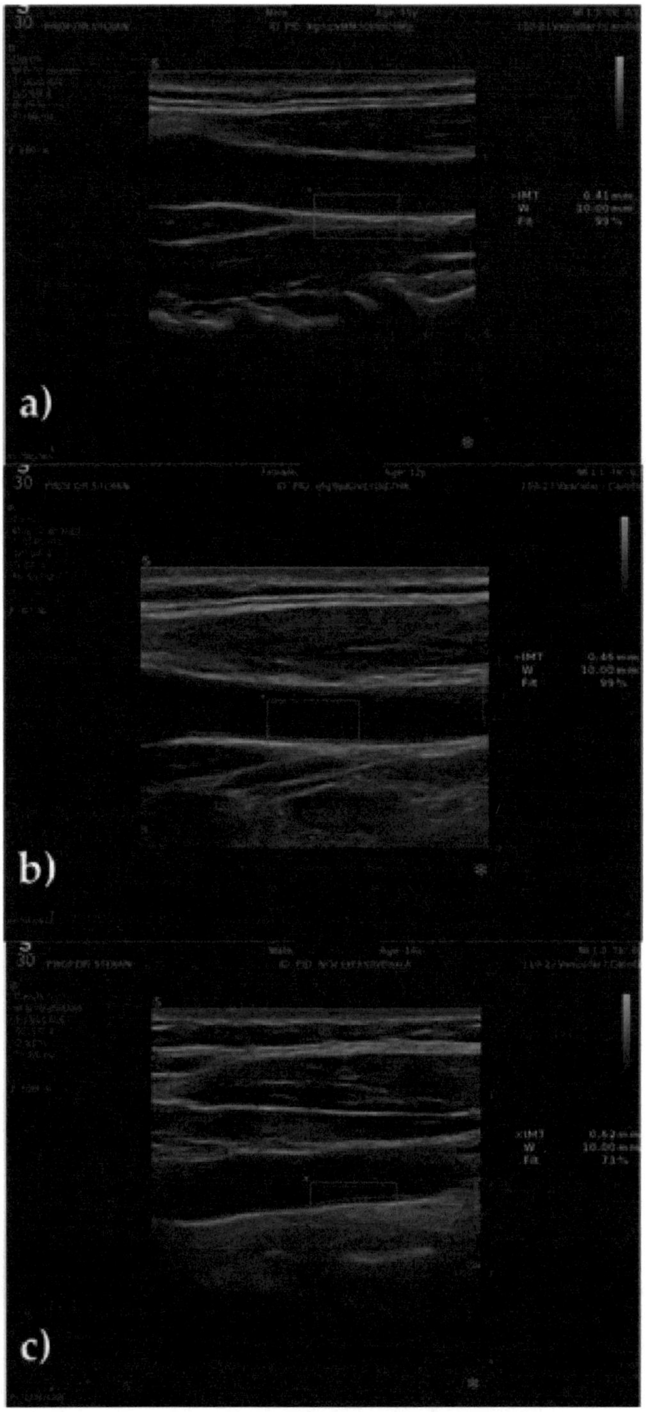

Figure 1.
Examples of CIMT measurements made with the Aixplorer MACH 30 echography device (automated software): (a) an 11-year-old normal-weight boy; (b) a 12-year-old overweight girl; (c) a 16-year-old obese boy (source: Dr. D Medical Centre, Timisoara, Romania).

9. Impactful comorbidities and complications of childhood obesity leading to atherosclerosis

9.1 Insulin resistance and type 2 diabetes mellitus

Insulin resistance (IR) associated with obesity is a key contributor to the onset of type 2 diabetes mellitus and cardiovascular diseases [79]. Essentially, IR signifies a diminished ability of insulin to facilitate glucose utilization by muscle and adipose cells, while also inhibiting hepatic glycogenesis and glycogenolysis. It affects protein and lipid metabolism, endothelial function, and gene expression [80]. The fundamental mechanism involves the liver's increased production of acetyl-coenzyme-A, leading to inflammation in adipose tissue [79]. Excessive fatty acids play a pivotal role in inducing IR in obese children [79]. Accumulation of excess fat in the liver, muscles, and β-cells leads to increased IR in these organs [81]. Children with obesity often exhibit increased intramyocellular lipid content, exacerbating IR [82]. Lipotoxicity, induced by elevated circulating free fatty acids, disrupts insulin signaling pathways, contributing to insulin resistance in skeletal muscle. This abnormal insulin signaling is responsible for defects in glucose transport [81]. In states of IR or insulin deficiency, increased free fatty acid production can worsen hepatic glucose production [83]. Additionally, chronic low-grade inflammation caused by obesity triggers the production of pro-inflammatory chemokines and cytokines, further aggravating IR. Mitochondrial dysfunction is also implicated in IR development. In the liver and skeletal muscle, impaired fatty acid oxidation by mitochondria contributes to IR, impacting the normal insulin signaling pathway in peripheral tissues [84].

Substantial evidence supports the link between IR and vascular disease, leading to the widespread recognition of metabolic syndrome. IR contributes to dyslipidemia and other metabolic irregularities, creating a pro-atherogenic environment. Furthermore, impaired insulin signaling affects the utilization of glucose by peripheral tissue, resulting in elevated serum glucose levels and hyperinsulinemia [85].

9.1.1 Practical aspects

The 2023 guideline [2] stresses the need to assess prediabetes in obese children to prevent future diabetes. For those at risk of type 2 diabetes, a comprehensive evaluation is crucial, considering factors such as gestational size, family history, maternal diabetes, insulin resistance complications, and the use of obesity-related psychotropic drugs [2]. The American Diabetes Association's criteria for detecting glucose metabolism changes are outlined in **Table 1** [86].

Confirmation of hyperglycemia requires either two different tests or the same test on two separate occasions, with an essential 8-hour fasting period [86]. While fasting plasma glucose is an early indicator in adults, its reliability in obese children is diminished due to varying insulin resistance levels, impacting glucose fluctuations [87].

Despite the reproducibility of the oral glucose tolerance test (OGTT), it may not be suitable for ambulatory clinical practices, being time-consuming and potentially limited by unpalatable glucose solutions in certain situations [88].

The glycosylated hemoglobin test (HbA1c), not requiring fasting, provides a measure of chronic hyperglycemia and enhances type 2 diabetes evaluation in primary

Type of analysis	Impaired glucose tolerance	Diabetes mellitus
Fasting glucose (mg/dL)	100–125	≥126
2-h plasma glucose (mg/dL) – OGTT	140–199	≥200
Random plasma glucose	Not applicable	≥200
HbA1c (%)	5.7–6.4	≥6.5

Table 1.
According to the American Diabetes Association, impaired glucose tolerance and diabetes mellitus is diagnosed as such [86].

care settings [89]. Although recommended for monitoring prediabetes, it has lower sensitivity in children compared to adults, and its efficacy may be limited in detecting early glucose anomalies due to significant variations in children with obesity [88].

For a more precise assessment of insulin resistance, the HOMA-IR is a reliable proxy, predicting the risk of type 2 diabetes. Despite its value, insulin measurement is not standard, potentially not covered by insurance in many countries, and requires adjusted HOMA-IR cut-offs based on puberty, race, sex, genetics, and environment [80]. The formula used for calculating HOMA-IR is *[glucose (mg/dl) × insulin (μU/mL)]/405* [90]. Due to the influence of puberty development on HOMA-IR, cut-off values for HOMA-IR remain a subject of debate. For Caucasian children, different researchers have proposed cut-off values according to their Tanner stage.

- For pre-pubertal children, the HOMA-IR cut-off can be considered 2.3, and for pubertal children, 3.4, as defined in a large study on Italian Caucasian obese children aged 8–15 [91].

- For post-pubertal children, the HOMA-IR cut-off can be considered 3.4. A study on normal-weight and obese children aged 2–17.8 years old placed the cut-off value for obese children at 3.42, as the 75% percentile, for individuals who may develop cardiovascular risk factors very early in life [92].

Two other indexes that may be useful in assessing insulin resistance are the Visceral Adiposity Index (VAI) and the triglyceride-glucose index (TyG). VAI, an indicator of "visceral adipose function" and insulin sensitivity, is calculated using sex-specific formulas. In these calculations, WC is measured in cm, and triglycerides and HDL-c are measured in mmol/l. Proposed cut-off values for VAI are 8.8 for men and 8.7 for women. In children, although precise cut-off values are not established, studies propose more or less the same values [91, 93]. The formulas are as follows:

- for males, *VAI = {WC / [39.68 + (1.88 × BMI)]} × (triglycerides/1.03) × (1.31/HDL-c);*

- for females, *VAI = {WC / [36.58 + (1.89 × BMI)]} × (triglycerides /0.81) × (1.52/HDL-c).*

The TyG index, a marker of muscular resistance to insulin, can be obtained using the formula *Ln [(triglycerides × glucose/2]*, with triglycerides and glucose measured in mg/dl. The cut-off value for TyG is 1 [94].

9.2 Dyslipidemia

As mentioned before, weight excess can induce lipid metabolism changes, leading to dyslipidemia characterized by elevated total cholesterol (TC), low-density lipoprotein cholesterol, non-high-density lipoprotein cholesterol, and triglycerides, along with reduced high-density lipoprotein cholesterol levels [95]. Lipoprotein levels vary based on age and sex, and reference values have been established through population-based studies [95–98]. Hyperlipidemia is often unrelated to lipoprotein metabolism disorders, with the consumption of high saturated and trans fats elevating LDL-c levels, and excessive intake of refined carbohydrates and sugars increasing triglycerides [99]. Obesity-related conditions like insulin resistance and metabolic-associated fatty liver disease (MAFLD) contribute to dyslipidemia [99]. LDL-c and other apo-B-containing lipoproteins play a crucial role in atherosclerosis development, particularly when associated with low HDL-c [100, 101]. The presence of both alterations negatively impacts the long-term cardiovascular prognosis in children [101].

HDL-c exhibits an inverse association with cardiovascular risk, acting as an anti-inflammatory agent by transporting excess cholesterol from arterial walls to hepatic cells [101]. In sedentary children with lower HDL-c levels, there is an increased susceptibility to atherosclerosis progression and arterial stiffness within the metabolic syndrome [100].

Non-HDL-c, encompassing all atherogenic lipoproteins, is calculated as the difference between total cholesterol and HDL-C, showing a strong relationship with cardiovascular risk comparable to LDL-C [102]. Triglycerides, reflecting lifestyle and dietary habits, exhibit personal variability but are important in evaluating cardiovascular health in high-risk patients [103].

The TG-to-HDL-c ratio is suggested as a reliable indicator of cardiovascular, metabolic, and dysglycemia risks [103, 104]. In adults, the TC-to-HDL-c ratio is an independent predictor of ischemic coronary events, particularly potent when associated with larger waist circumferences, insulin resistance, and dyslipidemia [105].

Research links blood lipoprotein levels to vascular damage, where HDL-c negatively correlates with arterial elasticity loss, while triglycerides, LDL-c, and total cholesterol show positive correlations [106]. Maintaining a healthy weight, adopting a nutritious diet, and engaging in physical activity since childhood can effectively prevent vascular damage in adulthood, potentially obviating the need for lipid-lowering therapy.

9.2.1 Practical aspects

The 2023 guideline [2] underscores the significance of assessing dyslipidemia in children with excess weight. It is crucial to obtain a fasting lipid panel, especially considering that the triglyceride level may be inaccurate otherwise [95]. In situations where a blood test is conducted under non-fasting conditions, the measurement of non-HDL-c (the mathematical difference between total cholesterol and HDL-c) can provide guidance for further investigations. If the non-HDL-c value exceeds the normal range, obtaining a fasting lipid panel promptly is recommended [2, 95]. The cutoff criteria for lipid fractions, adapted from the National Heart, Lung, and Blood Institute (NHLBI) guidelines [95], are presented in **Table 2**. It is important to note that cut-off values for triglycerides vary across age groups.

Lipid fraction		Low	Normal	Borderline high	High
Total cholesterol (mg/dl)		—	<170	170–199	≥200
LDL-c (mg/dl)		—	<110	110–129	≥130
HDL-c (mg/dl)		<40	>45	—	—
non-HDL-c (mg/dl)		—	<120	120–144	≥145
Triglycerides(mg/dl)	< 9 years old	—	<75	75–99	≥100
	10–19 years old	—	<90	90–129	≥130

Table 2.
At risk and diagnostic values for dyslipidemia adapted from the NHLBI criteria [95].

Parameters such as the ratio of triglycerides to HDL-c or the ratio of total cholesterol to HDL-c also provide valuable insights into the assessment of dyslipidemia. The total cholesterol-to-HDL-c ratio is recognized as a robust predictor of ischemic coronary events, owing to its ability to capture the metabolic disturbances commonly observed in individuals with abdominal obesity, insulin resistance, and dyslipidemia. Consequently, its predictive efficacy is particularly pronounced in individuals exhibiting all these factors [106]. In the case of children, the triglyceride-to-HDL-c ratio may prove to be an even more effective predictor of cardiometabolic risk and insulin resistance compared to the traditional metabolic syndrome status. Numerous studies have suggested its superior predictive ability in this context [104, 105, 107].

9.3 Metabolic dysfunction-associated steatotic liver disease

Non-alcoholic fatty liver disease (NAFLD) is a complex and progressive condition influenced by factors like obesity, insulin resistance, and genetics [108]. With rising rates of obesity and diabetes, NAFLD has become the most common chronic liver disease in both adults and children (prevalent in nearly 80% of obese children), posing a significant global health concern due to its impact on cardio-metabolic health. It extends beyond a liver-specific ailment, representing a manifestation of a broader systemic metabolic disorder [108, 109]. Associations between NAFLD and cardio-metabolic abnormalities have been identified, even in childhood. In 2020, the term "metabolic-associated fatty liver disease" (MAFLD) was proposed as a new term for NAFLD [110, 111] to update the terminology according to today's standards: In June 2023, a consensus from multiple liver disease societies, including the American Association for the Study of Liver Diseases, introduced the new terminology: metabolic dysfunction-associated steatotic liver disease (MASLD) [112].

To diagnose MASLD, hepatic steatosis must be present (imagistic evidence), along with criteria such as weight excess, type 2 diabetes mellitus, or suggestive metabolic alterations [112, 113]. The association between hepatic steatosis and metabolic syndrome is mutual and bidirectional [114]. Studies have demonstrated connections between MASLD and early carotid atherosclerosis, with the presence of MASLD increasing cardiovascular risk, independent of traditional factors, especially in patients with type 2 diabetes. Liver fibrosis stage is an independent predictor of carotid intima-media thickness, confirming a strong connection between hepatic steatosis and both subclinical atherosclerosis and major cardiovascular events over the past two decades [115, 116].

9.3.1 Practical aspects

MASLD is characterized by elevated ALT and AST enzymes. Screening is recommended for all obese children aged nine or older, and those with personal or familial risk factors should also consider it. Initial screening with ALT, interpreted using sex-specific reference ranges, is advised. A sex-specific ALT over twice the upper limit showed 88% sensitivity for detecting MASLD, with specificity at 26% [117–120].

Metabolic dysfunction-associated steatohepatitis (MASH) is more common in obese children with ALT levels above 80 U/L. Further evaluation is recommended for those with ALT over 80 U/L [117–120]. Ultrasound is cost-effective but less sensitive for early-stage steatosis. European guidelines recognize it for screening obese children with elevated ALT or signs of insulin resistance [121].

Elastography assesses liver stiffness, with >9 kilopascals indicating advanced fibrosis. Biomarkers and scoring systems lack validation in children [122].

Magnetic resonance proton density fat fraction helps differentiate hepatic steatosis grades, but validation is pending for children [117].

9.4 Polycystic ovaries syndrome

Polycystic ovaries syndrome (PCOS), prevalent in young women of reproductive age, is often associated with obesity [123, 124]. Adolescents with PCOS and obesity commonly experience hyperinsulinemia, insulin resistance, and hyperandrogenism, with a reciprocal relationship between elevated androgen levels and insulin issues [125]. Hirsutism and acanthosis nigricans are more common in these cases [126]. Diagnosing PCOS in adolescents is challenging due to the lack of universally defined criteria. Fundamental criteria include unexplained ovulatory dysfunction and signs of hyperandrogenism. Menstrual irregularities and hirsutism are key indicators. Mild hirsutism is now considered sufficient evidence, and severe inflammatory acne may also prompt testing [127].

Biomarkers like anti-Müllerian hormone or testosterone-to-dihydrotestosterone ratio can be evaluated but are not standalone diagnostic criteria [127, 128].

Obesity in adolescence is linked to PCOS development in adulthood, as revealed by a longitudinal study showing increased likelihood of menstrual disorders and hirsutism in adulthood for those overweight or obese at age 14 [129]. PCOS is associated with an elevated risk of cardiovascular disease [130, 131], leading to increased risks of hypertension, type 2 diabetes, dyslipidemia, and non-fatal cerebrovascular events compared to those without PCOS [131]. Hyperandrogenism and hyperinsulinemia impact body mass distribution and glucose balance, contributing to an increased risk of coronary artery disease [132].

9.5 Disruptions of gut microbiota

The gut microbiota primarily includes five phyla: Bacteroidetes, Firmicutes, Actinobacteria, Proteobacteria, and Verrucomicrobia. Anaerobic Bacteroidetes and Firmicutes, constituting over 90% of bacterial species in a healthy gut, play roles in breaking down polysaccharides, regulating calorie absorption, and producing short-chain fatty acids for cardiovascular health [133].

Early-life factors like birth conditions, delivery mode, perinatal colonization, and family exposure shape gut microbiota composition, impacting immune and metabolic functions. Imbalances can contribute to conditions such as obesity, atherosclerosis, and cardiovascular diseases by influencing insulin resistance and fat accumulation [133].

Studies suggest that obese individuals often exhibit reduced gut microbiota diversity, with a higher proportion of Bacteroidetes and Firmicutes, contributing to enhanced energy extraction from food and potential mechanisms of hunger regulation. A low Bacteroidetes-to-Firmicutes ratio is linked to obesity, as observed in intervention studies with high-calorie diets [129, 131, 134–136].

The gut microbiota's specific composition has implications for obesity, insulin resistance, and type 2 diabetes mellitus, as evident in studies on germ-free mice. Additionally, connections have been identified between gut microbiota, inflammation, and various conditions like cancer, autoimmune disorders, and cardiovascular disease. Metabolites produced by the gut microbiome, including trimethylamin N-oxide (TMAO), may influence platelet hyper-reactivity and enhance thrombotic potential, suggesting a role in arterial disease [137, 138]. However, conclusive evidence on the associations with atherosclerotic and thrombotic components remains challenging, emphasizing the need for mechanistic investigations.

TMAO is derived from dietary sources like red meat, poultry, eggs, milk, and whole grains, containing precursors such as choline, L-carnitine, γ-butyrobetaine, trimethyllysine, betaine, and δ-valerobetaine. Upon digestion, these precursors are absorbed through the intestinal mucosa and metabolized by gut microbiota into trimethylamine, further oxidized in the liver to form TMAO [139–142]. The composition of the predominant gut microbiota, including Bacteroidetes, Firmicutes, Proteobacteria, and Fusobacteria, influences TMAO production, with modifications achievable through probiotics or antibiotics [143–145].

Elevated TMAO levels are observed in individuals with metabolic disorders, including obesity, type 2 diabetes mellitus [146], MAFLD [147], chronic kidney disease [148], and gastrointestinal cancers [149]. However, the precise mechanisms through which TMAO contributes to oxidative, osmotic, and hydrostatic stress are only partially understood. TMAO influences hepatic glucose metabolism, gluconeogenesis, hepatic glucose transport, and insulin resistance. It also affects vascular health by disturbing bile acid metabolism, inhibiting reverse cholesterol transport, inducing foam cell formation, activating platelets, and promoting oxidative stress and vascular inflammation [150–155].

Animal model studies reveal complex metabolic associations between TMAO and insulin resistance, atherosclerosis, and cardio-metabolic diseases, emphasizing the link between diet, gut microbiota changes, and these conditions [156–158]. In human adults, TMAO and its precursors are implicated in disorders related to insulin resistance, atherosclerosis, chronic kidney disease, cardiovascular disorders, MAFLD, psoriasis, cancer, and Alzheimer's disease [159–162].

However, limited data exist on the role of TMAO in children. Existing studies primarily focus on establishing links between TMAO levels (or its precursors) and dietary habits in children, with sparse research connecting TMAO to specific pathologies [163, 164]. Notably, a study on prepubertal obese children demonstrated that lifestyle interventions resulting in weight loss significantly reduced TMAO levels [165]. Compelling evidence that supports the connections between TMAO, obesity, and early vascular damage in children has been recently published [166]. The elevated TMAO levels observed in obese children suggest its potential as a biomarker for obesity. Furthermore, the positive correlations found between TMAO and CIMT, along with markers of arterial stiffness, underscore the adverse vascular effects of TMAO. These findings highlight the necessity for further research to unravel the underlying mechanisms and investigate TMAO as a potential target for addressing vascular issues associated with obesity. A comprehensive understanding of TMAO's role in obesity-related cardiovascular risk could inform tailored interventions for cardio-metabolic conditions in young individuals grappling with obesity [166].

10. Conclusions and future perspectives

Childhood obesity not only exacerbates arterial stiffness and subclinical atherosclerosis but also significantly heightens the risk of early-onset cardiovascular disorders in adulthood. In the assessment of vascular health in obese children, clinical markers like waist circumference and waist-to-height ratio play pivotal roles. Notably, insulin-resistant obese children are particularly susceptible to heightened arterial stiffness and subclinical atherosclerosis [167].

Risk factors such as excessive weight gain, smoking overall metabolic disturbances during pregnancy, family history of cardiovascular risk, and high blood pressure are linked to elevated CIMT in obese children. Reliable correlations with CIMT are observed in the lipid profile and lipid ratios, while fasting glucose does not show such associations [168]. Moreover, excessive weight-gain during pregnancy, exposure to cigarette smoke (both passive and active smoking), insufficient sleep, and sedentary behavior have been shown to aggravate arterial stiffness, an intermediate stage of early atherosclerosis [169, 170].

CIMT, arterial stiffness biomarkers and even metabolites such as TMAO offer valuable insights for clinicians managing the care of obese children. Understanding the mechanisms leading to irreversible cardiovascular damage in these patients, especially when preventable, becomes a critical undertaking. It is crucial to enhance our understanding of the metabolic and cardiovascular condition in children with obesity to effectively mitigate future cardiovascular risks. Evaluating vascular damage from childhood can significantly contribute to the management of future adults with cardiometabolic disorders. Additionally, measuring these markers facilitates communication among doctors, parents, and patients, promoting awareness of the risks associated with obesity and improving the effectiveness of actions necessary for weight loss.

11. Conclusions

Childhood obesity exacerbates the progression of subclinical atherosclerosis and arterial stiffness. Carotid intima-media thickness, serving as a marker for atherosclerosis, proves to be a valuable non-invasive tool for assessing early vascular damage in obese children. Serum trimethylamine N-oxide emerges as an intriguing biomarker with potential implications for addressing obesity-related vascular issues, given its associations with weight excess and vascular surrogate markers.

The critical objective lies in understanding how these patients undergo irreversible vascular damage, particularly when preventable, making early detection and intervention pivotal in averting further complications.

Acknowledgements

We express our gratitude to the authorship of this chapter for their valuable contributions and extend our appreciation to our affiliated centers for their support in facilitating this research. We would like to acknowledge VICTOR BABES UNIVERSITY OF MEDICINE AND PHARMACY TIMISOARA for their support in covering the costs of publication for this chapter.

Conflict of interest

The authors declare no conflict of interest.

Acronyms and abbreviations

ALT	alanine aminotransferase
AST	aspartate aminotransferase
BMI	body mass index
CDC	centers for disease control and prevention
CIMT	carotid intima-media thickness
H	height
HbA1c	glycosylated hemoglobin
HDL-c	high-density lipoprotein cholesterol
HOMA-IR	homeostatic model assessment for insulin resistance
IR	insulin resistance
LDL-c	low-density lipoprotein cholesterol
MAFLD	metabolic-associated fatty liver disease
MetS	metabolic syndrome
NAFLD	non-alcoholic fatty liver disease
NASH	non-alcoholic steatohepatitis
NHLBI	The National Heart, Lung, and Blood Institute
OGTT	oral glucose tolerance test
PCOS	polycystic ovary syndrome
TC	total cholesterol
TMAO	trimethylamine N-oxide
TyG	triglyceride-glucose index
VAI	Visceral Adiposity Index

Author details

Monica Simina Mihuta[1], Corina Paul[2]*, Andreea Borlea[3], Cristina Mihaela Roi[4], Denisa Pescari[4] and Dana Liana Stoian[3]

1 Center of Molecular Research in Nephrology and Vascular Disease, Faculty of Medicine, Victor Babes University of Medicine and Pharmacy, Timisoara, Romania

2 Department of Pediatrics, Victor Babes University of Medicine and Pharmacy, Timisoara, Romania

3 2nd Department of Internal Medicine and Center of Molecular Research in Nephrology and Vascular Disease, Victor Babes University of Medicine and Pharmacy, Timisoara, Romania

4 Department of Doctoral Studies and Center of Molecular Research in Nephrology and Vascular Disease, Victor Babes University of Medicine and Pharmacy, Timisoara, Romania

*Address all correspondence to: paul.corina@umft.ro

References

[1] Haslam DW, James WP. Obesity. Lancet. 2005;**366**(9492):1197-1209. DOI: 10.1016/S0140-6736(05)67483-1

[2] Hampl SE, Hassink SG, Skinner AC, Armstrong SC, Barlow SE, Bolling CF, et al. Clinical practice guideline for the evaluation and treatment of children and adolescents with obesity. Pediatrics. 1 Feb 2023;**151**(2):13-14

[3] Ogden CL, Freedman DS, Hales CM. CDC extended BMI-for-age percentiles versus percent of the 95th percentile. Pediatrics. 2023;**152**:1-3

[4] Anderson LN, Carsley S, Lebovic G, Borkhoff CM, Maguire JL, Parkin PC, et al. Misclassification of child body mass index from cut-points defined by rounded percentiles instead of Z-scores. BMC Research Notes. 2017;**10**(1):639

[5] WHO Regional Office for Europe. Report on the fifth round of data collection, 2018-2020: WHO European childhood obesity surveillance initiative (COSI). [Internet]. In: World Health Organization, editor. European Childhood Obesity Surveillance Initiative, Office for Prevention & Control of NCDs (MOS). Editors: Copenhagen: Regional Office for Europe; 2022. Available from: https://apps.who.int/iris/bitstream/handle/10665/353747/9789289057738-eng.pdf [Accessed: January 28, 2024]

[6] Stierman B, Afful J, Carroll MD, Chen TC, Davy O, Fink S, et al. National Health and Nutrition Examination Survey 2017–March 2020 Prepandemic Data Files—Development of Files and Prevalence Estimates for Selected Health Outcomes. National Health Statistics Reports; No 158. Hyattsville, MD: National Center for Health Statistics; 2021

[7] Lange SJ, Kompaniyets L, Freedman DS, Kraus EM, Porter R, Blanck HM, et al. Longitudinal trends in body mass index before and during the COVID-19 pandemic among persons aged 2-19 years — United States, 2018-2020. MMWR. Morbidity and Mortality Weekly Report. 2021;**70**(37):1278-1283

[8] Janssen I, Katzmarzyk PT, Boyce WF, et al. Comparison of overweight and obesity prevalence in school-aged youth from 34 countries and their relationships with physical activity and dietary patterns. Obesity Reviews. 2005;**6**:123

[9] GBD 2015 Obesity Collaborators, Afshin A, Forouzanfar MH, et al. Health effects of overweight and obesity in 195 countries over 25 years. The New England Journal of Medicine. 2017;**377**:13

[10] World Obesity Federation. World Obesity Atlas 2024. London: World Obesity Federation; 2024. Available from: https://data.worldobesity.org/publications/?cat=22

[11] Yoo S. Dynamic Energy Balance and Obesity Prevention. Journal of Obesity & Metabolic Syndrome. 2018;**27**(4):203-212

[12] Duffey KJ, Gordon-Larsen P, Jacobs DR, Williams OD, Popkin BM. Differential associations of fast food and restaurant food consumption with 3-y change in body mass index: The coronary artery risk development in young adults study. The American Journal of Clinical Nutrition. 2007;**85**(1):201-208

[13] Obri A, Claret M. The role of epigenetics in hypothalamic energy balance control: Implications for obesity. Cell Stress. 2019;**3**(7):208-220

[14] Fitzgerald MP, Hennigan K, O'Gorman CS, McCarron L. Obesity, diet and lifestyle in 9-year-old children with parentally reported chronic diseases: Findings from the growing up in Ireland longitudinal child cohort study. Irish Journal of Medical Science (1971-). 2019;**188**(1):29-34

[15] Romero-Ibarguengoitia ME, Vadillo-Ortega F, Caballero AE, Ibarra-González I, Herrera-Rosas A, Serratos-Canales MF, et al. Family history and obesity in youth, their effect on acylcarnitine/aminoacids metabolomics and non-alcoholic fatty liver disease (NAFLD). Structural equation modeling approach. PLoS One. 2018;**13**(2):e0193138

[16] Balasundaram P, Krishna S. Obesity effects on child health. In: StatPearls [Internet]. Treasure Island, FL, USA: StatPearls Publishing; 2022. Available from: https://www.ncbi.nlm.nih.gov/books/NBK570613/ [Accessed: January 28, 2024]

[17] Velea IP, Albulescu R, Arghirescu ST. Obezitatea la copil. In: Velea IP, editor. Pediatrie-Curs pentru Studentii Facultatii de Medicina. Timisoara, Romania: Editura Victor Babes; 2016. pp. 289-297

[18] Hale PM, Cushman TT, Kimball ES, Nair A, Shaffer RG. Secondary causes of obesity in childhood. In: Ferry R Jr, editor. Management of Pediatric Obesity and Diabetes Nutrition and Health. Totowa, NJ, USA: Humana Press; 2011

[19] Soliman A, Yasin M, Kassem A. Leptin in pediatrics: A hormone from adipocyte that wheels several functions in children. Indian Journal of Endocrinology and Metabolism. 2012;**16**(9):577

[20] Warner M, Wesselink A, Harley KG, Bradman A, Kogut K, Eskenazi B. Prenatal exposure to dichlorodiphenyltrichloroethane and obesity at 9 years of age in the CHAMACOS study cohort. American Journal of Epidemiology. 2014;**179**(11):1312-1322

[21] Lustig RH, Collier D, Kassotis C, Roepke TA, Kim MJ, Blanc E, et al. Obesity I: Overview and molecular and biochemical mechanisms. Biochemical Pharmacology. 2022;**199**:115012

[22] Bliss ES, Whiteside E. The gut-brain axis, the human gut microbiota and their integration in the development of obesity. Frontiers in Physiology. 12 Jul 2018;**9**:900

[23] Torres-Fuentes C, Schellekens H, Dinan TG, Cryan JF. The microbiota–gut–brain axis in obesity. The Lancet Gastroenterology & Hepatology. 2017;**2**(10):747-756

[24] Kim KN, Yao Y, Ju SY. Short chain fatty acids and fecal microbiota abundance in humans with obesity: A systematic review and meta-analysis. Nutrients. 2019;**11**(10):2512

[25] Majka SM, Barak Y, Klemm DJ. Concise review: Adipocyte origins: Weighing the possibilities. Stem Cells. 2011;**29**(7):1034-1040

[26] Coppack SW. Adipose tissue changes in obesity. Biochemical Society Transactions. 2005;**33**(5):1049-1052

[27] Després JP, Lemieux I. Abdominal obesity and metabolic syndrome. Nature. 2006;**444**(7121):881-887

[28] Spalding KL, Arner E, Westermark PO, Bernard S, Buchholz BA, Bergmann O, et al. Dynamics of fat cell turnover in humans. Nature. 2008;**453**(7196):783-787

[29] Martos-Moreno GÁ, Barrios V, Martínez G, Hawkins F, Argente J. Effect

of weight loss on high-molecular weight adiponectin in obese children. Obesity. 2010;**18**(12):2288-2294

[30] Rupérez FJ, Martos-Moreno GÁ, Chamoso-Sánchez D, Barbas C, Argente J. Insulin resistance in obese children: What can metabolomics and adipokine modelling contribute? Nutrients. 2020;**12**(11):3310

[31] Sone M, Osamura RY. Leptin and the pituitary. Pituitary. 2001;**4**(1/2):15-23

[32] Nishimura R, Sano H, Matsudaira T, Miyashita Y, Morimoto A, Shirasawa T, et al. Childhood obesity and its relation to serum adiponectin and leptin: A report from a population-based study. Diabetes Research and Clinical Practice. 2007;**76**(2):245-250

[33] Jeffery AN, Murphy MJ, Metcalf BS, Hosking J, Voss LD, English P, et al. Adiponectin in childhood. International Journal of Pediatric Obesity. 2008;**3**(3):130-140

[34] Cirulli ET, Guo L, Leon Swisher C, Shah N, Huang L, Napier LA, et al. Profound perturbation of the metabolome in obesity is associated with health risk. Cell Metabolism. 2019;**29**(2):488-500.e2

[35] Menni C, Migaud M, Kastenmüller G, Pallister T, Zierer J, Peters A, et al. Metabolomic profiling of long-term weight change: Role of oxidative stress and urate levels in weight gain. Obesity. 2017;**25**(9):1618-1624

[36] Caleyachetty R, Thomas GN, Toulis KA, Mohammed N, Gokhale KM, Balachandran K, et al. Metabolically healthy obese and incident cardiovascular disease events among 3.5 million men and women. Journal of the American College of Cardiology. 2017;**70**(12):1429-1437

[37] Zaman AG, Helft G, Worthley SG, Badimon JJ. The role of plaque rupture and thrombosis in coronary artery disease. Atherosclerosis. 2000;**149**(2):251-266

[38] Powell-Wiley TM, Poirier P, Burke LE, Després JP, Gordon-Larsen P, Lavie CJ, et al. Obesity and cardiovascular disease: A scientific statement from the American Heart Association. Circulation. 25 May 2021;**143**(21):e984-e1010

[39] Harris RA, Nishiyama SK, Wray DW, Richardson RS. Ultrasound assessment of flow-mediated dilation. Hypertension. 2010;**55**(5):1075-1085

[40] Green D. Point: Flow-mediated dilation does reflect nitric oxide-mediated endothelial function. Journal of Applied Physiology. 2005;**99**(3):1233-1234

[41] Lacolley P, Regnault V, Laurent S. Mechanisms of arterial stiffening. Arteriosclerosis, Thrombosis, and Vascular Biology. 2020;**40**(5):1055-1062

[42] Laurent S, Boutouyrie P. The structural factor of hypertension. Circulation Research. 2015;**116**(6): 1007-1021

[43] Bornfeldt KE, Tabas I. Insulin resistance, hyperglycemia, and atherosclerosis. Cell Metabolism. 2011;**14**(5):575-585

[44] Zieske AW, Malcom GT, Strong JP. Natural history and risk factors of atherosclerosis in children and youth: The Pday study. Pediatric Pathology & Molecular Medicine. 2002;**21**(2):213-237

[45] Shirwany NA, Zou M, hui. Arterial stiffness: A brief review. Acta Pharmacologica Sinica. 2010;**31**(10):1267-1276

[46] Zieman SJ, Melenovsky V, Kass DA. Mechanisms, pathophysiology, and therapy of arterial stiffness. Arteriosclerosis, Thrombosis, and Vascular Biology. 2005;**25**(5):932-943

[47] Wolinsky H, Glagov S. Structural basis for the static mechanical properties of the aortic media. Circulation Research. 1964;**14**(5):400-413

[48] Tounian P, Aggoun Y, Dubern B, Varille V, Guy-Grand B, Sidi D, et al. Presence of increased stiffness of the common carotid artery and endothelial dysfunction in severely obese children: A prospective study. The Lancet. 2001;**358**(9291):1400-1404

[49] Toth PP. Subclinical atherosclerosis: What it is, what it means and what we can do about it. International Journal of Clinical Practice. 2008;**62**(8):1246-1254

[50] Hansson GK. Inflammation, atherosclerosis, and coronary artery disease. New England Journal of Medicine. 2005;**352**(16):1685-1695

[51] Al-Shorman A, Al-Domi H, Faqih A. Markers of subclinical atherosclerosis in schoolchildren with obesity and metabolic syndrome. Swiss Medical Weekly. 30 Dec 2020;**147**:w14446

[52] Al-Shorman A, AlKhatib B, Abusalma B, Al-Domi H. The association between fat mass and subclinical atherosclerosis in healthy schoolchildren. Clinical Nutrition ESPEN. 2020;**37**:87-92

[53] Abraham TM, Pedley A, Massaro JM, Hoffmann U, Fox CS. Association between visceral and subcutaneous adipose depots and incident cardiovascular disease risk factors. Circulation. 2015;**132**(17):1639-1647

[54] Beauloye V, Zech F, Tran Thi Mong H, Clapuyt P, Maes M, Brichard SM. Determinants of early atherosclerosis in obese children and adolescents. The Journal of Clinical Endocrinology and Metabolism. 2007;**92**(8):3025-3032

[55] Farello G, Antenucci A, Stagi S, Mazzocchetti C, Ciocca F, Verrotti A. Metabolically healthy and metabolically unhealthy obese children both have increased carotid intima media thickness: A case control study. BMC Cardiovascular Disorders. 2018;**18**(1):140

[56] van den Oord SCH, Sijbrands EJG, ten Kate GL, van Klaveren D, van Domburg RT, van der Steen AFW, et al. Carotid intima-media thickness for cardiovascular risk assessment: Systematic review and meta-analysis. Atherosclerosis. 2013;**228**(1):1-11

[57] Qiu H, Zhu Y, Sun Z, Trzeciakowski JP, Gansner M, Depre C, et al. Short communication: Vascular smooth muscle cell stiffness As a mechanism for increased aortic stiffness with aging. Circulation Research. 2010;**107**(5):615-619

[58] Patro Golab B, Santos S, Voerman E, Lawlor DA, Jaddoe VWV, Gaillard R, et al. Influence of maternal obesity on the association between common pregnancy complications and risk of childhood obesity: An individual participant data meta-analysis. The Lancet. Child & Adolescent Health. 2018;**2**(11):812-821

[59] Crispi F, Miranda J, Gratacós E. Long-term cardiovascular consequences of fetal growth restriction: Biology, clinical implications, and opportunities for prevention of adult disease. American Journal of Obstetrics and Gynecology. 2018;**218**(2):S869-S879

[60] Di Bernardo S, Mivelaz Y, Epure AM, Vial Y, Simeoni U, Bovet P,

et al. Assessing the consequences of gestational diabetes mellitus on offspring's cardiovascular health: MySweetHeart cohort study protocol, Switzerland. BMJ Open. 2017;7:e016972

[61] Benschop L, Schalekamp-Timmermans S, Roeters van Lennep JE, Jaddoe VWV, Steegers EAP, Ikram MK. Cardiovascular risk factors track from mother to child. Journal of the American Heart Association. 2 Oct 2018;**7**(19):S18

[62] Jølving LR, Nielsen J, Kesmodel US, Nielsen R, Norgard BM, Beck-Nielsen SS. Chronic diseases in the children of women with maternal thyroid dysfunction: A nationwide cohort study. Clinical Epidemiology. 2018;**10**:1381-1390

[63] İşgüven P, Gündüz Y, Kılıç M. Effects of thyroid autoimmunity on early atherosclerosis in Euthyroid girls with Hashimoto's thyroiditis. Journal of Clinical Research in Pediatric Endocrinology. 2016;**8**(2):150-156

[64] Belbasis L, Savvidou MD, Kanu C, Evangelou E, Tzoulaki I. Birth weight in relation to health and disease in later life: An umbrella review of systematic reviews and metaanalyses. BMC Medicine. 2016;**14**(1):147

[65] Oddy WH, Mori TA, Huang RC, Marsh JA, Pennell CE, Chivers PT, et al. Early infant feeding and adiposity risk: From infancy to adulthood. Annals of Nutrition & Metabolism. 2014;**64**(3-4):262-270

[66] de Giorgis T, Giannini C, Scarinci A, D'Adamo E, Agostinelli S, Chiarelli F, et al. Family history of premature cardiovascular disease as a sole and independent risk factor for increased carotid intima–media thickness. Journal of Hypertension. 2009;**27**(4):822-828

[67] Li S, Yun M, Fernandez C, Xu J, Srinivasan SR, Chen W, et al. Cigarette smoking exacerbates the adverse effects of age and metabolic syndrome on subclinical atherosclerosis: The Bogalusa Heart study. PLoS One. 2014;**9**(5):e96368

[68] Khalil A, Huffman MD, Prabhakaran D, Osmond C, Fall CHD, Tandon N, et al. Predictors of carotid intima–media thickness and carotid plaque in young Indian adults: The New Delhi Birth Cohort. International Journal of Cardiology. 2013;**167**(4):1322-1328

[69] da Silva AC, do Carmo AS, dos Santos LC. Associations between sleep practices and social behavior of children and adolescents: A systematic review. Journal of Public Health (Bangkok). 2022;**30**(5):1101-1112

[70] Bots ML, Hofman A, De Jong PTVM, Grobbee DE. Common carotid intima-media thickness as an indicator of atherosclerosis at other sites of the carotid artery the Rotterdam study. Annals of Epidemiology. 1996;**6**(2):147-153

[71] Downing R, Michael T, Place R, Hoffman E, Visich P. The influence of metabolic syndrome risk factors on carotid intima media thickness in children. Global Pediatric Health. 2021;**8**:2333794X2098745

[72] Zhang Y, Guallar E, Qiao Y, Wasserman BA. Is carotid intima-media thickness as predictive as other noninvasive techniques for the detection of coronary artery disease? Arteriosclerosis, Thrombosis, and Vascular Biology. 2014;**34**(7):1341-1345

[73] Rudd JHF, Narula J, Strauss HW, Virmani R, Machac J, Klimas M, et al. Imaging atherosclerotic plaque inflammation by fluorodeoxyglucose with positron emission tomography.

Journal of the American College of Cardiology. 2010;**55**(23):2527-2535

[74] Vanoli D, Wiklund U, Lindqvist P, Henein M, Naslund U. Successful novice's training in obtaining accurate assessment of carotid IMT using an automated ultrasound system. European Heart Journal Cardiovascular Imaging. 2014;**15**(6):637-642

[75] Gómez-Marcos MA, Recio-Rodríguez JI, Patino-Alonso MC, Agudo-Conde C, Gómez-Sanchez L, Gómez-Sanchez M, et al. Protocol for measuring carotid intima-media thickness that best correlates with cardiovascular risk and target organ damage. American Journal of Hypertension. 2012;**25**(9):955-961

[76] Polak JF, Meisner A, Pencina MJ, Wolf PA, D'Agostino RB. Variations in common carotid artery intima-media thickness during the cardiac cycle: Implications for cardiovascular risk assessment. Journal of the American Society of Echocardiography. 2012;**25**(9):1023-1028

[77] Vermeersch SJ, Rietzschel ER, De Buyzere ML, Van Bortel LM, D'Asseler Y, Gillebert TC, et al. Validation of a new automated IMT measurement algorithm. Journal of Human Hypertension. 2007;**21**(12):976-978

[78] Meiburger KM, Zahnd G, Faita F, Loizou CP, Carvalho C, Steinman DA, et al. Carotid ultrasound boundary study (CUBS): An open multicenter analysis of computerized intima–media thickness measurement systems and their clinical impact. Ultrasound in Medicine & Biology. 2021;**47**(8):2442-2455

[79] Tagi VM, Chiarelli F. Obesity and insulin resistance in children. Current Opinion in Pediatrics. 2020;**32**(4):582-588

[80] Chiarelli F, Marcovecchio ML. Insulin resistance and obesity in childhood. European Journal of Endocrinology. 2008;**159**(Suppl. 1):S67-S74

[81] DeFronzo RA. From the triumvirate to the ominous octet: A new paradigm for the treatment of type 2 diabetes mellitus. Diabetes. 2009;**58**(4):773-795

[82] Weiss R, Dufour S, Taksali SE, Tamborlane WV, Petersen KF, Bonadonna RC, et al. Prediabetes in obese youth: A syndrome of impaired glucose tolerance, severe insulin resistance, and altered myocellular and abdominal fat partitioning. The Lancet. 2003;**362**(9388):951-957

[83] Bergman RN, Iyer MS. Indirect regulation of endogenous glucose production by insulin: The single gateway hypothesis revisited. Diabetes. 2017;**66**(7):1742-1747

[84] Sivitz WI, Yorek MA. Mitochondrial dysfunction in diabetes: From molecular mechanisms to functional significance and therapeutic opportunities. Antioxidants & Redox Signaling. 2010;**12**(4):537-577

[85] Semenkovich CF. Insulin resistance and atherosclerosis. Journal of Clinical Investigation. 2006;**116**(7):1813-1822

[86] Amer DA. Diagnosis and classification of diabetes mellitus American Diabetes Association. Diabetes Care. 2011;**34**:S62-S69

[87] Chakarova N, Dimova R, Grozeva G, Tankova T. Assessment of glucose variability in subjects with prediabetes. Diabetes Research and Clinical Practice. 2019;**151**:56-64

[88] Roman R, Zeitler PS. Oral glucose tolerance testing in asymptomatic obese

children: More questions than answers. The Journal of Clinical Endocrinology and Metabolism. 2008;**93**(11):4228-4230

[89] Love-Osborne KA, Sheeder J, Svircev A, Chan C, Zeitler P, Nadeau KJ. Use of glycosylated hemoglobin increases diabetes screening for at-risk adolescents in primary care settings. Pediatric Diabetes. 2013;**14**(7):512-518

[90] Matthews DR, Hosker JP, Rudenski AS, Naylor BA, Treacher DF, Turner RC. Homeostasis model assessment: Insulin resistance and beta-cell function from fasting plasma glucose and insulin concentrations in man. Diabetologia. 1985;**28**(7):412-419

[91] Vizzuso S, Del Torto A, Dilillo D, Calcaterra V, Di Profio E, Leone A, et al. Visceral adiposity index (VAI) in children and adolescents with obesity: No association with daily energy intake but promising tool to identify metabolic syndrome (MetS). Nutrients. 2021;**13**(2):413

[92] Shashaj B, Luciano R, Contoli B, Morino GS, Spreghini MR, Rustico C, et al. Reference ranges of HOMA-IR in normal-weight and obese young Caucasians. Acta Diabetologica. 2016;**53**(2):251-260

[93] Amato MC, Giordano C, Galia M, Criscimanna A, Vitabile S, Midiri M, et al. Visceral adiposity index. Diabetes Care. 2010;**33**(4):920-922

[94] Nayak SS, Kuriyakose D, Polisetty LD, et al. Diagnostic and prognostic value of triglyceride glucose index: A comprehensive evaluation of meta-analysis. Cardiovascular Diabetology. 2024;**23**:310. DOI: 10.1186/s12933-024-02392-y

[95] National Heart L, BI. Expert panel on integrated guidelines for cardiovascular health and risk reduction in children and adolescents: Summary report. Pediatrics. 2011;**128**(Suppl. 5):S213-S256

[96] Jolliffe CJ, Janssen I. Distribution of lipoproteins by age and gender in adolescents. Circulation. 2006;**114**(10):1056-1062

[97] Dai S, Yang Q, Yuan K, Loustalot F, Fang J, Daniels SR, et al. Non–high-density lipoprotein cholesterol: Distribution and prevalence of high serum levels in children and adolescents: United States National Health and nutrition examination surveys, 2005-2010. The Journal of Pediatrics. 2014;**164**(2):247-253

[98] Kit BK, Carroll MD, Lacher DA, Sorlie PD, DeJesus JM, CyntjL O. Trends in serum lipids among US youths aged 6 to 19 years, 1988-2010. Journal of the American Medical Association. 8 Aug 2012;**308**(6):591-600

[99] Cook S, Kavey REW. Dyslipidemia and pediatric obesity. Pediatric Clinics of North America. 2011;**58**(6):1363-1373

[100] Hatami M, Tohidi M, Mohebi R, Khalili D, Azizi F, Hadaegh F. Adolescent lipoprotein classifications according to National Health and Nutrition examination survey (NHANES) vs. National Cholesterol Education Program (NCEP) for predicting abnormal lipid levels in adulthood in a Middle East population. Lipids in Health and Disease. 2012;**11**(1):107

[101] Kosmas CE, Martinez I, Sourlas A, Bouza KV, Campos FN, Torres V, et al. High-density lipoprotein (HDL) functionality and its relevance to atherosclerotic cardiovascular disease. Drugs Context. 2018;**7**:1-9

[102] Frontini MG, Srinivasan SR, Xu J, Tang R, Bond MG, Berenson GS.

Usefulness of childhood non–high density lipoprotein cholesterol levels versus other lipoprotein measures in predicting adult subclinical atherosclerosis: The Bogalusa Heart Study. Pediatrics. 2008;**121**(5):924-929

[103] Boullart ACI, de Graaf J, Stalenhoef AF. Serum triglycerides and risk of cardiovascular disease. Biochimica et Biophysica Acta (BBA) - Molecular and Cell Biology of Lipids. 2012;**1821**(5):867-875

[104] Krawczyk M, Rumińska M, Witkowska- Sędek E, Majcher A, Pyrżak B. Usefulness of the triglycerides to high-density lipoprotein cholesterol ratio (TG/HDL-C) in prediction of metabolic syndrome in polish obese children and adolescents. Acta Biochimica Polonica. 19 Nov 2018;**65**(4):605-611

[105] Nur Zati Iwani AK, Jalaludin MY, Wan Mohd Zin RM, Fuziah MZ, Hong JYH, Abqariyah Y, et al. TG: HDL-C ratio is a good marker to identify children affected by obesity with increased cardiometabolic risk and insulin resistance. International Journal of Endocrinology. 2019;**2019**:1-9

[106] Lemieux I, Lamarche B, Couillard C, Pascot A, Cantin B, Bergeron J, et al. Total cholesterol/HDL cholesterol ratio vs LDL cholesterol/HDL cholesterol ratio as indices of ischemic heart disease risk in men. Archives of Internal Medicine. 2001;**161**(22):2685

[107] Iwani NAKZ, Jalaludin MY, Zin RMWM, Fuziah MZ, Hong JYH, Abqariyah Y, et al. Triglyceride to HDL-C ratio is associated with insulin resistance in overweight and obese children. Scientific Reports. 2017;**7**(1):40055

[108] Castillo-Leon E, Cioffi CE, Vos MB. Perspectives on youth-onset nonalcoholic fatty liver disease. Endocrinology, Diabetes and Metabolism. 17 Oct 2020;**3**(4):e00184

[109] Morandi A, Di Sessa A, Zusi C, Umano GR, El Mazloum D, Fornari E, et al. Nonalcoholic fatty liver disease and estimated insulin resistance in obese youth: A Mendelian randomization analysis. The Journal of Clinical Endocrinology and Metabolism. 2020;**105**(11):e4046-e4054

[110] Di Bonito P, Valerio G, Licenziati MR, Miraglia del Giudice E, Baroni MG, Morandi A, et al. High uric acid, reduced glomerular filtration rate and non-alcoholic fatty liver in young people with obesity. Journal of Endocrinological Investigation. 2020;**43**(4):461-468

[111] Manco M. Insulin resistance and NAFLD: A dangerous liaison beyond the genetics. Children. 2017;**4**(8):74

[112] Di Sessa A, Guarino S, Umano GR, Arenella M, Alfiero S, Quaranta G, et al. MAFLD in obese children: A challenging definition. Children. 2021;**8**(3):247

[113] Eslam M, Newsome PN, Sarin SK, Anstee QM, Targher G, Romero-Gomez M, et al. A new definition for metabolic dysfunction-associated fatty liver disease: An international expert consensus statement. Journal of Hepatology. 2020;**73**(1):202-209

[114] Hanley AJG, Williams K, Festa A, Wagenknecht LE, D'Agostino RB, Haffner SM. Liver markers and development of the metabolic syndrome. Diabetes. 2005;**54**(11):3140-3147

[115] Targher G, Bertolini L, Padovani R, Zenari L, Zoppini G, Falezza G. Relation of nonalcoholic hepatic steatosis to early carotid atherosclerosis in healthy men. Diabetes Care. 2004;**27**(10):2498-2500

[116] Targher G, Bertolini L, Poli F, Rodella S, Scala L, Tessari R, et al. Nonalcoholic fatty liver disease and risk of future cardiovascular events among type 2 diabetic patients. Diabetes. 2005;**54**(12):3541-3546

[117] Hunter AK, Lin HC. Review of clinical guidelines in the diagnosis of pediatric nonalcoholic fatty liver disease. Clinical Liver Disease (Hoboken). 2021;**18**(1):40-44

[118] Schwimmer JB, Newton KP, Awai HI, Choi LJ, Garcia MA, Ellis LL, et al. Paediatric gastroenterology evaluation of overweight and obese children referred from primary care for suspected non-alcoholic fatty liver disease. Alimentary Pharmacology & Therapeutics. 2013;**38**(10):1267-1277

[119] Vos MB, Abrams SH, Barlow SE, Caprio S, Daniels SR, Kohli R, et al. NASPGHAN clinical practice guideline for the diagnosis and treatment of nonalcoholic fatty liver disease in children: Recommendations from the expert committee on NAFLD (ECON) and the North American Society of Pediatric Gastroenterology, Hepatology and Nutrition (NASPGHAN). Journal of Pediatric Gastroenterology and Nutrition. 2017;**64**(2):319-334

[120] American Association for the Study of Liver Diseases. The diagnosis and management of nonalcoholic fatty liver disease: Practice guidance from the American Association for the Study of Liver Diseases. Clinical Liver Disease (Hoboken). 2018;**11**(4):81-81

[121] Shannon A, Alkhouri N, Carter-Kent C, Monti L, Devito R, Lopez R, et al. Ultrasonographic quantitative estimation of hepatic steatosis in children with NAFLD. Journal of Pediatric Gastroenterology and Nutrition. 2011;**53**(2):190-195

[122] Nobili V, Alisi A, Valenti L, Miele L, Feldstein AE, Alkhouri N. NAFLD in children: New genes, new diagnostic modalities and new drugs. Nature Reviews. Gastroenterology & Hepatology. 2019;**16**(9):517-530

[123] Aboeldalyl S, James C, Seyam E, Ibrahim EM, Shawki HED, Amer S. The role of chronic inflammation in polycystic ovarian syndrome—A systematic review and meta-analysis. International Journal of Molecular Sciences. 2021;**22**(5):2734

[124] Calcaterra V, Verduci E, Cena H, Magenes VC, Todisco CF, Tenuta E, et al. Polycystic ovary syndrome in insulin-resistant adolescents with obesity: The role of nutrition therapy and food supplements as a strategy to protect fertility. Nutrients. 2021;**13**(6):1848

[125] Trent M, Gordon CM. Diagnosis and management of polycystic ovary syndrome inbAdolescents. Pediatrics. 2020;**145**(Suppl. 2):S210-S218

[126] Yetim Şahin A, Baş F, Yetim Ç, Ucar A, Poyrazoglu Ş, Bundak R, et al. Determination of insulin resistance and its relationship with hyperandrogenemia, anti-Müllerian hormone, inhibin A, inhibin B, and insulin-like peptide-3 levels in adolescent girls with polycystic ovary syndrome. Turkish Journal of Medical Sciences. 2019;**49**(4):1117-1125

[127] Teede HJ, Misso ML, Costello MF, Dokras A, Laven J, Moran L, et al. Recommendations from the international evidence-based guideline for the assessment and management of polycystic ovary syndrome. Fertility and Sterility. 2018;**110**(3):364-379

[128] Ibáñez L, Oberfield SE, Witchel S, Auchus RJ, Chang RJ, Codner E, et al. An international consortium update: Pathophysiology, diagnosis,

and treatment of polycystic ovarian syndrome in adolescence. Hormone Research in Pædiatrics. 2017;**88**(6):371-395

[129] Laitinen J, Taponen S, Martikainen H, Pouta A, Millwood I, Hartikainen AL, et al. Body size from birth to adulthood as a predictor of self-reported polycystic ovary syndrome symptoms. International Journal of Obesity. 2003;**27**(6):710-715

[130] Aziz M, Sidelmann JJ, Faber J, Wissing M, Louise M, Naver KV, et al. Polycysticovarysyndrome:Cardiovascular risk factors according to specific phenotypes. Acta Obstetricia et Gynecologica Scandinavica. 2015;**94**(10):1082-1089

[131] Kandaraki E, Chatzigeorgiou A, Piperi C, Palioura E, Palimeri S, Korkolopoulou P, et al. Reduced ovarian glyoxalase-I activity by dietary glycotoxins and androgen excess: A causative link to polycystic ovarian syndrome. Molecular Medicine. 2012;**18**(8):1183-1189

[132] Mani H, Levy MJ, Davies MJ, Morris DH, Gray LJ, Bankart J, et al. Diabetes and cardiovascular events in women with polycystic ovary syndrome: A 20-year retrospective cohort study. Clinical Endocrinology. 2013;**78**(6):926-934

[133] Musso G, Gambino R, Cassader M. Obesity, diabetes, and gut microbiota. Diabetes Care. 2010;**33**(10):2277-2284

[134] Ley RE, Turnbaugh PJ, Klein S, Gordon JI. Human gut microbes associated with obesity. Nature. 2006;**444**(7122):1022-1023

[135] Ley RE, Bäckhed F, Turnbaugh P, Lozupone CA, Knight RD, Gordon JI. Obesity alters gut microbial ecology. National Academy of Sciences of the United States of America. 2005;**102**(31):11070-11075

[136] Bäckhed F, Ding H, Wang T, Hooper LV, Koh GY, Nagy A, et al. The gut microbiota as an environmental factor that regulates fat storage. National Academy of Sciences of the United States of America. 2004;**101**(44):15718-15723

[137] Tang WHW, Bäckhed F, Landmesser U, Hazen SL. Intestinal microbiota in cardiovascular health and disease. Journal of the American College of Cardiology. 2019;**73**(16):2089-2105

[138] Yang Q, Vijayakumar A, Kahn BB. Metabolites as regulators of insulin sensitivity and metabolism. Nature Reviews. Molecular Cell Biology. 2018;**19**(10):654-672. DOI: 10.1038/s41580-018-0044-8

[139] Yonemori KM, Lim U, Koga KR, Wilkens LR, Au D, Boushey CJ, et al. Dietary choline and betaine intakes vary in an adult multiethnic population. The Journal of Nutrition. 2013;**143**(6):894-899

[140] Yu Z, Zhang L, Jiang X, Xue C, Chi N, Zhang T, et al. Effects of dietary choline, betaine, and L-carnitine on the generation of trimethylamine-N-oxide in healthy mice. Journal of Food Science. 2020;**85**(7):2207-2215

[141] Zhang AQ, Mitchell SC, Smith RL. Dietary precursors of trimethylamine in man: A pilot study. Food and Chemical Toxicology. 1999;**37**(5):515-520

[142] Zeisel SH, Warrier M. Trimethylamine N-oxide, the microbiome, and heart and kidney disease. Annual Review of Nutrition. 2017;**37**(1):157-181

[143] Fu BC, Hullar MA, Randolph TW, Franke AA, Monroe KR, Cheng I, et al.

Associations of plasma trimethylamine N-oxide, choline, carnitine, and betaine with inflammatory and cardiometabolic risk biomarkers and the fecal microbiome in the multiethnic cohort adiposity phenotype study. The American Journal of Clinical Nutrition. 2020;**111**(6):1226-1223

[144] Qiu L, Tao X, Xiong H, Yu J, Wei H. *Lactobacillus plantarum* ZDY04 exhibits a strainspecific property of lowering TMAO via the modulation of gut microbiota in mice. Food & Function. 2018;**9**(8):4299-4309

[145] Cantero MA, Guedes MRA, Fernandes R, Lollo PCB. Trimethylamine N-oxide reduction is related to probiotic strain specificity: A systematic review. Nutrition Research. 2022;**104**:29-35

[146] Dambrova M, Latkovskis G, Kuka J, Strele I, Konrade I, Grinberga S, et al. Diabetes is associated with higher trimethylamine N-oxide plasma levels. Experimental and Clinical Endocrinology & Diabetes. 2016;**124**(04):251-256

[147] Li X, Hong J, Wang Y, Pei M, Wang L, Gong Z. Trimethylamine-N-oxide pathway: A potential target for the treatment of MAFLD. Frontiers in Molecular Biosciences. 1 Oct 2021;**8**:733507

[148] Dong F, Jiang S, Tang C, Wang X, Ren X, Wei Q, et al. Trimethylamine N-oxide promotes hyperoxaluria-induced calcium oxalate deposition and kidney injury by activating autophagy. Free Radical Biology & Medicine. 2022;**179**:288-300

[149] Xu R, Wang Q, Li L. A genome-wide systems analysis reveals strong link between colorectal cancer and trimethylamine N-oxide (TMAO), a gut microbial metabolite of dietary meat and fat. BMC Genomics. 2015;**16**(S7):S4

[150] Paul B, Barnes S, Demark-Wahnefried W, Morrow C, Salvador C, Skibola C, et al. Influences of diet and the gut microbiome on epigenetic modulation in cancer and other diseases. Clinical Epigenetics. 2015;**7**(1):112

[151] Gao X, Liu X, Xu J, Xue C, Xue Y, Wang Y. Dietary trimethylamine N-oxide exacerbates impaired glucose tolerance in mice fed a high fat diet. Journal of Bioscience and Bioengineering. 2014;**118**(4):476-481

[152] Tong M, Neusner A, Longato L, Lawton M, Wands JR, de la Monte SM. Nitrosamine exposure causes insulin resistance diseases: Relevance to type 2 diabetes mellitus, nonalcoholicsteatohepatitis, and Alzheimer's disease. Journal of Alzheimer's Disease. 2009;**17**(4):827-844

[153] de la Monte SM, Tong M, Lawton M, Longato L. Nitrosamine exposure exacerbates high fat diet-mediated type 2 diabetes mellitus, non-alcoholic steatohepatitis, and neurodegeneration with cognitive impairment. Molecular Neurodegeneration. 2009;**4**(1):54

[154] Ming CY, Liu Y, Fen ZR, Ling CX, Wang C, Ying TX, et al. Associations of gut-flora-dependent metabolite trimethylamine-N-oxide, betaine and choline with nonalcoholic fatty liver disease in adults. Scientific Reports. 2016;**6**(1):19076

[155] Stols-Gonçalves D, Hovingh GK, Nieuwdorp M, Holleboom AG. NAFLD and atherosclerosis: Two sides of the same dysmetabolic coin? Trends in Endocrinology & Metabolism. 2019;**30**(12):891-902

[156] Lindskog Jonsson A, Caesar R, Akrami R, Reinhardt C, Fåk Hållenius F, Borén J, et al. Impact of gut microbiota

and diet on the development of atherosclerosis in Apoe −/−mice. Arteriosclerosis, Thrombosis, and Vascular Biology. 2018;**38**(10):2318-2326

[157] DiNicolantonio JJ, McCarty M, OKeefe J. Association of moderately elevated trimethylamine N-oxide with cardiovascular risk: Is TMAO serving as a marker for hepatic insulin resistance. Open Heart. 2019;**6**(1):e000890

[158] Zhu T, Goodarzi MO. Metabolites linking the gut microbiome with risk for type 2 diabetes. Current Nutrition Reports. 2020;**9**(2):83-93

[159] Eyileten C, Jarosz-Popek J, Jakubik D, Gasecka A, Wolska M, Ufnal M, et al. Plasma trimethylamine-N-oxide is an independent predictor of long-term cardiovascular mortality in patients undergoing percutaneous coronary intervention for acute coronary syndrome. Frontiers in Cardiovascular Medicine. 29 Oct 2021;**8**:728724

[160] Yu D, Shu X, Rivera ES, Zhang X, Cai Q, Calcutt MW, et al. Urinary levels of trimethylamine-N-oxide and incident coronary heart disease: A prospective investigation among urban Chinese adults. Journal of the American Heart Association. 8 Jan 2019;**8**(1):e010606

[161] Xu J, Cheng A, Song B, Zhao M, Xue J, Wang A, et al. Trimethylamine N-oxide and stroke recurrence depends on ischemic stroke subtypes. Stroke. 2022;**53**(4):1207-1215

[162] Nam HS. Gut microbiota and ischemic stroke: The role of trimethylamine N-oxide. Journal of Stroke. 2019;**21**(2):151-159

[163] Dai Y, Zhang J, Wang Z, Xu S, Zhang Q, Duan Z, et al. Associations of diet with urinary trimethylamine-N-oxide (TMAO) and its precursors among free-living 10-year-old children: Data from SMBCS. Nutrients. 2022;**14**(16):3419

[164] Hsu CN, Lu PC, Lo MH, Lin IC, Chang-Chien GP, Lin S, et al. Gut microbiota-dependent trimethylamine N-oxide pathway associated with cardiovascular risk in children with early-stage chronic kidney disease. International Journal of Molecular Sciences. 2018;**19**(12):3699

[165] Leal-Witt MJ, Llobet M, Samino S, Castellano P, Cuadras D, Jimenez-Chillaron JC, et al. Lifestyle intervention decreases urine trimethylamine N-oxide levels in prepubertal children with obesity. Obesity. 2018;**26**(10):1603-1610

[166] Mihuta MS, Paul C, Borlea A, Roi CM, Pescari D, Velea-Barta O-A, et al. Connections between serum trimethylamine N-oxide (TMAO) a gut derived metabolite vascular biomarkers evaluating arterial stiffness subclinical atherosclerosis in children with obesity. Frontiers in Endocrinology. 2023;**14**:1253584

[167] Mihuta MS, Paul C, Borlea A, Roi CM, Velea-Barta OA, Mozos I, et al. Unveiling the silent danger of childhood obesity: Non-invasive biomarkers such as carotid intima-media thickness, arterial stiffness surrogate markers, and blood pressure are useful in detecting early vascular alterations in obese children. Biomedicine. 2023;**11**(7):1841

[168] Mihuta MS, Paul C, Ciulpan A, Dacca F, Velea IP, Mozos I, et al. Subclinical atherosclerosis progression in obese children with relevant cardiometabolic risk factors can be assessed through carotid intima media thickness. Applied Sciences. 2021;**11**(22):10721

[169] Mihuta MS, Paul C, Borlea A, Cepeha CM, Velea IP, Mozos I, et al. The oscillometric pulse wave analysis is useful in evaluating the arterial stiffness of obese children with relevant cardiometabolic risks. Journal of Clinical Medicine. 2022;**11**(17):5078

[170] Mihuta MS, Stoian D, Borlea A, Roi CM, Velea-Barta OA, Mozos I, et al. Evaluating the arterial stiffness as a useful tool in the Management of Obese Children. Children. 2023;**10**(2):183